Examples of how to describe the clinical features of lesions or rash

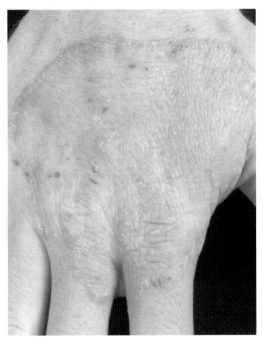

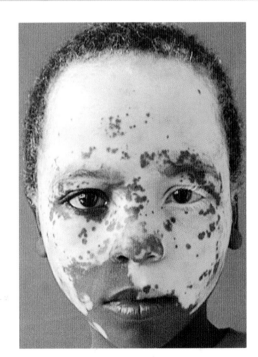

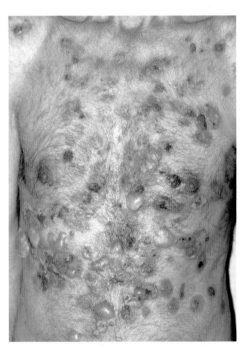

1. Dorsum hand
2. Erythematous
3. Chronic
4. Surface scale
5. Raised lesion – plaque

1. Face
2. Non-erythematous
3. Chronic
4. Surface normal
5. Flat lesion – patch
6. Colour – white

1. Trunk
2. Erythematous
3. Chronic
4. Surface crust
5. Lesions – bullae & erosions

For Jim, Louise, Nicholas, Felicity, Simon, Christopher and Camilla

Differential Diagnosis in Dermatology

Third Edition

Richard Ashton

*Consultant Dermatologist to the Royal Navy and
Portsmouth NHS Trust, Royal Hospital Haslar, Gosport, Hampshire*

Barbara Leppard

*Consultant Dermatologist, Southampton University NHS Trust,
Royal South Hants Hospital, Southampton*

RADCLIFFE PUBLISHING

Radcliffe Publishing Ltd
18 Marcham Road
Abingdon
Oxon OX14 1AA
United Kingdom

www.radcliffe-oxford.com
Electronic catalogue and worldwide online ordering facility.

British Library Cataloguing in Publication Data

A catalogue record for this book is available from the British Library

ISBN 185775 660 6

Typeset by Advance Typesetting Ltd, Long Hanborough, Oxon
Printed and bound by Nuffield Press Ltd, Abingdon, Oxon

Contents

Preface to third edition

Like its predecessors this book has been written to help the primary care physician reach the correct diagnosis of a rash or lesion with the patient sitting in front of him. The three interlocking components of the book – the algorithms, the descriptive text and the colour photographs – should be used together in reaching a diagnosis. The chapters are divided into the different body areas, and the algorithms deal with the differential diagnosis of similar lesions or rashes. Common conditions (ones you will see at least once a year) are printed in white text in a dark blue box, uncommon ones are printed in black on the pale blue background. In this edition we have included treatment for the first time, not in as much detail as in our other book *Treatment in Dermatology*, but enough to manage most everyday problems.

We would like to thank Galderma for their generous financial support for this edition, all the patients who have allowed us to use their photographs, Professor Peter Friedman for Figs 8.61 & 8.62, Dr Peter Goodwin for Fig. 1.90, Dr Raj Mani for Fig. 12.29 and the graphics department of Haslar Hospital for the line drawings. We would also like to thank our spouses and children for their patience while we have been busy writing.

October 2004

Richard Ashton
Barbara Leppard

Introduction to dermatological diagnosis

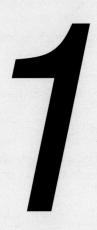

Basic biology of the skin

Diagnosis of skin disease

History taking

Describing skin lesions

Special investigations

BASIC BIOLOGY OF THE SKIN

THE EPIDERMIS

As the outside layer of the skin, the function of the epidermis is to produce keratin and melanin. Pathology in the epidermis produces a rash or a lesion with abnormal scale, change in pigmentation, or loss of surface integrity (exudate or erosion).

Keratin

Keratin is the end product of maturation of the epidermal cells; its function is to make the skin waterproof.

Melanin

Melanin is produced by melanocytes in the basal layer. Packets of melanin (melanosomes) are transferred from the melanocytes through their dendritic processes into the surrounding epidermal cells (Fig. 1.02). Melanosomes protect the nucleus from the harmful effects of ultraviolet radiation; without this protection skin cancer may develop.

THE DERMIS

The bulk of the dermis is made up of connective tissue: collagen which gives the skin its strength and elastic fibres which allow it to stretch. Here are also the blood vessels, lymphatics, cutaneous nerves and the skin appendages (hair follicles, sebaceous glands and sweat glands) (Fig. 1.01). Diseases of the dermis usually result in change in elevation of the skin (i.e. papules, nodules, atrophy), and if the pathology is restricted to the dermis, there will be no surface changes such as scale, crust or exudate. Loss or necrosis of the dermis results in an ulcer (as opposed to an erosion which is due to loss of epidermis alone).

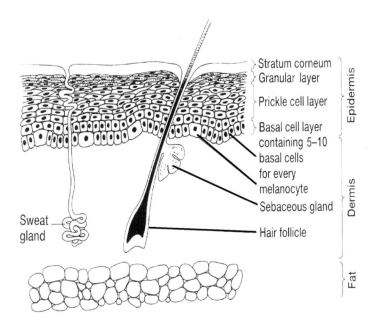

Fig. 1.01 The structure of the skin.

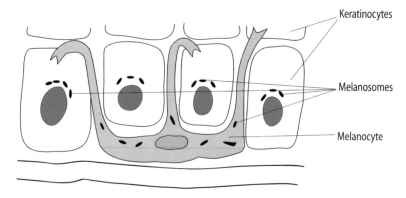

Fig. 1.02 Melanocyte in basal layer inserting melanosomes into keratinocytes.

DIAGNOSIS OF SKIN DISEASE

The diagnosis of skin disease is made by following the same general principles as in any other branch of medicine. Begin by taking a history. This is followed by careful physical examination. If at this stage the diagnosis has not been made, further investigations can be carried out. Very often the non-dermatologist tends to look at a rash or skin lesion and 'guess' the diagnosis. This is quite unnecessary. Below we have outlined a scheme to enable you to make the correct diagnosis.

HISTORY OF PRESENTING COMPLAINT

Duration of individual lesions

How long have the lesion(s) been present? This is the most important question in the history. Acute lesions present for less than 2 weeks need to be distinguished from chronic ones.

Do the lesions come and go? Do they occur at the same site or at different sites? This question is particularly important if the diagnosis of urticaria or herpes simplex is being considered. Urticaria (p. 150) can be diagnosed by a history of lesions coming and going within a 24-hour period. To establish the transitory nature of urticarial weals, draw a line around a weal and ask the patient to return the next day. You will see that the site and shape will have changed. Herpes simplex (p. 91) and fixed drug eruptions (p. 160) last around 7–14 days and usually reoccur at the same site.

Relationship to physical agents

A past history of living or working in a hot climate may be the clue you need for the diagnosis of skin cancer. Determine the

---

Skin types (Table 1.01)

Type 1:	Always burns, never tans
Type 2:	Always burns, tans minimally
Type 3:	Sometimes burns, tans gradually
Type 4:	Rarely burns, tans well
Type 5:	Asian skin
Type 6:	Black skin

Those with fair skin (types 1 and 2) are more liable to develop skin cancers.

---

patient's skin response to sun exposure. Six skin types are recognised depending on how well a patient develops a skin tan (Table 1.01). In rashes on the face and backs of the hands ask about relationship to sun exposure. The important questions to ask are the time interval after sun exposure before the rash occurs and whether the patient gets the rash through window glass on a sunny day. In solar urticaria, the rash occurs within five minutes of sun exposure and is gone in an hour. In polymorphic light eruption (p. 83), the rash occurs several hours after sun exposure and lasts several days. In porphyria (which is very rare, *see* p. 361) the rash occurs within a few minutes and lasts several days. Rashes that occur through window glass are due to UVA and will need a sunblock containing titanium dioxide or zinc oxide (*see* p. 33).

Ask about irritants on the skin in hand eczema, e.g. detergents and oils, and about working practices and hobbies. Are the hands protected by rubber gloves or in direct contact with irritants?

Itching

Itching is a nuisance to the patient but may not help you in making a diagnosis. Severe itching – especially at night – bad enough to prevent sleep should make you think of scabies (p. 218) or rarely dermatitis herpetiformis (p. 216).

PAST, FAMILY & SOCIAL HISTORY

Past history

Has the patient had a rash before and, if so, was it the same as now? If eczema is present, a history of infantile eczema, asthma or hay fever may suggest a diagnosis of atopic eczema.

Family history

Does anyone else in the family have a skin problem and is it the same as the patient's? This will indicate either that the skin disease is genetically determined, e.g. atopic eczema, ichthyosis or psoriasis, or that it is contagious, e.g. scabies or impetigo.

Social history

This should include family relationships and work practices which may give you a clue as to the cause of the problem. For instance, in cases of hand dermatitis, does the condition improve at weekends or when away on holiday?

PREVIOUS TREATMENT

What topical agents have been used and did they help? Establish whether these are ointments or creams because the base may be as important as the active agent. Remember that topical local anaesthetics, antibiotics and antihistamines may induce allergic contact dermatitis. A drug history is important if a drug-induced rash is considered, e.g. if there is a sudden onset of a widespread rash. If the patient has been on the drug for more than 2 months, the likelihood of it being the cause of the rash is low.

DESCRIBING SKIN LESIONS

LOOK first and identify:–
1. Sites involved
2. Number of lesions
3. Distribution
4. Arrangement

FEEL the lesions by:–
5. Surface palpation with finger tips and
6. Deep palpation by squeezing between finger and thumb

DESCRIBE a typical lesion under the following headings:–
7. Type of lesion
8. Surface features/texture
9. Colour, including erythematous or non-erythematous
10. Border of rash/lesions
11. Size and shape of individual lesions

CHECK other sites, e.g. scalp, nails, mouth & genitalia.

1. SITES INVOLVED Describe body areas involved.

2. NUMBER OF LESIONS

Single (Fig. 1.03 – Lymphoma)

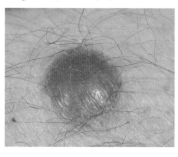

Multiple (Fig. 1.04 – Lichen planus)

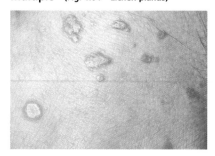

3. DISTRIBUTION

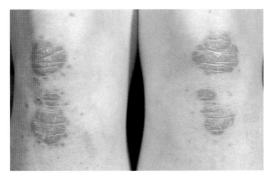

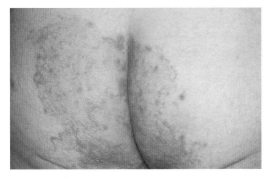

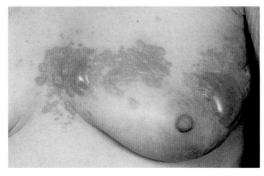

Symmetrical   (Fig. 1.05 – Psoriasis)
Involving both sides of body to a similar extent; usually due to endogeneous causes, e.g. acne, eczema, psoriasis.

Asymmetrical   (Fig. 1.06 – Tinea corporis on buttocks)
Involving predominantly one side of the body, usually due to exogeneous cause, e.g. infections or contact dermatitis.

Unilateral   (Fig. 1.07 – Herpes zoster)
Restricted to one side of body only.

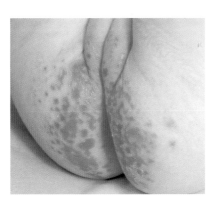

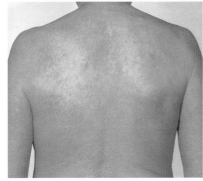

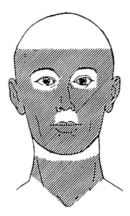

Localised   (Fig. 1.08 – Nappy/diaper rash)
Restricted to one area of skin.

Generalised
(Fig. 1.09 – Erythrodermic psoriasis)
Covering most of the body surface.

Sun exposed   (Fig. 1.10)   (Fig. 1.11)
Involving the face ,'V' and back of the neck, dorsum of hands and forearms.
N.B. Behind ears and under chin and/or eyebrows will be spared.

4. ARRANGEMENT

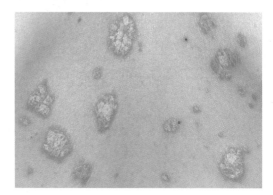

Discrete (Fig. 1.12 – Psoriasis)
Individual lesions separated from each other by normal skin.

Coalescing (Fig. 1.13 – Eczema)
Similar lesions merging together.

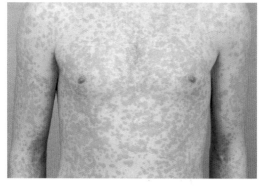

Disseminated (Fig. 1.14 – Psoriasis)
Widespread discrete lesions.

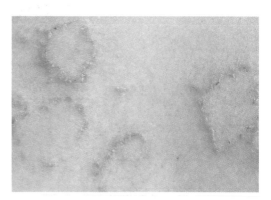

Annular (Fig. 1.15 – Eczema)
Arranged in ring (see p. 176).

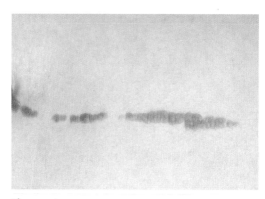

Linear (Fig. 1.16 – Epidermal naevus)
Arranged in line (see p. 179).

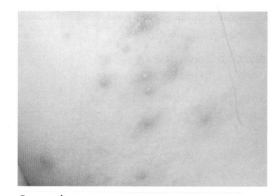

Grouped (Fig. 1.17 – Insect bites)
Multiple similar lesions grouped together in one area.

FEEL THE LESIONS

5. SURFACE PALPATION

Feel the surface with your finger tips.

Smooth: Feels like normal skin

Uneven: Found with fine scaling or some warty lesions

Rough: Feels like sandpaper, and is characteristic of keratin/horn or crust.

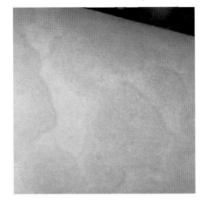

Smooth (Fig. 1.18 – Urticaria)

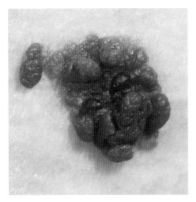

Uneven (Fig. 1.19 – Compound naevus)

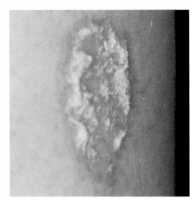

Rough (Fig. 1.20 – Solar keratosis)

6. DEEP PALPATION

Compress the lesion between thumb and index finger.

Normal: Feels the same as the normal surrounding skin

Soft: Easily compressible – feels like the lips

Firm: Only slightly compressible – feels like the tip of nose

Hard: Not compressible – feels like bone.

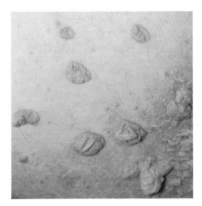

Soft (Fig. 1.21 – Skin tags)

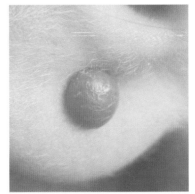

Firm (Fig. 1.22 – Keloid scar)

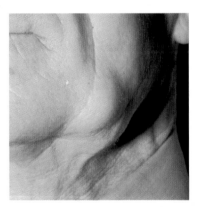

Hard (Fig. 1.23 – Osteoma on jaw)

7. TYPE OF LESION

Assess whether the lesions are flat or raised, solid or fluid filled, or have a broken surface.

a. Flat lesions

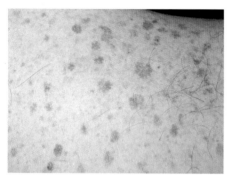

Macule ≤ 1cm diameter   (Fig. 1.24 – Lentigines)

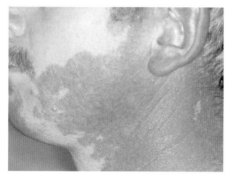

Patch > 1cm diameter   (Fig. 1.25 – Port wine stain)

b. Raised solid lesions

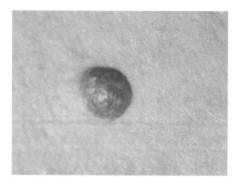

Papule ≤ 1cm diameter
(Fig. 1.26 – Compound naevus)

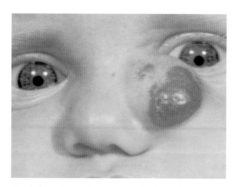

Nodule > 1cm diameter (= thickness)
(Fig. 1.27 – Strawberry naevus)

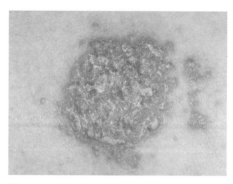

Plaque > 1cm diameter (>>thickness)
(Fig. 1.28 – Discoid eczema)

Flat lesions Any area of colour or surface change which cannot be felt on palpation.

Raised solid lesions

Papule Any solid lesion (≤1cm size) that is raised above the surface or can be felt on palpation.

Nodule Any elevated lesion (>1cm diameter) which is palpable between finger and thumb, i.e. there is substance to the lesion. Often due to dermal pathology but there may be surface change.

Plaque Any lesion (size > 1cm) where the diameter is >> than the thickness, i.e. the lesion can be felt only with finger tips. Usually due to epidermal pathology with surface scale, crust or keratin.

c. Fluid filled lesions

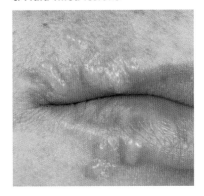

Vesicle ≤ 1cm diameter
(Fig. 1.29 – Herpes simplex)

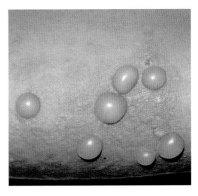

Bulla > 1cm diameter
(Fig. 1.30 – Bullous pemphigoid)

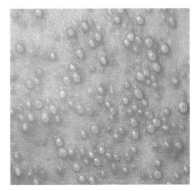

Pustule ≤ 1cm diameter   (Fig. 1.31)

d. Lesions due to a broken surface

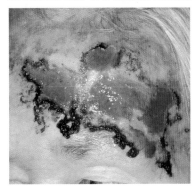

Erosion   (Fig. 1.32)
Loss of epidermis only.

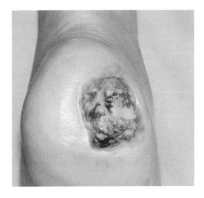

Ulcer   (Fig. 1.33 – Neuropathic ulcer)
Loss of epidermis and dermis.

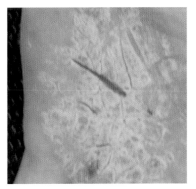

Fissure   (Fig. 1.34 – Hand psoriasis)
Linear split in skin.

Blisters (vesicles and bullae) contain clear fluid (serum) and last for a few days only. The presence of fluid can be confirmed by pricking with a needle. The site of the blister can be within the epidermis or at the dermo-epidermal junction.

Intra-epidermal blisters break easily to form erosions, while **sub-epidermal** ones can persist for several days and may contain blood.

Pustule (≤1cm) Contains opaque fluid (pus). Prick the lesion and pus comes out.

Loss of some or all of the epidermis results in an **erosion**, which will heal without scarring. Erosions can be due to:–

1. A blister which has burst, or
2. Trauma.

Loss of dermis (from any cause) will result in an **ulcer** which will heal with scar tissue formation. There will be surface exudate, crust or slough.

Splitting of the skin (**fissure**) is due to abnormal keratin (usually secondary to eczema or psoriasis).

e. Other terms used

Weal (Fig. 1.35 – Urticaria)
Transient swelling (i.e. papule or plaque) due to dermal oedema – should last for less than 24 hours. Usually synonymous with urticaria.

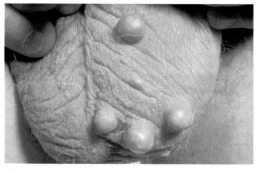

Cyst (Fig. 1.36 – Scrotal epidermoid cysts)
A fluctuant papule or nodule lined by epithelium containing fluid, pus or keratin.

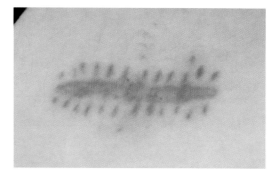

Scar (Fig. 1.37 – Surgical scar)
A healed dermal lesion (macule/papule/plaque/nodule) secondary to trauma, surgery, infection or loss of blood supply.

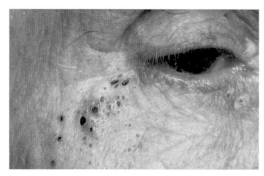

Comedone (Fig. 1.38 – Solar elastosis)
Papule due to a plugged sebaceous follicle containing altered sebum and keratin.

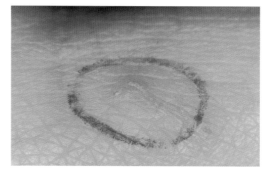

Burrow (Fig. 1.39 – Scabies)
Linear 'S'-shaped papule 3–5mm long found on the hands and fingers of a patient with scabies.

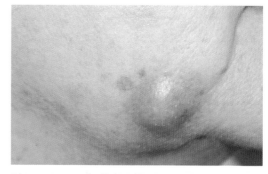

Abscess (Fig. 1.40 – Boil on angle of jaw)
A large collection of pus.

8. SURFACE FEATURES/TEXTURE

b. Abnormal keratinization

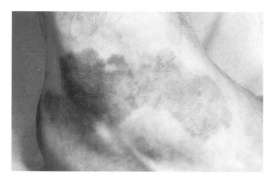

a. Normal (Fig. 1.41 – Granuloma annulare)
Surface not different from surrounding skin and feels smooth. Change in elevation and/or colour.

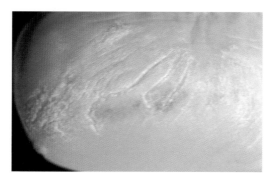

Hyperkeratotic (Fig. 1.42 – Foot psoriasis)
Rough uneven surface due to increased formation of keratin. Seen usually on palms and soles.

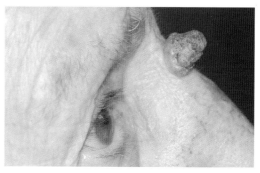

Keratin horn (Fig. 1.43 – Keratoacanthoma)
Accumulation of compact keratin on the surface. Feels rough and is adherent so difficult to pick off.

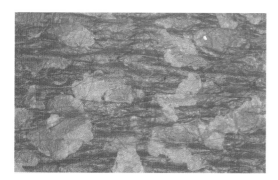

Scale (Fig. 1.44 – Erythrodermic psoriasis)
Dry/flaky surface due to abnormal stratum corneum with increased shedding of keratinocytes.

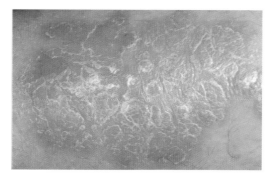

Scratch test – before (Fig. 1.45 – Psoriasis)
If surface is scaly, scratch surface of scale vigorously with finger nail.

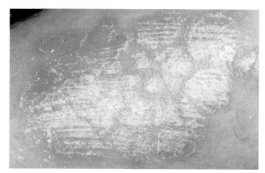

Scratch test – after (Fig. 1.46 – Psoriasis)
Profuse silver scale indicates that the diagnosis is psoriasis.

c. Broken surface

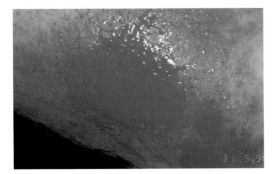

Exudate (Fig. 1.47 – Acute eczema)
Serum, blood or pus that has accumulated on the surface.

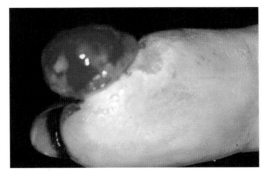

Friable (Fig. 1.48 – Pyogenic granuloma)
Surface bleeds easily after minor trauma.

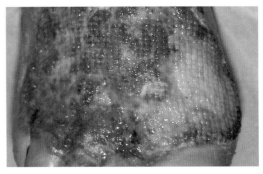

Slough (Fig. 1.49 – Foot ulcer)
A combination of exudate and necrotic tissue.

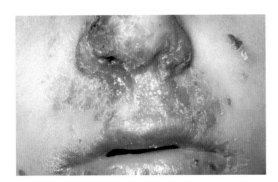

Crust (Fig. 1.50 – Impetigo)
Dried exudate. There should be a history of weeping, pus or bleeding.

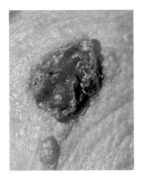

(Fig. 1.51 – Basal cell carcinoma)　　(Fig. 1.52)
To find the cause of a crust pick it off to see what is underneath. There will either be an ulcer or an erosion. Under the crust in Fig. 1.51 there is an ulcer due to a basal cell carcinoma (Fig. 1.52).

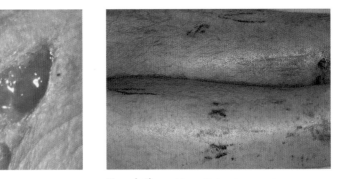

Excoriation (Fig. 1.53 Atopic eczema)
Localised damage to the skin due to scratching: linear erosions and crusts.

d. Changes in thickness

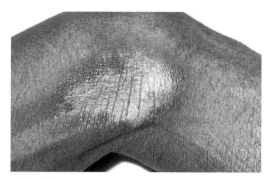

Lichenification (Fig. 1.54 – Lichen simplex)
Thickening of the epidermis with increased skin markings due to persistent scratching (found in atopic eczema or lichen simplex).

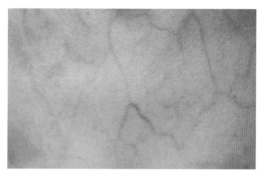

Dermal atrophy (Fig. 1.55 – due to topical steroids)
Depression of the surface due to thinning of the dermis. Blood vessels are easily seen under the skin.

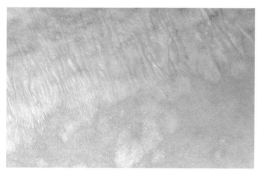

Epidermal atrophy (Fig. 1.56 – Lichen sclerosus)
Fine surface wrinkling like 'cigarette paper'.

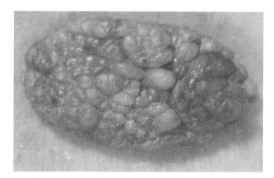

Papillomatous (Fig. 1.57 – Intradermal naevus)
Surface consisting of minute finger-like or round projections.

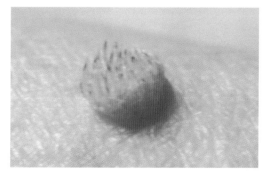

Warty (Fig. 1.58 – Filiform wart)
Surface consisting of rough finger-like projections.

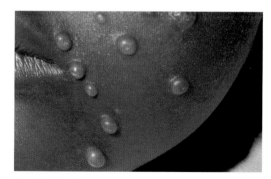

Umbilicated (Fig. 1.59 – Molluscum contagiosum)
Papule with central depression. Characteristically seen in molluscum contagiosum.

9. COLOUR OF LESION

a. Red, pink or purple

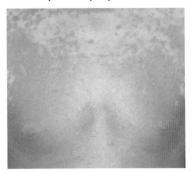

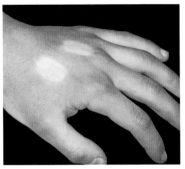

Erythema (Fig. 1.60 – Psoriasis)   (Fig. 1.61 – Chilblains)
Redness due to dilated blood vessels which blanche (become white) on pressure.
It is the result of inflammation and is seen most easily in white-skinned individuals.

b. Brown

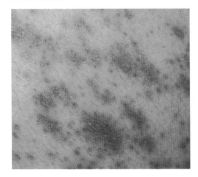

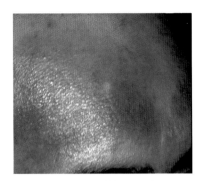

Hyperpigmentation (Fig. 1.65 – Lichen planus)   (Fig. 1.66 – Atopic eczema)
Increase in melanin pigmentation. It usually follows inflammation in the epidermis.
In pigmented skin it can be the first sign of inflammation.

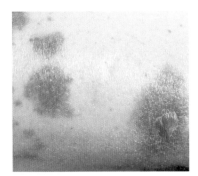

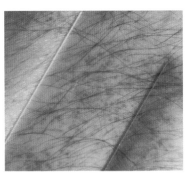

Telangiectasia (Fig. 1.62)
Redness due to individually visible dilated blood vessels.

Purpura (Fig. 1.63)   (Fig. 1.64)
Red, purple or orange colour due to blood that has leaked out of blood vessels. Purpura does not blanche on pressure and remains the same colour.

Haemosiderin pigment (Fig. 1.67)
Orange-brown due to breakdown of haemoglobin following purpura.

c. Blue-black

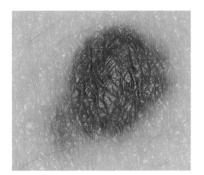

Melanin pigment
(Fig. 1.68 – Blue naevus)
Melanin pigment situated deep within dermis, seen in malignant melanoma and blue naevus.

d. White

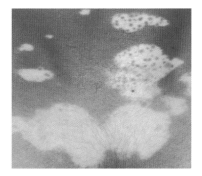

Depigmentation
(Fig. 1.69 – Vitiligo)
Complete loss of melanin due to loss of melanocytes in the epidermis.

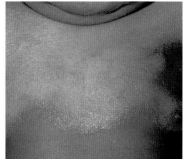

Hypopigmentation
(Fig. 1.70 – Eczema)
Partial loss of melanin secondary to inflammation in the epidermis.

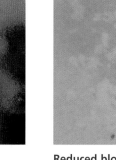

Reduced blood supply
(Fig. 1.71 – Naevus anaemicus)
White colour due to reduced blood supply.

e. Black-purple

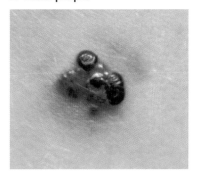

Stagnant blood
(Fig. 1.72 – Angioma)
Black-purple colour from dilated blood vessels within the skin.

f. Yellow

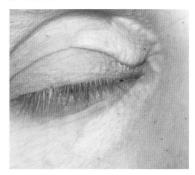

Lipid deposition
(Fig. 1.73 – Xanthelasma)
Yellow colour seen in xanthelasma on inner eyelids.

g. Blue-grey

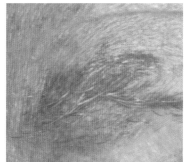

Minocycline pigmentation
(Fig. 1.74)
Grey-blue colour on eyebrow due to deposition of iron.

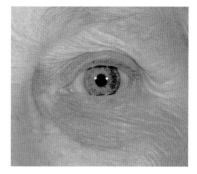

Gold pigment
(Fig. 1.75 – Chrysiasis)
Grey-blue colour seen in patients on gold therapy.

10. BORDER OF LESION OR RASH

Well defined or circumscribed

Able to draw a line around the lesion with confidence

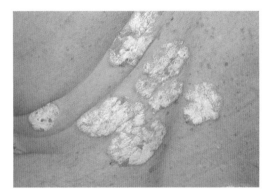

Psoriasis: well defined plaques   (Fig. 1.76)

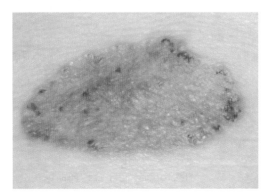

Superficial BCC: single well defined plaque (Fig. 1.79)

Poorly defined

Lesions have a border that merges into normal skin

Eczema: poorly defined plaques   (Fig. 1.77)

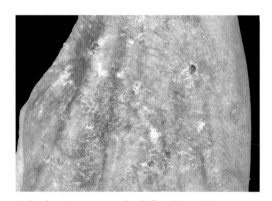

Solar keratoses: poorly defined papules (Fig. 1.80)

Accentuated edge

Border of lesion shows increased scaling with relative clearing in the centre

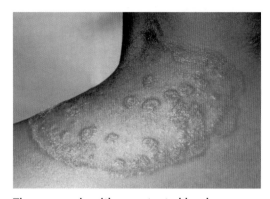

Tinea corporis with accentuated border (Fig. 1.78)

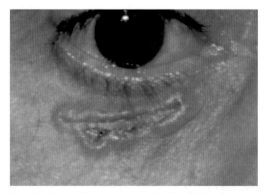

Basal cell carcinoma with raised rolled edge (Fig. 1.81)

11. SHAPE OF LESION

a. From above

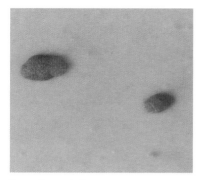

Round or oval
(Fig. 1.82 – Benign moles)

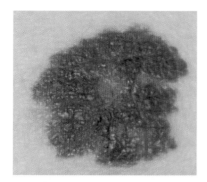

Irregular
(Fig. 1.83 – Malignant melanoma)

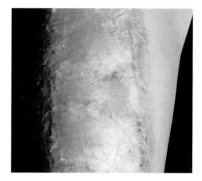

Square or rectangular
(Fig. 1.84 – Straight sides – dermatitis artefacta)

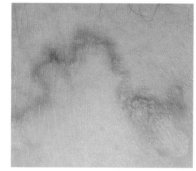

Serpiginous
(Fig. 1.85 – 'S' shaped – larva migrans)

b. In profile

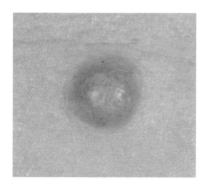

Dome shaped
(Fig. 1.86 – Benign intradermal naevus)

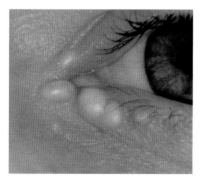

Spherical
(Fig. 1.87 – Epidermoid cysts/milia)

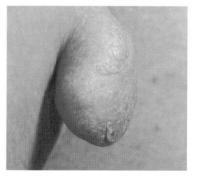

Pedunculated
(Fig. 1.88 – Fibroepithelial polyp – skin tag)

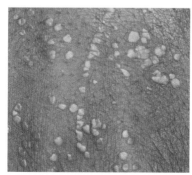

Flat topped   (Fig. 1.89 – Plane warts)

SPECIAL INVESTIGATIONS

WOOD'S LIGHT

This is a source of ultraviolet light where visible light is excluded by a nickel oxide filter. It is useful in identifying scalp ringworm due to *Microsporum* species which fluoresce green, and erythrasma which fluoresces bright pink. Porphyrins in urine and faeces also fluoresce a bright-pink colour.

In pigmentary disorders, the Wood's light will help distinguish complete loss of pigment in vitiligo (the skin is completely white) from hypopigmentation in pityriasis versicolor or post-inflammatory hypopigmentation (the skin is paler than normal).

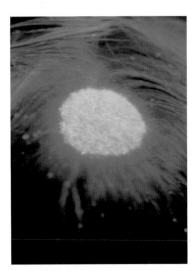 

Fluorescence seen under Wood's (ultra-violet) light:–
Fig. 1.90 (left) Green fluorescence of *Microsporum* species in scalp ringworm.
Fig. 1.91 (right) Coral pink of erythrasma.

DERMATOSCOPY

Applying oil to the surface and looking at pigmented lesions through the magnifying lens of a dermatoscope (Fig. 1.92) is a useful way of looking at the pigment pattern. Benign junctional naevi have a fine network pattern while in malignant melanoma the pigment is globular or streams outwards. Blood filled lesions (angiomas) show obvious dilated blood vessels.

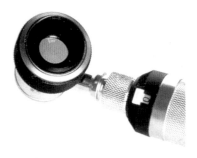 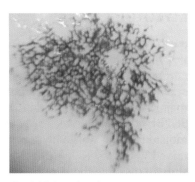

Fig. 1.92 Dermatoscope.

Fig. 1.93 Junctional naevus seen under the dermatoscope.

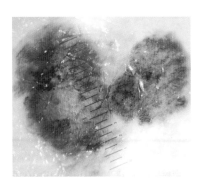 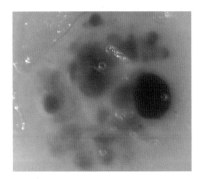

Fig. 1.94 Malignant melanoma seen under the dermatoscope.

Fig. 1.95 Angioma seen under the dermatoscope (lesion red, not brown).

BACTERIOLOGY CULTURES

Swabs can be taken from vesicles, pustules, erosions or ulcers to identify the causative bacteria by Gram stain and culture. Viruses can be identified by electron microscopy or culture. If you suspect herpes simplex or zoster you can do a PAP stain on blister fluid and see multinucleate giant cells.

MYCOLOGY

Superficial fungal infections caused by dermatophytes (ringworm/ tinea), and yeasts (candidiasis and pityriasis versicolor) all live on keratin and can be identified in scales taken from the edge of a scaly lesion. Use a blunt scalpel blade (e.g. banana-shaped – Swann major shape 'U', obtainable from Swann-Morton Ltd, Sheffield, S6 2BJ, UK). If the scales are too dry and do not stick to the blade, moistening the skin with surgical spirit helps. The scales can be mixed with 20% KOH (potassium hydroxide) solution on a glass slide to dissolve the keratin; heat the mixture gently until the solution bubbles. You can then look under the microscope to see the fungal hyphae or yeast spores (*see* Figs 10.3 and 10.12 on pp. 299 and 305).

Alternatively the skin scales may be sent to the mycology laboratory in special envelopes (Dermpak, PO Box 470, Toddington, Beds, LU5 6BF, England, or Mycotrans, PO Box 1172, Biggar, NL12 6NN, Scotland) where direct microscopy and culture can be performed.

SKIN BIOPSY

If the diagnosis is in doubt an ellipse of skin can be taken through the edge of the lesion, so that both normal and abnormal skin are included in the specimen. It should include epidermis, dermis and fat.

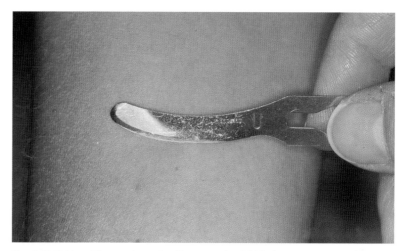

Fig. 1.96 Taking skin scraping using Swann major 'U' blade.

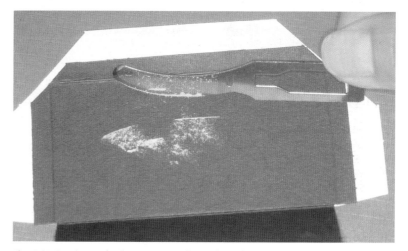

Fig. 1.97 Putting scales into a Dermpak envelope (black paper so scales show up) which can be sent to the mycology laboratory through the post.

Immune complexes can be identified by immunofluorescence. The sample needs to be sent to the laboratory in Michel's medium. In some instances a 'punch biopsy' can be used which takes a 3–6mm core of tissue, but this technique produces only a limited sample which may be inadequate for proper histological examination.

If a skin tumour is present, the whole lesion should be excised as an ellipse so that the wound can be sewn up in a straight line.

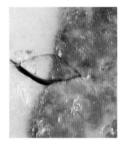

Fig. 1.98
Incisional biopsy.

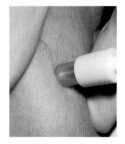

Fig. 1.99
Excisional biopsy.

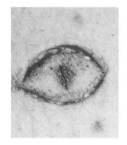

Fig. 1.100
Punch biopsy.

PRICK TESTING

This identifies an immediate hypersensitivity reaction in asthma, hay fever or contact urticaria. It is not of any use in the diagnosis of atopic eczema or idiopathic urticaria. It is useful in identifying natural rubber latex allergy. A drop of latex protein is placed on the forearm, and the skin surface is broken by pricking the skin. A weal indicates a positive reaction. A saline (negative) and histamine (positive) control should also be used. The risk of anaphylaxis is low but resuscitation drugs and equipment should be available. If latex prick testing is negative do a 'use test' wearing a finger of a latex glove on wet skin for 15 minutes with a finger of a vinyl glove as control.

PATCH TESTING

This is used to identify a type IV hypersensitivity reaction in the skin, i.e. allergic contact dermatitis. The allergens are suspended in white soft paraffin or aqueous solution and placed on aluminium discs, ten mounted on micropore tape (Finn chambers). These are applied to the back and left in place for 48 hours. The tapes are removed and a small circular plaque of eczema at the site of the aluminium disc at 48 and 96 hours indicates an allergic response to a specific allergen.

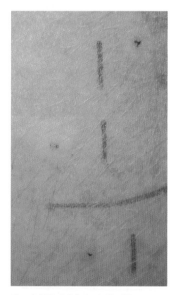

Fig. 1.101 Prick test. Positive result shows a weal around the needle prick after a few minutes.

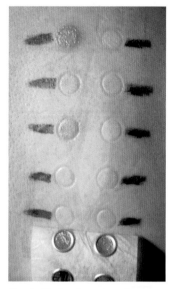

Fig. 1.102 Patch testing: 48 hour reading. The patches have just been removed and a single test (top left) is +ve. Erythema/vesicles = eczema.

Introduction to dermatological treatment

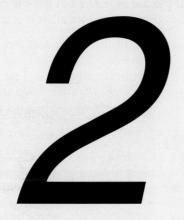

GENERAL PRINCIPLES OF TREATMENT

1. **Make a diagnosis before embarking on treatment.** Never think of treating a patient without first making a diagnosis or putting in hand the necessary investigations so that a diagnosis can be reached.

2. **Be realistic about what is possible.** Because skin disease is visible the patient will often assume that it must be easy to cure. Generally speaking skin disease can be put into three groups with regard to this:–

i. Those diseases that have a specific cause and hence a specific treatment. Once this has been given correctly, this should be the end of the problem. Such conditions include:–

- allergic contact dermatitis
- fungal and bacterial infections
- infestations such as scabies and lice
- skin tumours.

ii. Those diseases where no cure is possible, but spontaneous remissions and exacerbations occur. These may be helped considerably by treatment, but a cure is not possible and should not be sought. Examples include:–

- atopic eczema
- pemphigus and pemphigoid
- psoriasis
- rosacea.

iii. Those diseases which persist for a limited period of time and then disappear on their own. This group may require symptomatic treatment, but not always, and the patient should be reassured of their benign nature. Examples of these are:–

- alopecia areata
- erythema multiforme
- guttate psoriasis
- lichen planus
- pityriasis rosea.

The patient should be made aware of which of these categories their skin disease is in, so that they have a better idea of response to treatment and prognosis.

3. **Look at the whole person and not just at their rash.** Often the problem that presents itself is quite straightforward but at the same time there may be deeper needs shouting for attention. Body language speaks louder than words.

Patients with widespread skin disease often feel dirty, ashamed or guilty, thinking that somehow it is their own fault that they are ill. They may be afraid that their skin disease is contagious, or that they have cancer or AIDS; women with hirsutism may fear that they are turning into men; teenagers with acne lose their self-confidence.

Patients may also be embarrassed about having a rash because:–

- It is on a part of the body which shows such as the face or the hands. They will notice people looking at it and assume that they will think it is contagious. They will often wear clothes that will hide it and limit their activities so that others will not see it (e.g. not going swimming or to the beach on holiday).
- The treatment makes a mess. Grease on the clothes and bedding, and the smell and mess of tar preparations are not popular with patients or their families.
- The shedding of scales makes a mess, particularly in psoriasis.
- It smells, especially in patients with ulcerated legs.
- It is present on the genital area. It may interfere with sexual activity because of embarrassment and the patient may be afraid that their partner will think that it is catching (that they have an STD or AIDS).

It is important that you understand how the patient feels about having a skin problem as well as what to do about it.

4. Listen to what the patient has to say. Very often the patient will tell you what is wrong if you give them the opportunity.

5. Understand that not everyone wants to get well. Some patients get a lot of attention because of their illness which they do not want to give up by getting well. For others it is somehow respectable to have a rash (which will not go away) but not to own up to guilt about some person or event, a poor self image or conflict in the family. Using one ointment or pill after another will not resolve any of these and it is better to face up to reality sooner rather than later.

6. Treatment of acute rashes.

- Resting the skin is important in any acute or extensive skin disease. Going to bed is a helpful treatment in its own right. It is the basis for most in-patient treatments but can often be done just as well at home (by this we mean actually going to bed and not just lying down on the sofa as the latter will not stop the patient from pottering about). Sedation with alimemazine or promethazine may be needed to keep the patient resting in bed.
- Localised acute rashes should also be rested. If the patient has an acute blistering rash on the feet, it will not get better unless he stops walking around. A patient with an acute hand eczema is unlikely to get better while continuing to do the washing up.
- The more acute the rash, the more bland the treatment needs to be. If in doubt white soft paraffin is unlikely to do any harm and will keep the patient comfortable.

7. Explain to the patient what is going on. It is important to explain to the patient what is wrong with him, what the treatment is and how to use it. Time spent at the first consultation explaining the nature of the problem and the correct use of the treatment will be time well spent.

TOPICAL TREATMENT

Any applied agent contains two components:–

1. The vehicle or base.
2. The active constituent.

Both are equally important, but often the right type of vehicle is not taken into consideration when prescribing a treatment. The function of the base is to transport the active constituent into the skin so that it is delivered to where it is needed. Generally speaking the base is determined by the hydration of the skin at the particular site, while the active constituent is determined by the pathological process.

THE BASE

All bases are made up from one or more of the following:–

- Powders, e.g. zinc oxide, starch, calamine (zinc carbonate and ferric oxide).
- Liquids, e.g. water, alcohol, propylene glycol.
- Oils and greases, e.g. liquid paraffin, yellow and white soft paraffin[UK]/petrolatum[USA], lanolin (wool alcohols), polyethylene glycols (synthetic waxes).

These may be mixed together to produce lotions, ointments, creams and pastes:–

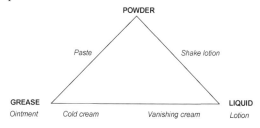

CREAMS

Creams are a mixture (emulsion) of an ointment with water. In order to prevent the two elements separating from one another, stabilisers and emulsifiers have to be added. There are 2 types of cream:–

1. **A water-in-oil emulsion** (like butter). These are the cold creams. They behave like oils in that they do not mix with any exudate from the skin. They are easier to apply than ointments, and more cosmetically acceptable, although they are greasier than the vanishing creams (*see* below). Many of them contain lanolin as the oil which can cause an allergic contact dermatitis in some patients. Examples include:–

- Oily cream/hydrous ointment[UK] (lanolin 50%, water 50%).
- Pond's Dry Skin cream[USA] (mineral oil 56%, white wax 12%, spermaceti 12%, sodium borate 0.5%, water 19%).

2. **An emulsion of oil-in-water** (like milk and cream). These are the vanishing creams. They rub into the skin easily and mix readily with water so they are very popular with patients. They contain a high proportion of water and the oil component is kept in suspension by using an emulsifying agent such as glycerol or sodium lauryl sulphate. Examples of oil-in-water creams are:–

- Aqueous cream[UK] (emulsifying ointment 30%, water 69.9% and chlorocresol 0.1%).
- Cetomacrogol A cream[UK] (cetomacrogol 1.8%, cetostearyl alcohol 7.2%, white soft paraffin 15%, liq. paraffin 6%, water 69.9% and chlorocresol 0.1%) is used as a diluent for many steroid creams.
- Hydrophilic ointment[USA] (sodium lauryl sulphate 0.6%, propylene glycol 12%, stearyl alcohol 25%, white petrolatum 25%, water 37% and parabens 0.4%).

One of the main disadvantages of creams is that they tend to make dry skin even drier because the water in them evaporates. If the skin is dry (e.g. in atopic eczema), a vanishing cream may make the condition worse; a cold cream or ointment will be better. A further disadvantage is that they must contain preservatives, such as parahydroxybenzoic acid esters (parabens), chlorocresol, propylene glycol or ethylene diamine, to prevent the cream from becoming contaminated by bacteria. All these preservatives can act as sensitisers and cause an allergic contact dermatitis in some patients.

OINTMENTS

Ointments contain little or no water and consist of organic hydrocarbons, alcohols and acids. These are greasy and form an impermeable layer over the skin which prevents evaporation of water. Examples include:–

- White soft paraffin[UK]/petrolatum[USA] (*Vaseline*).
- Emulsifying ointment[UK] (emulsifying wax 30%, liquid paraffin 20%, white soft paraffin 50%) [emulsifying wax = cetostearyl alcohol, sodium lauryl sulphate and water].
- Hydrophilic petrolatum[USA] (cholesterol 3%, stearyl alcohol 3%, white wax 8%, petrolatum 86%).
- Lanolin (wool fat purified from sheep wool 6%, paraffins 94%).

Organic hydrocarbons are sub-divided by their melting points:–

- Liquid paraffin[UK]/liquid petrolatum[USA] is liquid at room temperature and is used in bath oils.
- White soft paraffin[UK] (WSP)/petrolatum[USA] is semi-solid at room temperature, but melts at body temperature, so rubs in easily.
- A mixture comprising equal parts of liquid paraffin and white soft paraffin is useful for covering large areas of the body with grease.

- Waxes have high melting points and are useful for stiffening up an ointment base.

Some ointments may be water soluble, and consist of polyethylene glycols such as fatty acid propylene glycol (FAPG). These compounds are semi-solids similar to WSP, so they spread well on the skin and wash off with water.

PASTES

Pastes are a mixture of a powder in an ointment. They stay where you put them and do not spread away from that site as the skin warms up (like creams and ointments do). Zinc oxide paste[USA] is the one which is most commonly used. It contains 25% starch, 25% zinc oxide, and 50% white soft paraffin. Lassar's paste[UK] contains 2% salicylic acid as well.

Cooling pastes are preparations which contain a powder (zinc oxide), water (lime water) and an oil (arachis oil). They are called creams rather than pastes in the UK, e.g. zinc cream B.P. (zinc oxide 32g, oleic acid 0.5ml, arachis oil 32ml, wool fat 8g, calcium hydroxide 45mg, water to 100g).

LOTIONS

A lotion is any liquid. It may be a straightforward liquid such as normal saline or a solution of potassium permanganate, or a shake lotion consisting of a suspension of an insoluble powder in a liquid.

Shake lotions, such as calamine lotion (calamine 15%, zinc oxide 5%, glycerine 5%, water 75%) have a cooling effect because the liquid evaporates leaving the inert powder on the skin. In practice these are hardly ever used except to cool sunburn.

GELS

Gels are transparent semisolid emulsions of organic polymers (e.g. methylcellulose, agar or gelatine) in a liquid (e.g. water). They have the property of being solid (or semisolid) in the cold and becoming liquid on warming up (like a jelly).

When to use which kind of vehicle

Ointments and creams are used most of the time. Which you use depends mainly on the patient's preference and the hydration of the skin. Start with a cream on normal or moist skin and an ointment on dry skin. Creams are much more cosmetically acceptable, particularly on the face (patients do not like walking around with a shiny face), in the flexures and when the medicament has to be applied all over (so that the clothes are not covered with grease), but may be too drying if the skin is itself dry (e.g. in patients with atopic eczema and ichthyosis). In general ointments are more effective than creams, but you may have to try both to see which suits the patient best. Because creams contain water, they must also contain preservatives to prevent contamination by bacteria and fungi; these can cause an allergic contact dermatitis. In patients with an acute eczema or allergic contact dermatitis where you do not know the cause, always use an ointment (which does not contain lanolin) rather than a cream until you have discovered the cause.

Pastes are used where you want to apply a noxious chemical to a particular part of the skin without getting it onto the surrounding normal skin, e.g. dithranol[UK]/anthralin[USA] in psoriasis. They are not used very much because they are unsightly. They have to be applied with a gloved hand or a spatula and they have to be cleaned off with oil (e.g. arachis oil) rather than soap and water.

Lotions are used on wet surfaces and on hairy areas, e.g:–

- In the mouth as a mouth wash.
- On the scalp so that it does not make a mess.
- On wet rashes (e.g. weeping eczema). Use an astringent which will coagulate protein and dry up the exudate. The two which are commonly used are:–

1. Potassium permanganate (KMnO₄)

This is dispensed as crystals, as a tablet (*Permitab*), or as a 1:1000 solution. The crystals or tablets are best dissolved in a jar of water to produce a dark purple solution. This then needs to be diluted so that the final colour of the liquid is light pink (Fig. 2.01). If the solution used is too strong (i.e. purple), then the skin and nails will be stained brown (Fig. 2.02).

2. Aluminium acetate (Burow's solution)

It is made by mixing 5 parts of a 13% solution of aluminium acetate in 100 parts of sterile water, or by dissolving a packet or tablet of *Domeboro* or *Bluboro* in 1 pint of water. This is used as a soak. The neat 13% solution may be used as ear drops to treat exudative otitis externa.

Gels are used as alternatives to lotions mainly on hairy parts of the body. For example, since all topical steroid lotions are in an alcoholic base they are not suitable for applying to excoriated eczematous skin because they will sting. A steroid gel (which does not contain alcohol) can be rubbed into the scalp without causing stinging. It becomes liquid when it is rubbed in and is therefore cosmetically acceptable (like a lotion).

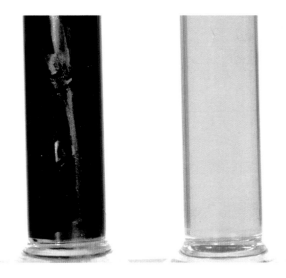

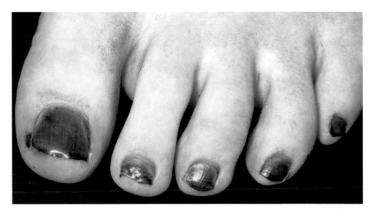

Fig. 2.01 (above) Potassium permanganate solution. On the right, the pale pink colour is the correct dilution. On the left the solution is too strong and if used like this will stain the skin and nails brown (**Fig. 2.02** below).

ACTIVE INGREDIENTS

TOPICAL STEROIDS

Topical steroids are extremely useful in inflammatory conditions of the skin, particularly in eczema but they are not the treatment for everything (they are contraindicated in acne, rosacea, all infections [bacterial, viral and fungal] and infestations, and on leg ulcers).

Topical steroids are divided into 4 groups in the UK and 7 groups in the USA according to their potency (*see* table on page 409).

UK group	USA group	Strength
Weak^{UK}	Group 6–7 ^{USA}	= to hydrocortisone
Moderately potent^{UK}	Group 4–5 ^{USA}	2.5 × stronger
Potent^{UK}	Group 2–3 ^{USA}	10 × stronger
Very potent^{UK}	Group 1 ^{USA}	50 × stronger

Table 2.01

There are a very large number to choose from and it is best to become familiar with a few (perhaps one or two from each group) rather than all of them. Relative potencies of the different groups compared with the potency of 1% hydrocortisone are important in deciding on which topical steroid to use. As a general rule, use the weakest possible steroid that is effective.

We would recommend that you only use 1% hydrocortisone* or equivalent (weak^{UK}/group 6–7^{USA}) topical steroid on the face, and start with this elsewhere, and only use something stronger if it does not work. Remember that in the flexures absorption of the steroid will be increased because of occlusion. In practice we rarely find it necessary to use anything stronger than moderately potent^{UK}/group 4–5^{USA} steroids for extensive eczema on the trunk and

*Drug names which are underlined are those prescribable in the UK by specialist nurse practitioners.

limbs. The potent^{UK}/group 2–3^{USA} steroids are useful for localised persistent eczema.

There is little place for very potent^{UK}/group 1^{USA} steroids in general practice, and where you might be considering their use, systemic steroids might be safer. 50g of 0.05% clobetasol propionate (*Dermovate*^{UK}/*Temovate*^{USA})/week will suppress the patient's adrenal glands. Hydrocortisone is 50 times weaker so is obviously a lot safer; in theory a patient could use up to 2.5kg/week before getting the same side effects.

Application of topical steroids

Although topical steroids are traditionally applied twice a day, there is no evidence that this is the best way to use them. Since the steroid molecule persists in the stratum corneum and is slowly absorbed, it may be that a single application at night would work just as well. Using a moisturiser frequently might be more effective than increasing the number of applications of a topical steroid.

Repeated application of potent topical steroids can result in a diminished effect (tachyphylaxis) sometimes after only one week of use. Recovery of response returns within a week of stopping. To prevent this happening use potent steroids in 5-day bursts only, followed by moisturisers for the other 2 days.

15g of ointment or cream is enough to cover the adult body surface once. To cover the whole body for a week if applied daily will require 100g. If a patient has widespread eczema adequate amounts of topical steroid should be prescribed or they are likely to relapse. A useful guide is the **finger-tip unit**, which is the amount of cream/ointment that is squeezed onto the index finger from tip to the distal IP joint. This amount of cream will cover the area of two palms.

Absorption of topical steroids

The potency of the steroid molecule can be enhanced by the base used, e.g. an ointment base makes the steroid more potent than a cream or lotion. Occlusion over the site of application increases the steroid potency 50-fold. Occlusion causes over hydration of the stratum corneum reducing the skin's natural barrier. It induces a reservoir effect so that the steroid can persist in the skin for several days. The site and degree of inflammation also affect absorption. The relative ability for a topical steroid to be absorbed at various sites is:–

Back < forearm < scalp < forehead < cheeks < axilla < scrotum

Normal skin < inflamed skin < erythrodermic skin

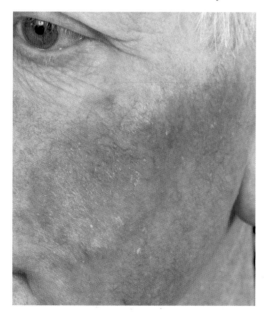

Fig. 2.03 Telangiectasia on the face caused by application of a potent topical steroid.

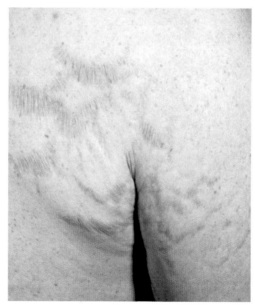

Fig. 2.04 Striae from application of a potent topical steroid in a patient with psoriasis.

Side effects of topical steroids

- Skin atrophy and striae (Fig. 2.04) from loss of dermal collagen.
- Tearing of the skin leading to odd shaped scars (stellate scars) due to loss of dermal collagen (Fig. 9.30, p. 245).
- Easy bruising due to loss of collagen support of the blood vessels in the dermis.
- Perioral dermatitis when steroids (moderately potent[UK]/groups 1–5[USA]) are applied to the face of young adults (*see* p. 97).
- Telangiectasia on the face when steroids from moderately potent [UK]/groups 1–5[USA] are applied to the face in middle and old age (Fig. 2.03).
- Rebound phenomenon causing worsening of the skin condition when the steroid is stopped, especially in psoriasis.
- Susceptibility to infection (bacterial, viral & fungal).
- Tachyphylaxis. Repeated use results in loss of effect.
- Allergic contact dermatitis. About 2% of patients being treated with topical steroids become allergic to the steroid itself (rather than the base).

- Cushing's syndrome when large amounts of potent or very potent[UK]/groups 1–3[USA] steroids are used. This includes a moon face and buffalo hump and all the systemic effects that you get with oral steroids (*see* p. 42).
- Pituitary axis depression when large amounts of potent steroids are being used, especially in young children.

TOPICAL IMMUNE-MODULATORS

1. Calcineurin inhibitors

These are macrolide lactones isolated from *Streptomyces tsukulaensis*. They block the activity of calcineurin and inhibit T-cell activation. Their action is very similar to that of ciclosporin, but because of their lower molecular weight they are absorbed through the skin.

Two agents are currently available:–

- 0.03% & 0.1% tacrolimus (*Protopic*) ointment.
- 1% pimecrolimus (*Elidel*) cream.

Their main use is in atopic eczema. Tacrolimus is as effective as a moderately potent[UK]/group 4–5[USA] steroid while pimecrolimus is equivalent to 1% hydrocortisone in potency. Because they have no effect on collagen synthesis, there is no thinning or bruising of the skin from long-term use. The only important side effect is itching and burning of the skin when they are first applied in up to 50% of patients. This lasts for 15–20 minutes but stops after the first few days.

2. Imiquimod (*Aldara*) cream is the first of a new group of compounds which stimulate the production of interferon and other cytokines by activation of TLR7 (Toll-like receptor 7) on monocytes, macrophages and dendritic cells. It has both anti-viral and anti-tumour activity and can be used for the treatment of genital warts, solar keratoses, Bowen's disease, superficial basal cell carcinomas and lentigo maligna. It is applied three times a week for up to 12 weeks and produces a marked inflammatory reaction (*see* Fig. 9.57a, p. 258).

TAR

Tar is not used very much these days because it is brown and smelly and patients do not like it. It is still used occasionally in both eczema and psoriasis. There are basically three types of tar available:–

1. Wood tars are produced by the destructive distillation of beech, birch, pine or juniper. In the UK the only one which is used therapeutically is Oil of Cade, which can be used to treat psoriasis of the scalp (*see* p. 75).

2. Bituminous tars were originally obtained from the distillation of shale deposits containing fossilised fish, hence the name ichthyol. They are mainly used today in paste bandages (e.g. ichthammol bandages, *Ichthopaste*[UK]) to soothe chronic eczema.

3. Coal tars are a mixture of about 10,000 different compounds, mainly aromatic hydrocarbons such as benzol, naphthalene and anthracene. Crude coal tar is what remains when coal is heated without air, originally to produce coal gas. Which compounds in tar actually work is not known. They reduce DNA synthesis and therefore epidermal proliferation and they are useful for stopping itching. Crude coal tar can be refined by boiling and then alcoholic extraction to produce coal tar solution (liquor picis carbonis[UK] [LPC]/liquor carbonis detergens[USA] [LCD]).

Crude coal tar is used in the treatment of both psoriasis and eczema. In patients with psoriasis tar should not be used if the disease is unstable (acutely erupting, erythrodermic or generalised pustular psoriasis) because it will make it worse. It should also be avoided in the flexures because it will make the patient sore. It can be used in stable plaque psoriasis, on scalp psoriasis or on pustular psoriasis of the palms and soles.

In eczema tar should not be used on acute weeping eczema but it is very useful in discoid eczema and lichen simplex.

It is usually prescribed as Coal tar and salicylic acid ointment BP^UK** (2% crude coal tar & 2% salicylic acid), White's tar ointment^USA (5%), or various strengths (2–10%) in WSP or Lassar's paste.

Coal tar solution is less messy but less effective. The messier the tar preparation the more effective it is, but less cosmetically acceptable for the patient. Coal tar solution can be dispensed as an ointment (2–10% coal tar solution in WSP) or as proprietary creams (_Clinitar_^UK, _Exorex_^UK, Fototar^USA, _Pragmatar_^UK, _Psoriderm_^UK, Tegrin^USA), as bath emollients (_Balnetar_^UK, Lavatar^USA, _Polytar_, _Psoriderm_^UK, T/Derm^USA, Zetar^USA) or as shampoos (Alphosyl 2in1^UK, Capasal^UK, _Clinitar_^UK, Estar^USA, _Psoriderm_^UK, _T-gel_).

Side effects of tar and problems with using it

- It is brown and smelly. Patients do not like the look of it (_see_ Fig. 8.53, p. 198) and it will stain the clothes and bedding. Some patients do not mind the smell but most do not like it.
- It can cause an irritant reaction on the skin.
- Occasionally it will cause a contact allergic eczema.
- It may cause a photosensitivity reaction.
- It will cause a folliculitis on hairy areas and is best avoided in patients who are very hairy.

*_Drug names_ which are underlined are those prescribable in the UK by specialist nurse practitioners.

**Available from Martindale Pharmaceuticals. Tel: 0800 137627.

DITHRANOL^UK/ANTHRALIN^USA

This is a synthetic anthracene derivative. It is a yellow powder which can be made up into a cream, ointment, stick or paste and is very effective in the treatment of stable plaque psoriasis (_see_ p. 198). Do not use it in acute eruptive psoriasis, erythrodermic psoriasis or generalised pustular psoriasis or the rash will get worse rather than better.

VITAMIN D$_3$ ANALOGUES

Calcitriol (_Silkis_), calcipotriol (_Dovonex_), and tacalcitol (_Curatoderm_) are vitamin D$_3$ analogues which are the first-line treatment for psoriasis (_see_ p. 198). They decrease epidermal proliferation and are effective in flattening the psoriatic plaques and removing the scale but not quite so good at getting rid of the redness. Only calcitriol and tacalcitol can be used on the face and flexures. Calcipotriol can cause redness and irritation at these sites. They do not cause hypercalcaemia and hypercalcuria, since less than 1% applied to the skin is absorbed.

They can be used in conjunction with a potent^UK/group 2–3^USA topical steroid (for a limited time only), UVB therapy or with a systemic retinoid for unresponsive psoriasis.

TOPICAL RETINOIDS

Topical retinoids act by increasing epidermal turnover and differentiation of corneocytes. Clinically they are useful for treatment of comedones in acne (_see_ p. 100) and psoriasis (_see_ p. 199). Retinoic acid also has an effect on the dermis whereby solar damage and solar elastosis may be reversed. The usefulness of retinoic acid is limited by its irritant effects – inflammation and exfoliation.

The topical retinoids available for acne are:–

- Adapalene (*Differin*) 0.1% cream and gel. A synthetic retinoid which avoids the irritancy of the retinoic acids.
- Isotretinoin (13-*cis*-retinoic acid) available as *Isotrex* 0.05% gel.
- Tretinoin (all-*trans*-retinoic acid) available as *Retin-A*, 0.01%–0.025% cream, lotion or gel.

The topical retinoid used for psoriasis is:–

- Tazarotene (*Zorac*). This causes some irritation of normal skin.

KERATOLYTIC AGENTS

These are used to remove hyperkeratosis in a whole variety of skin conditions including warts, hyperkeratotic eczema on the palms and soles, psoriasis and palmoplantar keratoderma. The ones most commonly used include:–

α-hydroxy acids (salicylic, lactic and benzoic acids). 2%, 5% or 10% salicylic acid ointment, applied twice a day, is useful for treating hyperkeratosis of the palms and soles or plane warts. It can be mixed with coal tar (Coal tar and salicylic acid ointment BP) for treating psoriasis (*see* p. 198), or with a topical steroid ointment for treating hyperkeratotic eczema (*see* p. 371). Lactic acid alone (*LactiCare*[UK]) or combined with urea (*Aquadrate*[UK], *Calmurid*[UK]) is a useful moisturiser. It is also combined with salicylic acid in proprietary wart paints (*see* p. 285). Benzoic acid is combined with salicylic acid (in Whitfield's ointment) for treating superficial fungal infections (*see* p. 203).

Propylene glycol. 50% propylene glycol in water is used under polythene occlusion at night to reduce excess keratin in hyperkeratotic eczema on the hands and feet (*see* p. 371). Normally a topical steroid will be used in the day time. Available as *Keralyt*[USA] gel & *Epilyt*[USA] solution.

Urea. A 40% solution of urea can be used for treating patients with hyperkeratotic eczema on the hands and feet or palmoplantar keratoderma. It is an alternative to propylene glycol but is more expensive. 10% urea cream (*Aquadrate*[UK], *Aquacare*[USA], *Carmel*[USA], *Cormel*[USA], *Eucerin*, *Neutraplus*[UK]) can be used to treat keratosis pilaris (p. 294) or mixed with 1% hydrocortisone cream (*Alphaderm*[UK], *Calmurid HC*[UK], *Carmol HC*[USA]) to treat atopic eczema (p. 208). It can be combined with lactic acid as a moisturiser (*Calmurid*[UK], *Ureacin*[USA]).

ANTIBIOTICS

As a general rule, topical antibiotics should not be used on the skin because most of them are potent skin sensitisers and will cause an allergic contact dermatitis. You do not want to sensitise someone to a drug which may at some future date be life saving. It is much easier to become allergic to an antibiotic applied to the skin than to one taken by mouth or given parenterally.

Virtually everyone will become sensitised to penicillin so this should never be used topically. Tetracyclines rarely cause problems and would be safe to use, but in practice they are not much use because the common skin pathogens, *Staphylococcus aureus* and *Streptococcus pyogenes* are not sensitive to tetracycline. Mupirocin (*Bactroban*) or fucidic acid (*Fucidin*) are the ones most commonly used and rarely cause problems.

Topical antibiotics should only be used in very superficial infections which will clear up in a matter of days, i.e. impetigo. They should not be used in infected eczema (because that is likely to be a recurrent problem and the patient may well become sensitised after using it several times) or on infected looking leg ulcers (almost all patients with chronic venous ulceration are allergic to a number of antibiotics on patch testing because they have been used inappropriately in the past).

Do not be tempted to use steroid–antibiotic mixtures because if the patient becomes allergic to the antibiotic in the mixture, the topical steroid will damp down the local reaction and you will only realise what has happened when the patient develops a widespread eczema. Most bacterial infections of the skin are more appropriately treated with systemic antibiotics.

ANTIVIRAL AGENTS

The only topical antiviral agents currently available are 5% aciclovir (_Zovirax_) cream and 1% penciclovir (_Vectavir_UK/ _Denavir_USA) cream. They are used for the treatment of herpes simplex (_see_ p. 91). They inhibit phosphorylation of viral thymidine kinase which prevents viral DNA synthesis and virus replication. There must be active viral replication to be effective so they need to be used immediately the first symptoms are noticed (usually tingling or paraesthesia). They are applied 5 times a day for 2–3 days until crusting has occurred.

ANTIFUNGAL AGENTS

These can be divided into 2 groups:–

1. Those active against dermatophyte fungi (which cause tinea). There are 6 groups of topical antifungal agents:–

i. **Keratolytic agents** act differently to all other antifungal agents. They remove the keratin on which the fungus lives rather than killing the fungus itself. The one which is most commonly used is Whitfield's ointment, a mixture of 6% benzoic and 3% salicylic acids in emulsifying ointment.

*_Drug names_ which are underlined are those prescribable in the UK by specialist nurse practitioners.

The others all interfere with the synthesis of ergosterol in the fungal cell membrane.

ii. **Undecanoate** as the acid zinc salt in _Mycota_UK or _Desenex_USA powder. These proprietary powders can be bought over the counter.

iii. **Tolnaftate** (_Mycil_UK, _Tinactin_UK, _Tinaderm_UK) is fungistatic. It is sold over the counter as a powder or cream.

iv. **Amorolfine** (_Loceryl_) is fungistatic. It is available as a nail lacquer or cream. The nail lacquer needs to be applied weekly after filing the surface of the nail. In the nail it also works against saprophytic moulds (such as _Hendersonula_ or _Scopulariopsis_).

v. **Imidazoles**. There are a large number of drugs in this group available as creams (_clotrimazole_, _econazole_, _ketoconazole_, _miconazole_, oxiconazole_USA, _sulconazole_). _Tioconazole_ (_Trosyl_UK) is another used as a nail lacquer. They are all fungistatic rather than fungicidal and of more or less equal efficacy. A number of imidazole–hydrocortisone mixtures are also made; these generally are not a good idea because it encourages treatment without first making a diagnosis on the mistaken belief that they will work for both fungal infections and eczema.

vi. **Allylamines**. Naftifine_USA and _terbinafine_ (_Lamisil_) are fungicidal and more effective than any of the other topical antifungal agents.

2. Those active against yeasts such as _Candida_ and _Pityrosporum_ species:–

i. **Imidazoles** are broad spectrum antifungal agents and work for yeasts as well as dermatophytes (_see_ above).

ii. **Polyenes.** Nystatin (named after the New York State Department of Health) is only effective against _Candida_. It is cheaper than the imidazoles but has the disadvantage that it stains everything it comes into contact with yellow. Amphotericin B is a broad spectrum polyene antifungal agent; it is mainly used as lozenges for treating *Candida* infections in the mouth.

3. Clioquinol is effective against *Candida* and various bacteria but not against dermatophytes. It is usually combined with a topical steroid (e.g. *Ala-Quin*[USA], *Betnovate C*[UK], *Locoid C*[UK], *Vioform HC*[UK]). It stains the skin and clothing yellow.

4. Rosaniline dyes. Gentian violet is effective against yeasts and Gram-positive organisms. It is used as a 0.5% aqueous solution but stains everything it comes into contact with purple. It is useful in wet areas, e.g. toe webs and flexures.

TOPICAL LOCAL ANAESTHETICS

Topical local anaesthetics are useful in children when applied before giving an injection of local anaesthetic, or in children or adults for providing anaesthesia to large areas of skin, e.g. before cautery of comedones or laser treatment.

The one most commonly used is *EMLA* cream (a eutectic mixture of local anaesthetics), which contains 2.5% lidocaine (lignocaine[UK]) and 2.5% prilocaine in an oil-in-water cream base. This combination allows penetration of local anaesthetic through the stratum corneum. It is applied under occlusion and left on for 90 minutes for maximum effect. Both are amides so do not cause contact sensitisation.

Tetracaine (amethocaine, *Ametop*) gel is an alternative and needs to be applied for only 45 minutes. Occlusion is not necessary but it can cause some local vasodilation and irritation. It may also cause an allergic contact dermatitis in some people.

SUNSCREENS

Sunscreens work either by absorbing or reflecting ultraviolet light.

Absorbent sunscreens contain chemicals that absorb UV light:–

1. Those which protect the skin from UVB. They are useful in protecting against sunburn, preventing solar urticaria or polymorphic light eruption (*see* p. 83). Examples include:–
- Para-aminobenzoic acid (PABA). Not commonly used because it causes allergic contact dermatitis.
- PABA esters, e.g. octyldimethyl PABA (Padimate-O). Only gives partial protection against UVB, but penetrates into the stratum corneum after ½–2 hours, so not easily removed by water. PABA preparations often sting the skin and stain the clothes yellow.
- Cinnamates, e.g. 2-ethylhexyl *p*-methoxycinnamate, octocrylene.
- Salicylates, e.g. octyl salicylate.

2. Those which protect against UVB and UVA up to 350nm:–
- Benzophenones, e.g. oxybenzone.

3. Those which protect only against UVA:–
- Dibenzoylmethanes, e.g. butyl methoxy dibenzoyl methane (avobenzone).

Reflectant sunscreens contain inert mineral pigments, either titanium dioxide or zinc oxide, which put an opaque barrier between the sun and the skin. They protect against both UVB and UVA but are unsightly for the patient because they are white. They are needed for patients with porphyria, photosensitive eczema or photosensitivity due to drugs.

The efficacy of sunscreens in protecting against UVB is measured by the sun protection factor (SPF). The higher the number the greater the protection. An SPF of 10 (for example) allows a person to remain in the sun 10× longer before burning.

TOPICAL AGENTS FOR WOUND CARE

Wound healing occurs in three stages:–

1. An influx of inflammatory cells to aid reabsorption of necrotic cells and prevent infection. This causes erythema and exudate.

2. The formation of granulation tissue and revascularisation. At this stage there is a reduction in exudate.

3. Migration of epidermal cells to cover the wound and growth of new connective tissue underneath.

Wound healing takes place most rapidly when:–

- There is a moist environment (not too wet, not too dry) and any excess fluid is able to evaporate.
- The wound is warm – a drop in temperature of 2°C significantly reduces healing.
- There is good blood perfusion. Dressings do not affect this although a suction pump may.

MANAGEMENT OF CHRONIC WOUNDS

Successful treatment of leg ulcers and other chronic wounds therefore depends on:–

1. Dealing with the underlying cause (e.g. compression bandages for venous hypertension, taking the weight off pressure sores etc.).

2. Attention to nutrition and correction of any deficiencies.

3. Management of the wound itself:–

- Removal of dead and necrotic tissue (*see* Table 2.03).
- Reduction of bacterial counts and treatment of clinical infection (*see* Table 2.04).
- Reduction of excessive exudate (*see* Table 2.05).
- Covering the wound to promote healing (*see* Table 2.06).

Type of wound surface	Dressing to use
1. Dry adherent black slough	Hydrogel (or surgical debridement)
2. Dirty superficial yellow slough – little exudate	Hydrocolloid Maggots
3. Clinical infection – low exudate	Iodine Silver
4. Clinical infection – high exudate	Silver based hydrofibre (*Aquacel AG*)
5. Smelly/fungating	Activated charcoal
6. Low exudate	Foam
7. Moderate exudate	Foam with high absorbance (*Allevyn*) Alginate
8. Excess exudate	Capillary – *Vacutex* Hydrofibre – *Aquacel* Hydroactive – *Cutinova*
9. Clean wound or one with healthy granulation tissue	Simple non-adherent dressing with padding for insulation and protection Biomaterial dressings (*Oasis* or *Promogran*)
10. Over granulation	Foam

Table 2.02 Type of wound and which dressing to use.

DEBRIDING AGENTS   (Table 2.03)

Wound cleansing for its own sake is not a good thing. The wound bed is disturbed and any new epithelium ripped off.
Any necrotic material should be removed. This can be done surgically with a pair of scissors or a scalpel, or by using a debriding agent.

Type	Brand names	Available as	Used on	How to use	Comments & contraindications
Hydrogel	*Aquaform*, *GranuGel*, *Intrasite*, *Nu-Gel*, *Purilon*, *Sterigel*	Gel Ointment	Dry sloughy or necrotic wounds	Squeeze gel onto wound & cover with a secondary dressing.	Do not use on wet wounds. Scarify dry necrotic tissue to allow gel to soak in.
	Aquaflo, *Curagel*, *Geliperm*, *Hydrosorb*, *Novogel*	Sheets		Apply sheet and cover with secondary dressing.	
Hydrocolloid	*Alione*, *Askina*, *CombiDERM*, *Comfeel*, *Cutinova*, *DuoDERM*, *Granuflex*, *Hydrocoll*, *Physiotulle*, *Replicare*, *Tegasorb*, *Ultec*	Sheets: hydrocolloid matrix backed with a waterproof polyurethane foam	Clean or sloughy wounds, with low to moderate exudate	Apply the hydrocolloid dressing with a 2cm overlap to hold in the exudate which is produced. The dressing is changed as soon as it begins to leak (approximately once or twice a week). There is a tendency for the exudate, as it accumulates, to force its way out of the dressing and run down the patient's leg particularly when walking about. *Cavilon* (*see* Table 2.06) can be used to protect the surrounding skin.	The hydrocolloid interacts with the ulcer exudate to form a soft moist gel which provides an acid environment allowing autolytic digestion of any necrotic material. Aerobic and anaerobic bacteria will flourish in this environment producing an unpleasant smell.
Maggots	*LarvE* from Biosurgical Research Unit, Princess of Wales Hospital, Bridgend, S.Wales, UK	Sterile maggots in small container or bag	Very sloughy wounds with mild to moderate exudate	Add saline to the maggots and tip them onto the fine mesh net provided. Place this with the maggots in contact with the ulcer inside a hydrocolloid sheet cut to the size of the ulcer. Cover the outside of the net with moistened swabs, an *NA dressing* and *Sleek* adhesive tape. The maggots should be left in place for 48–72 hours and then washed out with saline.	Maggots are extremely efficient debriding agents, feeding on necrotic tissue without affecting normal skin.
Acids	*Aserbine*	Cream and a solution	Sloughy wounds	Clean the ulcer with *Aserbine* solution, fill the ulcer with the cream and cover with a dry secondary dressing. The dressing will need changing every day.	Acid debriding agents are rarely used since they may damage the wound bed.
Enzymes	*Varidase*	Powder in saline	Sloughy wounds	Put solution on gauze or mix with KY jelly and apply to wound.	Rarely used since streptokinase is used for treating myocardial infaction.

REDUCING BACTERIAL COUNTS AND ODOUR (Table 2.04)

All wounds left open will become colonised by bacteria. Taking swabs is not usually helpful. Clinical signs of infection are cellulitis of the surrounding skin, a foul odour, or *increasing* levels of pain, exudate or capillary bleeding with pitted/spongy granulation tissue. The organisms that matter are:–

- A group A beta haemolytic streptococcus which causes cellulitis (*see* p. 331). This should be treated with iv or im benzyl penicillin.
- Pseudomonas which causes a green discoloration and has a distinctive foul smell. This can be treated with acetic acid or silver.

Do not use antibiotic impregnated tulle dressings because patients frequently become allergic to them.

Type	Brand names	Available as	Used on	How to use	Comments & contraindications
Activated charcoal dressings	*CarboFLEX*, *Lyofoam C*	Absorbent sheet	Smelly wounds	Apply direct and change when necessary.	*CarboFLEX* consists of 5 layers in the dressing. *Lyofoam C* is Lyofoam with added charcoal.
	Actisorb Silver 200, *Carbopad VC*, *CliniSorb*	Non-absorbent cloth		Needs absorbent pad and secondary dressing as well.	Charcoal absorbs odour but has no antibacterial activity. Not effective if wet.
Silver	*Flamazine*	Cream	Infected wounds	Apply direct onto wound or mix with a hydrogel.	Silver is effective against pseudomonas but needs moisture to activate it.
	Acticoat *Aquacel AG* *Avance* *Actisorb silver 200*	Sheet	Low exudate High exudate High exudate Low exudate	Direct to wound.	Rayon polyester core. Hydrofibre dressing with silver. Hydropolymer foam dressing, silver bonded polymer. Contains charcoal as well.
Metronidazole	*Metrotop*	Gel	Smelly wounds	Apply direct to wound.	Metronidazole useful for pseudomonas.
Natural products	Sugar paste* Manuka honey	Paste	Infected sloughy wounds	Need covering with film dressing.	Works by osmotic action, and by altering the pH to make the wound inhospitable for bacteria.
	5% acetic acid	Vinegar	Smelly wounds	Apply to gauze cut to shape of wound.	Useful for pseudomonas infection.
Iodine	*Inadine*, *Poviderm*	Fabric dressing	Low exudate	Apply direct to wound.	May cause allergic contact dermatitis.
	Iodoflex *Iodosorb*	Paste Ointment/powder	Moderate to high exudate		

Formula for sugar paste: Caster sugar (400g), icing sugar (600g), glycerol [glycerine] (480ml), hydrogen peroxide solution [30% BP] (7.5ml)

*__Drug names__ which are underlined are those prescribable in the UK by specialist nurse practitioners.

ABSORPTION OF EXUDATE (Table 2.05)

Venous ulcers produce serous exudate because of the high hydrostatic pressure. Exudate is a problem because it soaks through bandages and makes a mess of clothing and bedding. Drawing the exudate away from the wound surface will allow better healing.

Type	Brand names	Available	Used on	How to use	Comments & contraindications
Alginate	*Algisite M, Algosteril, Curasorb, Kaltostat, Melgisorb, SeaSorb, Sorbalgon, Sorbsan, Tegagen*	Sheet or ribbon	Moderately exuding wounds	Cut to the exact size and shape of the ulcer. They expand laterally when wet so can cause maceration of the surrounding skin. Leave in place for several days or up to a week at a time. Removed by squirting normal saline onto dressing or by lifting off with a pair of forceps.	Alginates are naturally occurring polysaccharides found only in brown seaweeds (*Phaeophycae*). The alginic acid is usually converted to calcium or sodium salts. Calcium alginate is insoluble in water; sodium alginate is very soluble in water.
Hydrofibre	*Aquacel*	Sheet or ribbon	Heavily exuding wounds	The sheet is not cut to size but put over the wound as a square. It should be changed according to the amount of exudate being produced (daily – weekly). The solid gel needs to be removed before a new sheet is applied.	The fibres absorb fluid and the material is drawn down into the ulcer to form a gel. The advantage over alginates is that it will lock in moisture, as well as absorbing 3× the amount of exudate that alginates do.
Hydroactive dressing	*Cutinova Hydro*	Sheet	Moderately exuding wounds	The dressing is placed over the wound or cut into strips to pack a deep wound. Cover with a secondary dressing. Change every 2–3 days initially, leave on longer as exudate diminishes.	A highly absorbent dressing made from a polyurethane matrix which absorbs water but leaves other molecules within the wound.
Capillary dressing	*Vacutex*	Sheet	Heavily exuding wounds	Vacutex can be cut to any shape for surface wounds or packed into deeper ones. It needs to be covered with a secondary permeable film.	*Vacutex* is a polyester and cotton sheet with its fibres arranged in such a way that fluid is drawn away from the wound.
Osmotic absorbents	*Debrisan, Iodosorb*	Beads	Moderately exuding wounds	The beads are poured into the ulcer and covered by a secondary dressing. They should be changed every 1–2 days depending on how much exudate is present. Clean out the old beads before replacing.	Dextranomer beads are able to absorb 4× their own weight of exudate.
Silastic foam	Cavi-Care Silastic foam BP	Foam	Deep cavities & bed sores	Mix liquid and catalyst. Mould foam into shape of cavity and leave for 48 hrs.	Allows wound to fill in from the bottom up. Needs a secondary dressing.

WOUND AND ULCER DRESSINGS (Table 2.06)

Type	Brand names	Available as	Used on	How to use	Comments & contraindications
Low contact primary dressings	*Atrauman*, *N-A dressing*, *Paratex*, *Setoprime*, *Tegapore*, *Tricotex*, *Urgotul*	Woven acrylic mesh dressing	Surgical wounds	Apply directly to wound.	
	Jelonet, *Paranet*, *Paratulle*	Paraffin gauze	Clean open wounds Low exudate		Large mesh allows epidermis to grow through resulting in trauma to epidermis on removal.
	Mepitel, *N-A Ultra* *Mepilex* (+foam backing)	Woven silicon mesh dressing	Clean open wounds Low exudate		These are more expensive but less adherent, so are less likely to damage the wound surface.
Film dressings	*Blisterfilm*, *Bioclusive*, *Central Gard*, *C-View*, *Hydrofilm*, *Mefilm*, *Opsite*, *Polyskin II*, *Tegaderm*, *Niko Gard*	Transparent film	Clean wounds with low exudate	Peel off backing and apply direct.	Waterproof and adhesive but lets vapour/air through. Have no insulating properties so wounds become cooled and heal more slowly.
	Cavilon, *SuperSkin*	Silicon liquid or spray	Protects normal skin around stomas, apply over pressure sores	Spray onto skin and allow to set.	Useful for skin in contact with faeces or urine, or skin onto which adhesive tape or a dressing is to be applied.
Absorbent pads	*Cutilin*, *Drisorb*, *Exu-Dry*, *Interpose*, *Mesorb*, *Release*, *Skintact*, *Solvadine-N*, *Telfa*		Any exuding wounds	Apply over a primary dressing.	Useful as a secondary dressing to absorb exudate.
Island dressings	*Ildress*, *Cosmporore E*, *Medipore*, *Mepore*, *Primapore*, *Sterifix*, *Telfa island*	Adhesive woven cloth with central pad	For protection of dry surgical wounds	Apply direct to wound.	Absorbs moisture but vapour permeable.
Foam dressings	*Allevyn*, *Biatain*, *Curafoam*, *FlexiPore*, *Hydrafoam*, *Lyofoam*, *Tielle*, *Transorbent*, *Trufoam*, *Mepilex* (+Silicon weave contact)	Sheet with or without adhesive border	As a secondary dressing As a pressure pad For insulation For over granulation	Apply direct to wound.	Polyurethane thin inner hydrophilic layer which absorbs limited amounts of exudate, and a thicker spongy outer hydrophobic breathable foamy layer which keeps wound moist, warm, protected from trauma, but allowing some evaporation.
Multi-layered dressings	*Transorbent*, *Versiva*	Sheet	Exuding wounds	Apply direct to wound.	Adhesive layer, non-adherent wound contact layer, hydrogel or hydrofibre absorptive layer, outer foam/polyurethane insulating layer.
New bio-engineered dressings	*Oasis* *Promogran*	Sheet	Clean, low exudate No infection, bleeding	Change 2–3 days when formed gel.	Derived from pig small intestine mucosa and containing collagen & regenerated cellulose.
	Hyalofill	Sheet	Deep exuding wounds	Apply direct.	Made from esterified hyaluronic acid.

*_Drug names_ which are underlined are those prescribable in the UK by specialist nurse practitioners.

SYSTEMIC TREATMENT

ANTIBIOTICS

Systemic antibiotics are used for:–

1. Staphylococcal infections in the skin, e.g. boils, carbuncles, ecthyma, staphylococcal scalded skin syndrome, sycosis barbae, and infected eczema and scabies. Flucloxacillin 250mg every 6 hours (double this for severe infections) is the drug of choice. For patients who are allergic to penicillin, erythromycin 500mg every 6 hours is an alternative. With this dose, gastrointestinal upsets occur in about 20% of patients. The cephalosporins are not as good as flucloxacillin against *Staphylococcus aureus* so should not be used as the first line of treatment.

2. MRSA (methicillin-resistant *Staphylococcus aureus*) infected wounds may need treatment with i.v. vancomycin. It is best to liaise with your local microbiologist or infection control team to check current sensitivities.

3. Streptococcal infections in the skin, e.g. erysipelas and cellulitis. Streptococci are always sensitive to penicillin so intravenous benzyl penicillin, 1200mg every 6 hours, is the drug of choice. Erythromycin 500mg every 6 hours orally is not as effective but is useful in patients who are allergic to penicillin. Streptococcal ecthyma, or eczema and scabies which are secondarily infected with *Streptococcus pyogenes* can be treated with phenoxymethyl penicillin 500mg every 6 hours.

4. Acne, perioral dermatitis and rosacea. These are not due to infection with bacteria but nevertheless respond well to low doses of broad spectrum antibiotics (*see* pp. 98–100, 105). How they work is not fully understood.

ANTIFUNGAL AGENTS

Normally superficial fungal infections of the skin are treated with topical antifungal agents. The exceptions are when the hair and nails are involved when it is not possible to get the antifungal agent to the site at which it is required. Four groups of antifungal agents are available for systemic use:–

1. Antibiotics – griseofulvin. This is the cheapest of the options and works well for tinea capitis; it is not very effective for nail infections. It is long acting so only has to be given once a day but it has to be taken with food because it is absorbed with fat.

Side effects are unusual – headache, irritability and nausea are the most common. Occasionally it can cause photosensitivity or a drug induced LE. If the patient is on warfarin, the INR will need to be checked because the anti-coagulant effect will be diminished. Do not use in patients with acute intermittent or variegate porphyria because it can induce acute attacks.

2. Allylamines – terbinafine. This is a fungicidal drug which is much more effective than griseofulvin and also much more expensive. It works well for any kind of dermatophyte infection but is particularly useful for tinea of the nails. It is taken once a day for 3 months for nail infections or for 2 weeks for infections on the skin or scalp. It occasionally causes mild gastrointestinal upsets – anorexia, nausea, diarrhoea, abdominal fullness. Do not use during pregnancy and lactation.

3. Imidazoles – ketaconazole. This is very effective for treating pityriasis versicolor where it is given as a single 400mg dose. It should not be used for longer periods of time because there is a small risk of liver toxicity.

4. Triazoles – itraconazole and fluconazole. They are used for infections with *Candida albicans*, *Cryptococcus* or *Histoplasmosis* in patients who are immunosuppressed (those with malignant disease, HIV or those on cytotoxic drugs).

Side effects of itraconazole include nausea, abdominal pain, dyspepsia and headache. As it is a potent inhibitor of cytochrome P450 enzymes it may elevate the blood levels of other drugs being taken concurrently such as ciclosporin, felodipine, digoxin, warfarin and oral hypoglycaemics. Fluconazole rarely causes hepatotoxicity.

Nystatin is not absorbed when given by mouth so the only reason for using it is if you want to clear the gut of *Candida albicans*.

ANTIVIRAL AGENTS

Aciclovir, famciclovir and valaciclovir are the systemic antiviral agents in current use. They all inhibit phosphorylation of viral thymidine kinase, which prevents viral DNA synthesis and virus replication. They are only effective while there is active viral replication and must therefore be given within 48 hours of the onset of vesicles in both herpes simplex and herpes zoster. They can be used for treating:–

1. Herpes simplex if the patient has disseminated disease, frequent recurrences, eczema herpeticum or recurrent erythema multiforme (*see* pp. 91, 92, 153).

2. Herpes zoster. This is much less sensitive to these drugs than herpes simplex so bigger doses need to be given (*see* p. 158).

ANTIHISTAMINES

Antihistamines act as competitive blockers of histamine receptors. They have a close structural resemblance to histamine. As there are two types of histamine receptor, H_1 and H_2, there are two types of antihistamines. Cutaneous blood vessels have both H_1 and H_2 receptors, but for skin disease H_1 antihistamines are the most effective.

NON-SEDATIVE ANTIHISTAMINES are the most useful drugs in urticaria and angio-oedema. Cetirizine, levocetirizine, fexofenadine, loratadine, desloratadine and mizolastine are the ones most commonly used. They are not useful in eczema.

SEDATIVE ANTIHISTAMINES are useful for sedating children with atopic eczema to ensure that they and their parents get a good night's sleep. It is essential to give a big enough dose to ensure the child sleeps through the night. They are also useful for adults with very widespread rashes who need to rest the skin, e.g. patients with erythrodermic eczema or psoriasis, and patients with acute blistering conditions on the feet who would otherwise find it difficult to rest in bed. Hydroxyzine (*Atarax*), promethazine (*Phenergan*) and alimemazine (trimeprazine, *Vallergan*) are the most useful. Chlorphenamine (*Piriton*) is short acting (4 hours). It can be used in acute urticaria and in patients with photosensitive eczema who may be allergic to the others.

H_2 ANTIHISTAMINES Cimetidine (*Tagamet*) and ranitidine (*Zantac*) are sometimes worth trying in patients with urticaria where H_1 antihistamines alone have not been effective. Cimetidine can also be given to reduce haemolysis and methaemoglobinaemia in patients taking dapsone (*see* p. 216).

---

*Drug names which are underlined are those prescribable in the UK by specialist nurse practitioners.

RETINOIDS

Retinoids are derivatives of Vitamin A. Their exact mode of action is unknown but they have many effects including:–

- Induction of differentiation of epidermal cells. This may be how they work in psoriasis, solar keratoses and Bowen's disease. In patients who have had organ transplants they may suppress the development of epithelial tumours (e.g. BCCs and SCCs), but they do not make established tumours go away.
- Shrinking of sebaceous glands causing decreased production of sebum.
- Anti-inflammatory effects by reducing prostaglandins and leukotrienes.
- Modulation of the immune response by enhancing T helper cells and stimulating interleukin 1.

There are two retinoids which are in current use:–

1. Isotretinoin, the 13-*cis* isomer of retinoic acid (*Roaccutane*[UK]/ *Accutane*[USA]), is used for the treatment of severe acne (*see* p. 101) at a dose of 0.5–1.0 mg/kg/day for 4 months.

2. Acitretin (*Neotigason*) is used to treat psoriasis and disorders of keratinization (Darier's disease, pityriasis rubra pilaris, severe types of ichthyosis). It can also be used in conjunction with PUVA (RePUVA) to decrease the amount of ultraviolet light that the patient is exposed to (*see* p. 49). Acitretin may help prevent the development of epithelial tumours (BCCs and SCCs) in patients who are immunosuppressed, especially those who have had renal transplants. It is given at a dose of 10–50 mg/day.

Some of it is converted to etretinate (an ester of acitretin) which has a long half-life of 2 years. It is recommended that female patients do not get pregnant whilst taking it or for 2 years after stopping it.

Side effects of retinoids

- Teratogenic (no effect on sperm). Must NOT be given to women of child bearing age unless on adequate contraception.
- Dryness of the lips. This always occurs and you can tell whether a patient is taking medication from this sign. *Vaseline* or a lip salve applied frequently will be necessary.
- Dryness of the nasal mucosa which can lead to nose bleeds.
- Musculoskeletal aches and pains especially after exercise. Those on long-term acitretin therapy can develop ossification of ligaments. Monitor by yearly X-ray of the lumbar spine.
- Conjunctivitis and dry eyes are usually not a problem unless the patient wears contact lenses. Hypromellose eye drops may help.
- Itching of the skin +/– an eczematous rash may need treatment with a moisturiser or 1% hydrocortisone ointment.
- Rise in serum triglycerides due to decreased extra-hepatic breakdown and increased secretion by the liver.
- Increase in liver enzymes. These resolve on stopping treatment.

Specific side effects of acitretin

- Peeling of palms and soles occurs at the beginning of treatment. When it stops the skin may feel sticky or clammy.
- Increased sweating does not usually cause problems.
- Poor wound healing. The skin easily bruises and cuts take longer to heal.
- Hair loss bad enough to be noticeable only occurs in a few patients and is reversible on stopping treatment.
- Paronychia. Painful swelling around finger and toe nails occurs in a minority of patients.
- Nausea, vomiting and abdominal pain are unusual complaints.

Long-term treatment requires monitoring of blood for liver function and lipids and X-ray of the spine for ossification of ligaments.

Specific side effects of isotretinoin

- Idiosyncratic depression. There seems to be no way of predicting this and in practice it is very uncommon (1:8000). Many patients who are already depressed benefit from the drug as this improves their acne, and it does not result in worsening of their depression.
- Irregularity or cessation of periods in women.

SYSTEMIC STEROIDS

Systemic steroids have a very limited use in the treatment of skin disease and are best restricted to use by a dermatologist. They should not be used in eczema or urticaria because, although the response may initially be dramatic, the disease is likely to flare badly when the tablets are stopped and it is then very difficult to get the patient off them. It is better to refer such a patient for an urgent dermatological opinion than to start him on prednisone.

Systemic steroids are essential and may be life saving in:–

- Pemphigus (*see* p. 226).
- Pemphigoid (*see* p. 224).
- Systemic lupus erythematosus (*see* p. 115).
- Dermatomyositis (*see* p. 115).

High doses are needed in all of these conditions and the risk of side effects is considerable. Interestingly such patients often do not show the typical steroid facies until the disease comes under control. For example, a patient can be on 60mg prednisolone for several weeks without any evidence of a moon face, but as soon as the disease comes under control the face fattens up.

Equivalent doses of different systemic steroids	
Cortisone	100mg
Hydrocortisone	80mg
Prednisone or prednisolone	20mg
Dexamethasone	2–4mg

Side effects of systemic steroids

- Increased fat deposition on the face, shoulders and abdomen causing a moon face, buffalo hump and enlarged abdomen.
- Acne and hirsutism.
- Easy bruising and tearing of the skin.
- Striae (Fig. 2.04, p. 28).
- Delayed tissue healing.
- Increased susceptibility to infections (bacterial, fungal and viral).
- Salt and water retention leading to oedema, hypertension and congestive cardiac failure.
- Diabetes.
- Peptic ulceration leading to bleeding and perforation.
- Proximal muscle weakness.
- Osteoporosis leading to fractures particularly of the vertebrae and ribs.
- Aseptic necrosis of the femoral head.
- Cataracts and glaucoma.
- Depression or euphoria (steroid psychosis).
- Growth retardation in young children; this is not usually a problem unless steroids are given for more than 6 months.
- Suppression of the pituitary–adrenal axis leading to adrenal insufficiency on withdrawal or if the patient has some intercurrent illness or needs surgery.

To prevent complications

1. Patients will need regular checking of:–

- Weight – to pick up fluid gain (weekly).
- Blood pressure – looking for hypertension (monthly).
- Urinalysis – looking for glycosuria (monthly).
- Dexascan if patient on steroids for more than 3 months (yearly).
- Chest X-ray – looking for re-activation of TB (yearly).

2. Patients should carry a STEROID CARD or MEDIC ALERT TAG with them all the time. If they have an accident or have some other illness extra steroids can be given to prevent an Addisonian crisis.

3. To prevent stomach ulceration either use enteric coated prednisolone which is absorbed in the small intestine, or prescribe a proton pump inhibitor in addition to the steroid.

4. To prevent osteoporosis give lifestyle advice – regular exercise, stop smoking, reduce alcohol intake. Do a base line Dexascan to look at bone mineral density before treatment. Start patient on *Calcichew D₃* forte, 2 tablets a day. Patients over the age of 45 with osteoporosis or at risk of osteoporosis should also be on a bisphosphonate to reduce bone turnover, e.g. alendronic acid (*Fosamax*) 70mg/week or risedronate (*Actonel*) 5mg/day.

IMMUNOSUPPRESSIVE AGENTS/BIOLOGICALS

A number of different immunosuppressive agents are used for severe skin disease, either in their own right or as steroid sparing agents. They are all potentially dangerous and should only be initiated by a dermatologist. The most important ones are methotrexate, ciclosporin, azathioprine, cyclophosphamide and hydroxyurea. Biologicals are antibodies that target specific cells, mediators or molecules, e.g. mycophenolate mofetil and the tumour necrosis factor antagonists infliximab, adilimumab and etanercept.

METHOTREXATE

Methotrexate is used for psoriasis, Hailey–Hailey disease (chronic benign familial pemphigus, *see* p. 302) and dermatomyositis (*see* p. 115). It inhibits dihydrofolate reductase and therefore cell division. It is probably the most effective of the systemic agents in use for the treatment of psoriasis and it works very quickly (within 48 hours).

Following routine blood tests (*see* below), a 5mg test dose is given. Provided no adverse reaction has occurred it is given as a single dose of 10–25mg orally or intramuscularly *once a week*. It is excreted unchanged principally through the kidneys, so the dose needs to be reduced if renal function is impaired or if the patient is elderly. It is continued long term at the lowest dose that keeps the psoriasis under control.

Serious side effects

- **Teratogenic** so must not be used in women who might become pregnant. In men it causes reversible oligospermia.
- **Bone marrow suppression**. Check FBC before starting, then weekly for 1 month and then every 2–3 months. If the MCV becomes elevated (over 100), reduce the dose.
- **Fibrosis of the liver** can occur after several years of treatment so do not give to a patient with pre-existing liver disease or anyone who has a history of alcohol abuse. Patients on methotrexate must not drink any alcohol. The development of liver fibrosis can be monitored by measuring blood levels of type 3 procollagen (P3NP) every 6 months.

P3NP levels		
	<4.2µg/l	normal
	>8.0µg/l	consider liver biopsy
	>10.0µg/l	stop methotrexate

Less serious side effects

- Nausea, vomiting, diarrhoea and abdominal discomfort. These effects can often be avoided by changing from oral to intramuscular methotrexate.
- Stomatitis and ulceration of the mouth.
- General malaise. Patients frequently feel generally unwell (headache, lethargy, irritability and depression) for about 24 hours after a dose of methotrexate.
- Extensive ulceration of the skin. This usually occurs at the same time as a profound fall in WBC.
- Hair loss. Theoretically this is possible but is extremely rare.
- Lung problems. When methotrexate is used for treating neoplastic disease, acute pneumonitis or diffuse interstitial fibrosis can occur. With the doses used for treating psoriasis, these changes do not seem to happen.

Most side effects can be prevented by giving 5mg folic acid once a week (*not* at the same time as the methotrexate) without stopping the therapeutic effect. Patients on methotrexate must not take aspirin, diuretics, hypoglycaemics, NSAIDs, phenytoin, probenecid, sulphonamides or trimethoprim. These increase the risk of pancytopenia.

CICLOSPORIN

Ciclosporin is an immuno-suppressive drug which is useful in the treatment of severe atopic eczema and psoriasis. The starting dose is 3–5mg/kg/day. Its effect is rapid (within 2 weeks). Once the disease is under control the dose can be reduced. It is not teratogenic so can be useful in severe skin disease in pregnancy.

Side effects

- The most important side effect is **nephrotoxicity**. Ciclosporin reduces renal blood flow and causes a rise in urea and creatinine. Keeping the maximum dose below 5mg/kg/day reduces toxicity. If the blood creatinine levels increase by 30% over baseline, the dose should be reduced.
- **Hypertension** secondary to reduced kidney blood flow. If blood pressure increases above 160/95 use a calcium channel blocker, e.g. nifedipine (5–10mg t.d.s.), to reduce it.
- Increased liver enzymes, serum uric acid and cholesterol.
- Nausea and vomiting.
- Gingival hyperplasia in patients with poor dental hygiene.
- Tiredness, headaches, paraesthesiae, tremor and convulsions are rare and reversible on reduction of the dose.
- Hypertrichosis (particularly a problem in women; may not be noticed in men).
- Increased risk of lymphoma and non-melanoma skin cancer.

To prevent complications

Ideally measure the GFR (glomerular filtration rate) before starting treatment. Always check blood pressure, potassium, blood creatinine, liver function and lipids before treatment. Monitor these fortnightly for 6 weeks, monthly for 3 months and then every 2–3 months. Repeat GFR if creatinine levels increase more than 30% above baseline.

CYCLOPHOSPHAMIDE

Cyclophosphamide is used in mucous membrane pemphigoid where it is the drug of first choice (*see* p. 128). It takes 6–8 weeks to work. It is given at a dose of 1–3mg/kg/day usually 50–100mg b.i.d.

Side effects

- Pancytopenia. The patient should have a full blood count measured regularly (weekly for a month and then 2 monthly).
- Hair loss.
- Haemorrhagic cystitis. Drink plenty of fluids to prevent this.

AZATHIOPRINE

Azathioprine is used for psoriasis, atopic and photosensitive eczema, and as a steroid-sparing drug in pemphigus, pemphigoid, dermatomyositis and SLE. It is given at a dose of 1–3mg/kg/day, usually 50–100mg b.i.d. Before starting check the thiopurine methyl transferase (TPMT) level (normal 25–50, carrier 10–25, deficiency <10 pmole/l/mg Hb), since if it is low, there is an increased risk of myelosuppression. It takes 6–8 weeks before there is any effect so it is no good as a first-line treatment in patients with pemphigus and pemphigoid. The patient is often started on azathioprine as well as the steroids; after 6–8 weeks, when the azathioprine will have begun to work, the dose of steroid is gradually reduced.

Side effects

- Nausea, vomiting and diarrhoea, particularly in the elderly. If this is going to occur it usually does so in the first week. It may be so severe that the drug must be stopped.
- Bone marrow depression. A full blood count should be measured regularly (once a week for the first month and then every 2–3 months).
- Teratogenicity. Do not give to pregnant women; safe in men.
- Mild cholestasis.
- Long term (>10 years) there is an increased risk of lymphoma.

HYDROXYCARBAMIDE (Hydroxyurea)

This is an antimetabolite which inhibits DNA synthesis without affecting RNA or protein synthesis. It is used for psoriasis in patients who have not responded to methotrexate and azathioprine but it takes 8–12 weeks to work. It is given at a dose of 500mg b.i.d.

Side effects are mainly on the bone marrow. It causes a macrocytic anaemia or pancytopenia. Patients should have a full blood count measured regularly (once a week for the first month and then every 2 months).

MYCOPHENOLATE MOFETIL

Mycophenolate is another drug used to prevent rejection of organ transplants. It is used for treating recalcitrant pemphigus vulgaris in conjunction with prednisolone, and for pyoderma gangrenosum. It takes about 8 weeks to work. The usual dose is 0.5–1.0g b.i.d.

Side effects are gastro-intestinal upsets (nausea, vomiting, diarrhoea), bone marrow suppression (check FBC weekly, then monthly) and an increased risk of infection, particularly in the elderly.

BIOLOGICAL THERAPIES

Four new agents, alefacept (*Amevive*), efalizumab (*Rapitiva*), etanercept (*Enbrel*) and infliximab (*Remicade*), have been, or will soon be released in Europe and the USA for the treatment of severe psoriasis.

Adalimumab (*Humira*) is available for severe psoriatic arthritis. Alefacept and efalizumab target T-cells or antigen-presenting cells, whilst etanercept, infliximab and adalimumab are TNF-α antagonists. They are all extremely expensive (£10,000 per year). They are likely to prove useful in cases of psoriasis and pemphigus which are unresponsive to other immunosuppressives.

There may be an acute influenza-like illness at the start of treatment with these drugs, but there is no liver or kidney toxicity. Long-term risks of immunosuppression may lead to the development of infection or lymphomas.

PHYSICAL TREATMENTS

CRYOTHERAPY WITH LIQUID NITROGEN

Freezing the skin produces changes similar to those caused by a burn:–

- erythema
- a blister at the dermo-epidermal junction
- necrosis of the skin

} depending on how long you freeze for.

For most skin lesions for which freezing is an appropriate treatment (viral and seborrhoeic warts, solar keratoses) you will want to cause a blister at the dermo-epidermal junction so that the abnormal tissue is lifted off in the blister roof.

For malignant lesions necrosis of the abnormal cells is required. Cell death occurs at a skin temperature of –40°C. At this temperature ice crystals form within the cells and disrupt the cells as they are rewarmed. Maximum damage occurs if the skin is frozen rapidly and allowed to thaw slowly. The thaw time should be at least 3 times as long as the freezing time. Repeated freeze-thaw cycles are more effective than a single long freeze.

Freezing can most easily be done using a *CRY-AC* or *CRYO-JEM* spray gun (Fig. 2.05). This is a stainless steel insulated vacuum flask with a side arm and a spray tip. Different tips are available depending on the size of lesion to be frozen. Spray liquid nitrogen onto the middle of the lesion to be treated. A white ball of ice will form and gradually expand. Keep freezing until it is 2mm outside the margin of the lesion you are treating. At that stage, stop freezing and give short sharp squirts of liquid nitrogen to hold the ice ball at a constant size for the period of time given in Table 2.07. After a time you will become experienced at estimating the amount of freeze that is necessary for treating a particular type of lesion. Do not

Skin condition	Approximate freeze time
Viral warts	
filiform	5 seconds
common	10 seconds
periungual	15–20 seconds
genital	10–30 seconds (dependent on size)
Molluscum contagiosum	5 seconds
Seborrhoeic warts	5–10 seconds
Solar keratoses	5–10 seconds
Bowen's disease	15 seconds × 2
Lentigo maligna	15–30 seconds × 2
Spider naevi	5 seconds

Table 2.07 Freeze times for various lesions treated with liquid nitrogen. On lower legs use half freeze time recommended.

freeze over enthusiastically at first, and *beware of freezing the lower legs* where a freeze time of half that recommended is adequate (excessive freezing on the lower legs can lead to ulceration).

The indications for using cryotherapy are limited. It is not a treatment to be used on any skin lesion that you think is probably benign. Do not use it on dermal lesions (e.g. melanocytic naevi) and malignant lesions (except Bowen's disease). It is essential therefore to make an accurate diagnosis before treatment; if there is any doubt, do a biopsy first. We would recommend that in general practice it is only used for treating viral warts, seborrhoeic warts and solar keratoses.

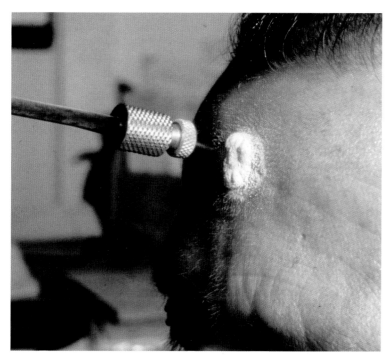

Fig. 2.05 Cryotherapy to solar keratosis.

Cryotherapy with dimethyl ether/propane

Dimethyl ether/propane gas can be obtained in an aerosol can (*Histofreezer* or *Wartner*). The gas is discharged through a cotton bud or directly onto the skin and can freeze the skin to −50°C. This is a useful method of freezing if you only wish to freeze warts very occasionally.

IONTOPHORESIS

Iontophoresis involves passing a low electric current into the skin. Skin resistance is lower through the sweat ducts than the skin so the current passes preferentially down them. This is a useful treatment for hyperhidrosis of the hands and feet, and is available in most dermatology or physiotherapy departments. Battery operated units are also commercially available from STD Pharmaceutical, Plough Lane, Hereford HR4 0EL, England; Tel. 01432–373555.

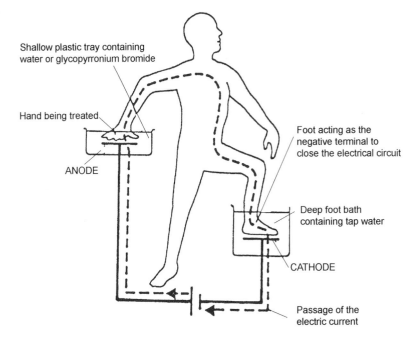

Fig. 2.06 Iontophoresis.

The hand/foot to be treated is placed in a container with only enough tap water or a solution of an anti-cholinergic agent (0.05% glycopyrronium bromide in distilled water) to cover the palmar or plantar surface. This is connected to the positive terminal of a DC unit producing up to 50 milliamps. The opposite foot/hand (not being treated) is placed in a deep bath of tap water connected to the –ve terminal (Fig. 2.06). A current of 10 milliamps is given for 10 minutes once a week until sweating stops. The current and time can be increased if the treatment is not effective. The sweating will gradually return after weeks – months, when the treatment can be repeated. Treatment response tends to be variable; not all patients respond well.

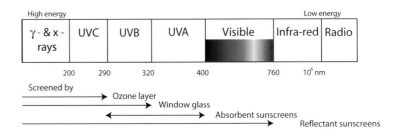

Fig. 2.07 The electromagnetic spectrum.

ULTRAVIOLET LIGHT

Many skin diseases improve in the summer and particularly on sun exposure. For some of these treatment with artificial ultraviolet light can be beneficial. The light is produced by banks of fluorescent lamps in stand-up booths (Fig. 2.08) or lie-down units. The lamps (whether UVB or UVA) must be of sufficient intensity (watts = joules/sec) to deliver a therapeutic dose (joules/cm^2) within a short period of time and it must also be possible to measure accurately the dose given.

UVC radiation (200–290nm) UVC from the sun is filtered out by the ozone in the atmosphere. It is not used therapeutically.

UVB radiation (290–320nm) is responsible for tanning and sunburn. UVB is present in sunlight but is filtered out by window glass. For treating psoriasis UVB (especially at 311–313nm) works much better than UVA. As a treatment UVB is given either by tubes emitting the whole UVB spectrum (broadband UVB) or in special TL01 tubes emitting at 311–313nm (narrowband UVB). Narrow band UVB is theoretically safer than broadband UVB because it is less carcinogenic and more effective for psoriasis. Narrowband UVB is given 3× a week and may eventually replace PUVA therapy. UV light therapy should not be given to children under the age of 10. Pregnant women can have UVB but not PUVA.

Although **tar** has traditionally been used in conjunction with UVB the reason for its apparent benefit is not clear. It has been assumed that the phototoxic agents in tar potentiate the effect of the UV radiation. In practice, if erythemogenic doses of UVB are used, there is no evidence that the topical application of tar is any better than using a simple lubricant (e.g. white soft paraffin). If a suberythema dose of UVB is used, tar is helpful.

UVA radiation (320–400nm) is ineffective on its own. Sunbeds bought commercially produce mainly UVA although a low dose of UVB is also emitted which probably produces the tan. Addition of a psoralen followed by UVA (**PUVA therapy**) has been found to be an effective treatment for several conditions (Table 2.08).

PUVA therapy (P = psoralen + UVA)

Psoralens are three-ringed compounds that can cross link DNA (through thymidine or cytosine in one chain of the double helix and pyrimidine in the other) in the presence of UVA light. The cross linking of DNA chains prevents cell division which is how it works in psoriasis. There may also be an effect on the immune system and increased production of melanin.

Either 8-methoxypsoralen (8-MOP) or 5-methoxypsoralen (5-MOP) can be used. Maximum photosensitivity occurs 2–3 hours after ingestion and exposure to the UVA is timed to coincide with this. UVA penetrates further into the dermis than UVB, and combined with the psoralen is more effective. The psoralen is taken 2 hours before irradiation at a dose dependent on weight – 8-MOP tablets, 0.6mg/kg body weight; 5-MOP tablets, 1.2mg/kg body weight. Alternatively the 8-MOP can be put in a bath and the patient soaks in the solution for 15 minutes immediately before UV exposure (bath PUVA), or applied directly to the skin as a gel (usually for hands and feet). Treatment is given twice weekly for 6–12 weeks until the skin is clear.

Determining the patient's sensitivity to PUVA or UVB

The dose of UVA or UVB is worked out in terms of light energy (joules/cm^2), and depending on the output of the machine (measured by an internal UV meter), the time of exposure is calculated. The reaction on the patient's skin induced by PUVA or UVB is a phototoxic one, i.e. erythema, oedema and as a maximum response, blistering. The erythema caused by PUVA differs from that produced by UVB in that it appears later, lasts longer, and is more intense. It does not peak until 48–72 hours (and sometimes not until 96 hours). The aim of UVB or PUVA therapy is to deliver to the patient as much UV as possible without producing more than a barely perceptible erythema, the **minimal erythematous dose** (MED). The MED for UVB or the **minimal phototoxic dose** (MPD) for PUVA are measured by applying a template with a number of 1 cm^2 cut-outs to the patient's skin (Fig. 2.09) and irradiating them with increasing doses of UV (the rest of the patient's skin being completely covered up). This is done in the same treatment booth that will be used for the treatment. For PUVA it is done 2 hours after the ingestion of 8-MOP. The tests are read at 72 hours and a barely perceptible erythema is the end point that you are looking for. The dose of UV (joules/cm^2) needed to produce this amount of erythema is the MED or MPD. The starting dose for treatment is 75% of the MED/MPD. Each dose is increased by 25% of the previous dose given until the disease is clear. Alternatively the starting dose can be assessed according to skin type (*see* p. 3).

It is recommended that the lifetime exposure to PUVA should be limited to 1000 joules/cm^2 or 200 treatments to reduce the long-term risk of skin cancer. No limit has been established as yet for narrowband UVB although every effort is made to keep the amount of radiation to a minimum.

In a UV machine the patient must protect his eyes against damage from ultraviolet light during, and with PUVA for 24 hours after the treatment, by wearing glasses which filter out both UVB and UVA.

RePUVA therapy

Some patients with psoriasis who do not respond to either PUVA or oral retinoids (*see* p. 41) will respond when they are given together. The retinoid (acitretin 20–50mg/day) is started two weeks before the PUVA therapy. Both are continued together (the retinoid taken daily, the PUVA given twice a week) until the skin is clear. The PUVA can then be stopped and the retinoid continued long term.

UVB	PUVA
Psoriasis	Psoriasis
Atopic eczema	Severe atopic eczema
Chronic superficial scaly dermatosis	Mycosis fungoides
Acne	Polymorphic light eruption
Pityriasis lichenoides chronica	Pityriasis lichenoides acuta
The itching of AIDS	Urticaria pigmentosum
Vitiligo – in conjunction with a topical steroid	Vitiligo especially in dark-skinned individuals
The itching of chronic renal failure	Alopecia areata

Table 2.08 Diseases which may respond to ultraviolet light treatment.

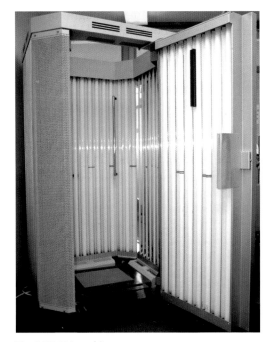

Fig. 2.08 UV machine.

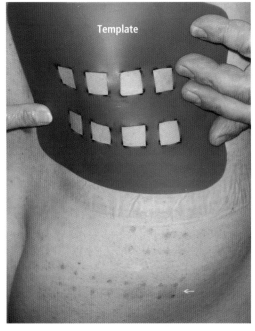

Fig. 2.09 Determining the MED. The MED dose is where the erythema fills the square seen on the right of the bottom row.

Short-term side effects of PUVA

- Nausea. This can be prevented by taking the 8-MOP tablets with food or a glass of milk. Occasionally an anti-emetic is required; we usually give 10mg metoclopramide hydrochloride (*Maxolon*) at the same time as the 8-MOP.
- Dryness and itching of the skin. This is very common and may need an antihistamine such as <u>chlorphenamine</u> 4–8mg given with the 8-MOP. Rarely severe persistent itching makes the patient stop treatment; it can persist for several days or even weeks afterwards.
- Erythema and tenderness. A few patients will get excessive erythema, oedema and tenderness of the skin 48–72 hours after treatment. This is the main reason why treatment is only given twice a week. If the patient gets burnt, the dose of irradiation is reduced for the next treatment. All patients are at risk of

*Drug names which are underlined are those prescribable in the UK by specialist nurse practitioners.

developing a phototoxic reaction after PUVA and should avoid direct sunlight for 8 hours after treatment (using a sunscreen which blocks out both UVB and UVA).
- PUVA pain. Severe skin pain is unusual but when it occurs treatment needs to be stopped. It can sometimes persist for several weeks after treatment is stopped.

Long-term side effects of PUVA

- Cataracts. The eyes are protected during treatment and for 24 hours afterwards by wearing sunglasses to prevent cataract formation.
- Skin cancer. There is an acceleration of the ageing process in the skin of patients who have been treated with PUVA and an increase in the incidence of basal and squamous cell carcinomas on the skin after 5–10 years. There have also been some reports of malignant melanoma occurring.
- Men must shield the genitalia during treatment because there is an increased risk of squamous cell carcinoma of the penis.

PHOTODYNAMIC THERAPY (PDT)

Photodynamic therapy (PDT) is a new treatment for pre-malignant lesions (solar keratoses & Bowen's disease) and non-melanoma skin cancers (superficial basal cell carcinomas). A photosensitising chemical, 5-amino-laevulinic acid (ALA), is converted to protoporphyrin-9 when irradiated with red light (630nm). The porphyrin accumulates in the abnormal cells and in the presence of oxygen releases singlet oxygen which causes cell death. Topical ALA is available as the methyl ester (methyl aminolaevulinate, *Metvix* cream) or the acid (*Levulan*USA only). The methyl ester has the advantage of being taken up preferentially into neoplastic cell (due to their defective stratum corneum).

Lesions to be treated have any scale or crust removed from the surface with saline, forceps or a curette. The *Metvix* cream is applied to the affected skin in a 1mm thick layer, covered with a non-adherent dressing and left in place for 3 hours. After this it is removed and the area irradiated with red light (Aktilight produces a continuous spectrum 570–670nm) for 8–10 minutes (37 J/cm^2). The patient feels a burning sensation which may last for a few hours. Bowen's disease and superficial BCCs are retreated a second time after an interval of 7 days; solar keratoses are treated only once.

The affected skin becomes inflamed, crusts after about a week, and heals within 4 weeks. Oedema, pain or redness can occur. Itching, ulceration, infection or pigmentary changes are less likely. In general PDT works very well on the scalp and face, but less well on the limbs. Patients for PDT should be referred to a dermatology department who have a lamp emitting the correct spectrum.

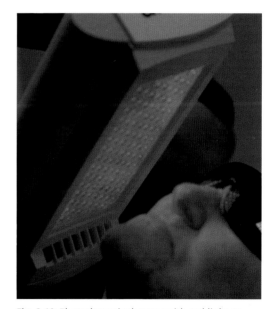

Fig. 2.10 Photodynamic therapy with red light to lesion on cheek.

LASERS

Laser is an acronym for light amplification by stimulated emission of radiation. It is a device which produces coherent light: an intense beam of pure monochromatic light which does not diverge and in which all the light waves are of the same polarity and travel in step in the same direction.

How lasers work

Various gases, liquids and solids will emit light when they are suitably stimulated or pumped. In a typical gas laser (CO_2 or argon), the gas is contained in a lasing tube which has a fully reflective mirror at one end and a partially reflective mirror at the other end (Fig. 2.11). The gas is stimulated by passing a high voltage electric current through it. A stimulated molecule of the gas emits a photon (a light particle), which strikes another stimulated molecule causing it to emit an identical photon (amplification). Emission of photons occurs in all directions but the light waves become aligned by resonance between the mirrors and the coherent light exits through the partially reflective mirror. The type of gas, liquid or solid in the lasing tube determines the wavelength of the coherent light that is produced.

The objective for any laser treatment is to restrict laser-induced injury to selected sites such as blood vessels or pigment cells with minimal damage to adjacent tissues. This effect is called **selective thermolysis**. It is achieved if the laser fulfils 3 requirements:–

1. The laser emits at the same wavelength that the target absorbs, e.g. for haemoglobin at 542 or 577nm (*see* Fig. 2.12).
2. The laser emits sufficient energy to damage the target tissue.
3. The duration of exposure of the tissue is short enough to limit damage to the target without excess heat diffusing outwards and damaging the surrounding tissues. This is determined by the **thermal relaxation time,** which is how long it takes for the target to dissipate half its thermal energy. For a blood vessel in a port wine stain this is 1–10 millisec (10^{-3}), while for tattoo pigment it is only 1–10 nanosecs (10^{-9}). The pulse duration of the lasers treating these targets must be of these magnitudes.

The **penetration into the skin** is determined by the wavelength of the light. The longer the wavelength the deeper the penetration; but longer wavelengths tend to have less energy so may be less effective. For hair removal, the laser must penetrate to the root of the hair follicle. The Alexandrite laser (755nm) will be able to deliver more energy to the dermal papilla than the Ruby (694nm) at the depth of a follicle (1mm). For port wine stains the highest peak of haemoglobin absorption at 418nm is no good as light of this wavelength will not penetrate very far. The light of the pulse dye laser at 585nm provides a compromise between penetration and energy absorption by haemoglobin.

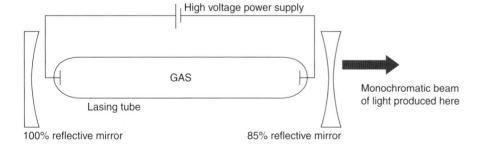

High voltage power supply

GAS

Lasing tube

Monochromatic beam of light produced here

100% reflective mirror

85% reflective mirror

Fig. 2.11 How a gas laser works.

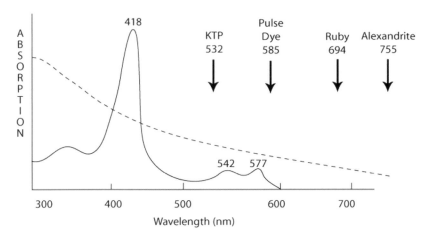

Fig. 2.12 Absorption spectrum of haemoglobin (continuous line) and melanin (dashed line).

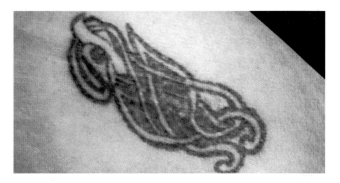

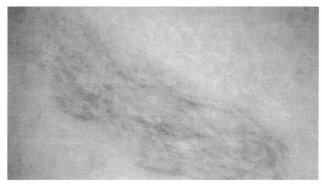

Fig. 2.13 (above) Tattoo before, and
Fig. 2.14 (below) after NdYag laser treatment.

There are three groups of skin lasers (*see* Table 2.09, p. 54) depending on the target tissue:–

- **Vascular lasers** target haemoglobin. Wavelengths selected are around the 577nm absorption peak (Fig. 2.12) to ensure adequate penetration. Pulse duration is selected depending on the diameter of the vessel being treated. If it is too long scarring may result; if it is too short it causes purpura without destroying the vessel.
- **Resurfacing or cutting lasers** target water and hence all tissue. A short pulse duration and high energy result in vaporisation of tissue with minimal damage to underlying structures. Healing comes from re-epithelisation from hair follicles.
- **Pigment lasers** target melanin and tattoo ink. Between 500 and 1100nm there is good penetration and preferred absorption by

melanin compared to haemoglobin. Some pigmented lesions such as lentigoes (not moles) and tattoos are treated by very short pulse widths (10^{-9} seconds) which are generated by 'Q-switching'. This causes a shock wave which breaks down melanin and tattoo pigments. For hair removal longer pulse widths and long wavelengths are needed to reach and damage the follicle.

Type of laser	Wavelength	Pulse time	Function	Comments
Vascular lasers Pulse dye (PDL)	585 or (595	0.45 msec @ 1.5 msec)	Port wine stains	Recommended – causes bruising which lasts 2 weeks.
			Strawberry naevi	Only useful for complications, e.g. bleeding, obstruction.
			Telangiectasia, spider naevi	Visible lesions on face. No good for erythema.
KTP	532	2–10 msec	Telangiectasia Port wine stains	Does not cause bruising so good for cosmetic lesions. Use if PDL not effective, since the longer pulse duration is better for larger vessels.
Pigment lasers Ruby or Alexandrite	694 755	25–40 nsec (Q-switched)	Lentigines & freckles	Good response.
			Café au lait & Becker's naevus	Variable to poor response.
			Naevus of Ota/Ito	Good to variable response.
NdYAG	532	6 nsec	Lentigines & freckles	Good response – short wavelength for surface lesions.
	1064	(Q-switched)	Café au lait & Becker's naevus	Variable to poor response.
			Naevus of Ota/Ito	Variable response – longer wavelength for deeper lesions.
Excimer	308	120 nsec	Psoriasis, vitiligo	Same wavelength as ultraviolet in phototherapy.
Tattoo removal NdYAG	1064	(Q-switched) 6 nsec	Blue-black tattoos	Useful laser as 2 options in 1 machine (1064 & 532nm).
	532		Red, orange, yellow tattoos	Preferred option due to fast repetition rate (10 Hz = shots/sec).
Ruby	694	25–40 nsec	Blue-black, green tattoos	Slower repetition rate (1 Hz), mainly useful for green.
Hair removal Ruby	694	270 µsec	Hair needs to be dark but	Slow repetition rate (1Hz) = long treatment times.
Alexandrite	755	2–20 msec	patient's skin type I or II	Preferred laser since penetrates deeper than Ruby.
NdYAG	1064	50 msec	Skin types IV–VI	Deeper penetration, very painful, better for darker skin types.
Intense pulsed light	590–1200			Not true coherent laser light.
Resurfacing lasers CO_2 (carbon dioxide)	10,600	10–20 msec	Resurfacing actinic damage & acne scarring	Thermal damage up to 100µm deep which stimulates collagen & elastic tissue regeneration.
Erbium-YAG	2940	200–400 msec	Resurfacing & removal of epidermal lesions	Thermal damage only 10µm deep – no deep damage. Quicker recovery time but less effective for marked scarring.

Table 2.09 Types of dermatological laser.

Hairy scalp

(For bald scalp *see* Chapters 5 & 9)

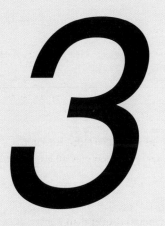

Hair physiology

Excess hair

Hair loss

Structural abnormalities of hair

Rashes and lesions in the hairy scalp

HAIR PHYSIOLOGY

WHAT IS HAIR?

Hair is a modified type of keratin produced by the hair matrix (equivalent to epidermis). On the scalp, apart from its social and cosmetic function, hair protects the underlying skin from sun damage.

Three types of hair occur in humans:–

1. Lanugo hair is the soft silky hair that covers the foetus *in utero*. It is usually shed before birth.

2. Vellus hair is the short fine unpigmented hair which covers the whole skin surface apart from the palms and soles.

3. Terminal hair is longer, coarser, and pigmented. Before puberty terminal hair is restricted to the scalp, eyebrows and eyelashes. After puberty secondary terminal hair develops in response to androgens in the axillae, pubic area and on the front of the chest in men.

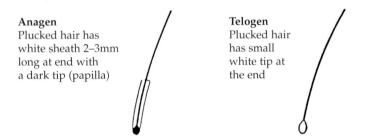

Anagen
Plucked hair has white sheath 2–3mm long at end with a dark tip (papilla)

Telogen
Plucked hair has small white tip at the end

Fig. 3.01 How to tell the difference between plucked anagen and telogen hairs.

HAIR CYCLE

There are between 100,000 and 150,000 hairs on the scalp. The hair cycle (Fig. 3.02) occurs randomly in each follicle over the scalp so that up to 100 hairs are being lost daily, but in normal circumstances moulting does not occur.

The three phases of the hair cycle are:–

Anagen (90% of hairs). This is the growing phase and on the scalp lasts 2–6 years.
Catagen. The hair matrix cells stop dividing and hair growth stops. It lasts about 2 weeks.
Telogen (10%). This is the resting phase. The hair shaft moves up in the dermis. It lasts 3 months and at the end of that time the hair is shed.

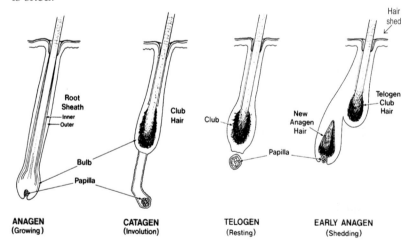

Fig. 3.02 The hair cycle.

EXCESS HAIR

Hair in the wrong place or hair which is coarser or longer than is socially acceptable is regarded as excessive. There are two different patterns, hirsutism and hypertrichosis.

HIRSUTISM

In women coarse terminal hair in the moustache or beard area, and on the chest or lower abdomen as in men, is known as hirsutism. It is extremely common, the amount of hair being genetically determined. How much facial and body hair is cosmetically acceptable in an individual is dependent on many factors, but particularly the patient's cultural and social background. What is considered normal in many parts of Southern Europe is deemed unacceptable in the UK or USA.

The amount of hair on the face, breasts and lower abdomen in women is under androgen control. Testosterone produced by the ovary is converted to dihydrotestosterone in the skin by the action of 5-alpha reductase and it is this which causes the increase in hair. If the periods are abnormal in any way it is always worth checking the serum testosterone level. If it is more than twice the upper limit of normal, the patient should be referred to an endocrinologist for a full endocrine work up. Many such patients have polycystic ovaries but this does not require any specific treatment unless associated with diabetes or ischaemic heart disease. As a rule if the periods are normal so are the hormone levels.

TREATMENT HIRSUTISM

By the time the patient seeks help from the doctor she will usually have tried all the simple things that do not require medical advice. If she has not, the following are available and may be helpful:–

1. **Bleaching the hairs** with lemon juice or hydrogen peroxide. For patients whose hair is very dark, bleaching will often disguise them enough to be cosmetically acceptable.

2. **Depilatory creams.** These mainly contain barium sulphide which dissolves keratin. In some patients these creams will make the skin sore by a direct irritant effect; they can also cause an allergic contact dermatitis and folliculitis. All of these will limit their usefulness.

3. **Waxing and sugaring.** These are basically methods of mass plucking of hairs. Hot wax or a thick sugar solution is applied to the hairy area of skin; it is allowed to cool, and then peeled off pulling the hairs out at the same time. Both methods are available from reputable beauticians. This method is suitable for removal of excess hair from the legs and body as well as the face.

Cont

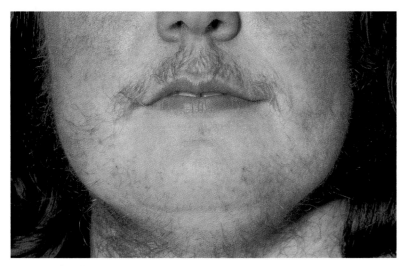

Fig. 3.03 Hirsutism.

4. **Plucking and shaving.** A surprising number of women still remove unwanted hair by plucking and shaving. Most do not like doing it but have found that other methods make their skin too sore.

5. **Electrolysis.** If the amount of unwanted hair is not too extensive, electrolysis and epilation using a short wave diathermy machine can provide a permanent answer. A fine sterile needle is placed into the hair follicle down to the level of the papilla. A high frequency alternating current is then passed through the needle for a microsecond. This destroys the papilla permanently and the hair is lifted out without pain. This process works well but is rather time consuming and expensive. Patients should be treated by practitioners who are members of the Institute of the Association of Electrologists. Some hospitals provide an electrolysis service under the NHS, but many do not.

6. **Lasers** are an effective method of removing hair. The light is absorbed by melanin in the hair shaft and the heat generated damages the follicle. The treatment works best on dark hair in a fair-skinned individual. Dark-skinned patients are likely to develop hyper-pigmentation after treatment. The best laser for hair removal is the Alexandrite (at 755nm). The Lyra (NdYAG at 1064nm) is preferred in patients with a darker skin type. Several treatments are necessary as only follicles in anagen respond. The hair loss is not permanent but a 60% reduction in hair density is seen after about 6 treatments spread over a year. Twice yearly 'top up' treatments will maintain things.

7. Eflornithine (Vaniqa) cream is an ornithine decarboxylase inhibitor which reduces hair growth over a 2–4 month period.

HYPERTRICHOSIS

Hypertrichosis is excessive hair all over the body. Either the foetal lanugo hair is not lost before birth or regrows at some later stage. When confined to the lumbosacral area (Fawn tail) it may be a marker of an underlying spina bifida.

Some drugs cause hyper-trichosis in all patients to a greater or lesser degree:–

- ciclosporin
- diazoxide
- minoxidil   .

The following drugs occasionally cause hypertrichosis:–

- diphenylhydantoin
- minocycline
- penicillamine
- psoralens

TREATMENT HYPERTRICHOSIS

There is no treatment which works. If it is due to a drug and it is possible to stop the drug, the hypertrichosis will be reversible, although it may take up to a year for the hairiness to disappear.

For other methods of hair removal – *see* hirsutism.

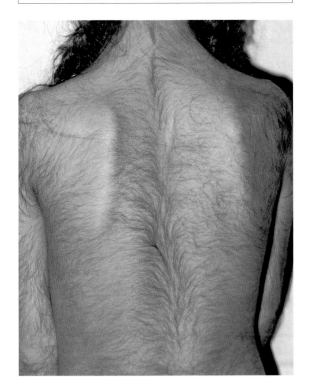

Fig. 3.04 Hypertrichosis.

HAIR LOSS

Hairy scalp
Discrete bald patches
a. Without scarring

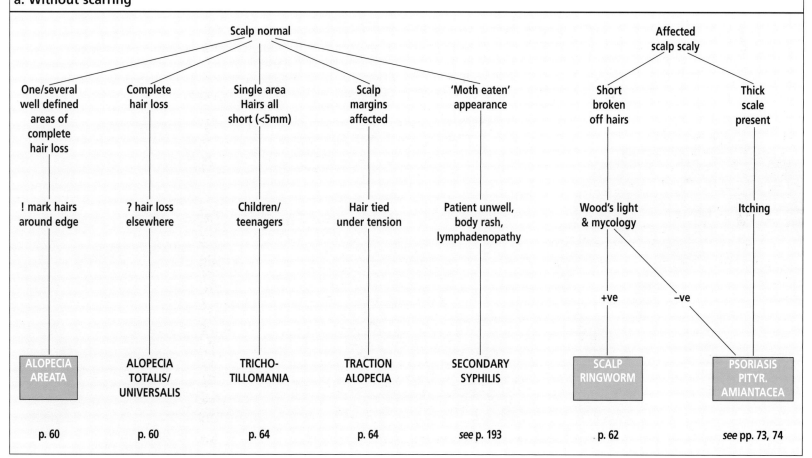

Scalp normal					**Affected scalp scaly**	
One/several well defined areas of complete hair loss	Complete hair loss	Single area Hairs all short (<5mm)	Scalp margins affected	'Moth eaten' appearance	Short broken off hairs	Thick scale present
! mark hairs around edge	? hair loss elsewhere	Children/ teenagers	Hair tied under tension	Patient unwell, body rash, lymphadenopathy	Wood's light & mycology	Itching
					+ve ─── ─ve	
ALOPECIA AREATA	ALOPECIA TOTALIS/ UNIVERSALIS	TRICHO-TILLOMANIA	TRACTION ALOPECIA	SECONDARY SYPHILIS	SCALP RINGWORM	PSORIASIS PITYR. AMIANTACEA
p. 60	p. 60	p. 64	p. 64	*see p. 193*	p. 62	*see pp. 73, 74*

ALOPECIA AREATA

This is the commonest cause of discrete hair loss in both children and adults. There is no redness or scaling of the underlying scalp. There may be one or several bald patches on the scalp or on any other hairy area (e.g. beard). While the disease is active, exclamation mark (!) hairs will be seen around the edge of the bald patches. These are short broken off hairs where the broken end is thicker and darker than where the hair emerges from the scalp. Only pigmented hairs are affected, so normal white/grey hairs will remain in the middle of a bald area. It usually lasts for 3–6 months and then the hair regrows spontaneously. It will usually regrow white or blonde initially, but goes back to its original colour after 6–8 weeks.

Alopecia areata is renamed **alopecia totalis** when all hair is lost from the scalp and **alopecia univeralis** if both scalp and body hair are absent.

Alopecia areata is thought to be an autoimmune disease so it is worth checking the urine for sugar and checking the autoimmune profile because some patients may have diabetes, pernicious anaemia or thyroid disease as well.

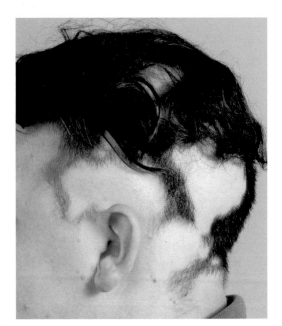

Fig. 3.05 Alopecia areata. Discrete bald patches with no evidence of erythema or scaling.

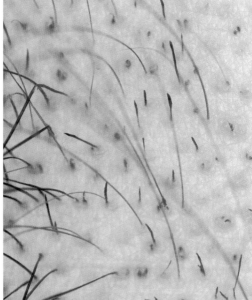

Fig. 3.06 Alopecia areata. ! hairs at edge of bald patch.

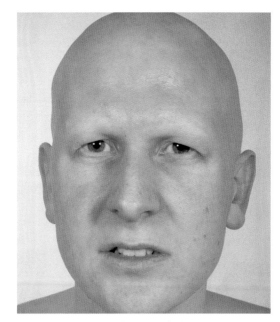

Fig. 3.07 Alopecia totalis. Loss of all hair on scalp, eyebrows, eyelashes and beard.

TREATMENT ALOPECIA AREATA

Reassure the patient that the hair will regrow spontaneously, usually in about 3–6 months. Warn the patient that the hair may regrow white or blonde until it is about 1.5cm long, but that it will go back to its normal colour after that.

A wig may be needed temporarily if the hair loss is extensive.

In a small minority of patients the hair will not regrow.

Treatment available by dermatologists is unsatisfactory but includes:–

1. **Intralesional injection of triamcinolone** (10mg/ml). This causes temporary regrowth of hair, but may cause atrophy of the skin.

2. **Application of potent skin sensitizers to the bald areas. Diphencyprone** is the drug most commonly used but only about 20% of patients do well with it, usually those whose hair loss has been present for less than 2 years. The scalp skin is sensitised by painting a 2% lotion to a small area which becomes eczematized over 2 weeks. The whole scalp is then painted with a diluted solution of the lowest concentration (0.001–0.1%) which will produce mild erythema. If it works, it has to go on being painted on the bald areas once a week until regrowth of hair is well established. Diphencyprone is degraded by light so patients have to keep their heads covered for 24 hours after treatment. Usually the eczema is too unpleasant for the patient to tolerate, and if the hair does regrow, it may fall out again when treatment is stopped.

The following are not very effective but may be worth a try:–

3. **PUVA** twice a week.

4. **Topical minoxidil** (5%) lotion. This is expensive. It is rubbed into the affected area twice a day.

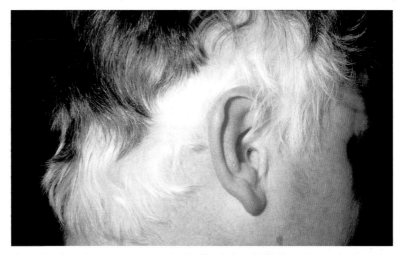

Fig. 3.08 Alopecia areata. Regrowth of white hair – this will repigment in due course.

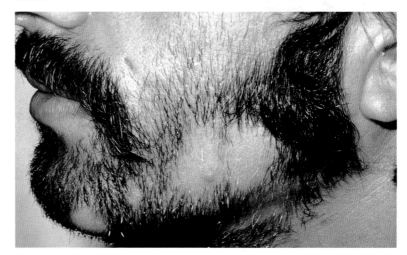

Fig. 3.09 Alopecia areata. Bald patches in the beard area.

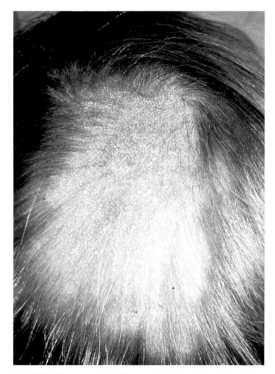

Fig. 3.10 Tinea capitis. Discrete bald patch with scaly surface.

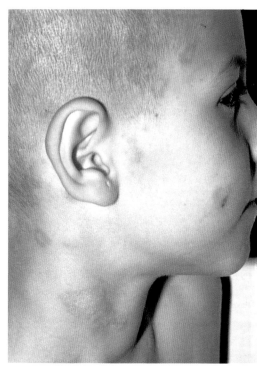

Fig. 3.11 Tinea capitis. Child with ringworm on scalp, face, and neck.

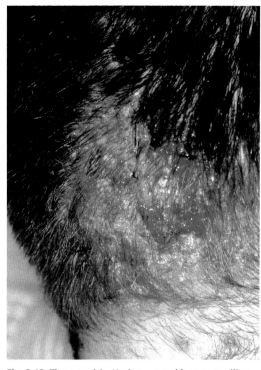

Fig. 3.12 Tinea capitis. Kerion – a red boggy swelling due to animal ringworm.

SCALP RINGWORM

Scalp ringworm only occurs in children; it is not a cause of hair loss in adults except those with HIV/AIDS. It is often due to *Trichophyton tonsurans* (caught from other children) or *Microsporum canis* (caught from kittens or puppies). Discrete bald areas occur with short broken off hairs in which the underlying skin is scaly and/or red. If the skin is red or if there is associated ringworm on the face or neck, it is more likely to be due to animal ringworm. There will be a history of other children with similar hair loss or a new kitten or puppy whose fur is falling out.

The diagnosis is confirmed by pulling out the short broken hairs, applying a drop of 20% potassium hydroxide (KOH) solution to the hair, heating it gently and looking for spores inside the hair shaft (Fig. 3.13). In addition scalp ringworm due to *M. canis* fluoresces green under the Wood's light (*see* p. 18). *T. tonsurans* does not fluoresce.

Animal ringworm of the scalp (due to *M. canis*) can sometimes produce a red boggy swelling discharging pus; this is called a **kerion**.

TREATMENT TINEA CAPITIS

Griseofulvin 15–20mg/kg body weight/day given as a single daily dose with food for 6 weeks. It can be given as tablets (125mg each) or as a suspension (125mg/5ml). Alternatively it can be given as a single large dose (5g) in ice cream. There is no need for topical treatment as well as this is ineffective since treatment applied to the surface cannot get into the hair shaft (*see* Fig. 3.14).

If it is due to *Microsporum canis*, the affected pet (kitten or puppy) must be treated with griseofulvin too. The pet should be taken to the local vet to get the treatment.

If the child has a **kerion**, the crusts should be softened with arachis oil and then removed. It is worth taking a bacteriology swab from under the crust or from a pustule. If *Staphylococcus aureus* is grown, treat with flucloxacillin as well as with griseofulvin.

Terbinafine (*Lamasil*) is an alternative to griseofulvin but is not as effective for infections with *M. canis*. The dose for 10–20kg body weight is 62.5mg/day; 21–40kg wt is 125mg/day and over 41kg wt is 250mg/day taken for 4 weeks.

Fig. 3.13 Tinea capitis. Direct microscopy showing small spores both inside the hair shaft and outside – typical of microsporum infection.

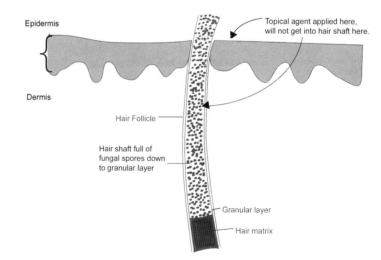

Fig. 3.14 Diagram showing hair shaft invaded with fungal spores which are inaccessible to topical treatment.

TRICHOTILLOMANIA

This is a well defined area of apparent hair loss. Close examination will reveal not a bald area, but an area where all the hairs are short, longer hairs having been pulled out. The remaining hair is just too short to twist around the fingers to pull out. It usually occurs in children as a habit tic or in teenagers who are unhappy.

If the diagnosis is in doubt, a biopsy from the abnormal area will show empty anagen follicles and melanin pigment casts.

TREATMENT TRICHOTILLOMANIA

Most cases in young children are due to a habit tic, but there may be an obvious emotional reason – one of the parents has left home or died, or some other major stress has occurred. Often the parent(s) have not noticed the child twisting the hairs around one of the fingers or pulling it out, but will do so once you tell them what is happening. It is best for them not to make a big thing of it, particularly not to punish the child for it, and to give them as much love and security as they can during the difficult time. Once the time of trauma is over, the child will nearly always stop pulling the hair out and the hair will regrow normally.

In teenagers the cause is often less obvious, but most will need psychiatric help to resolve the problem.

TRACTION ALOPECIA

This is a common condition in races with tight curly hair but much less common in Europeans. It is due to the hair being tightly pulled back, tied up, plaited, or straightened with hot combs. It causes hair loss at the temples but is reversible if the hair pulling is stopped.

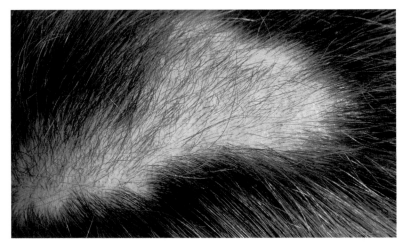

Fig. 3.15 Trichotillomania. Looks like a bald patch but in fact short hairs are present.

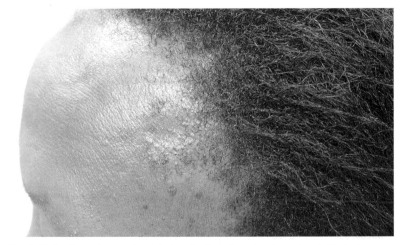

Fig. 3.16 Traction alopecia in a black lady. Note loss of hair on frontal hair line.

Hairy scalp
Discrete bald patches
b. With scarring
All of these are uncommon. The hair follicles are replaced by scar tissue so the hair loss is permanent.

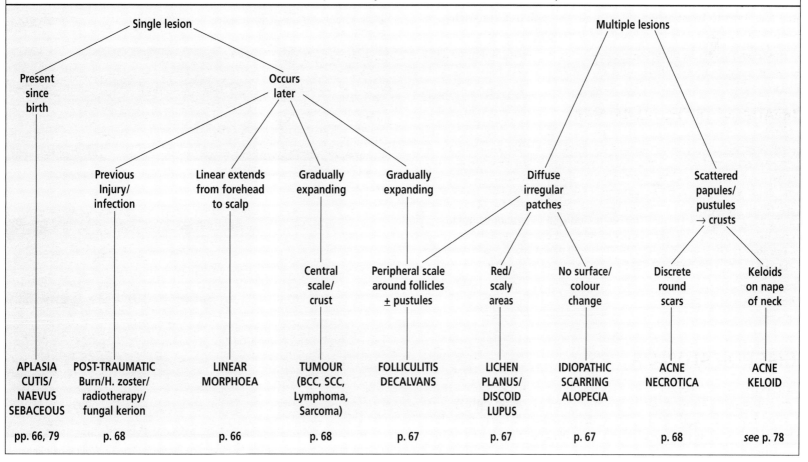

APLASIA CUTIS/ NAEVUS SEBACEOUS	POST-TRAUMATIC Burn/H. zoster/ radiotherapy/ fungal kerion	LINEAR MORPHOEA	TUMOUR (BCC, SCC, Lymphoma, Sarcoma)	FOLLICULITIS DECALVANS	LICHEN PLANUS/ DISCOID LUPUS	IDIOPATHIC SCARRING ALOPECIA	ACNE NECROTICA	ACNE KELOID
pp. 66, 79	p. 68	p. 66	p. 68	p. 67	p. 67	p. 67	p. 68	*see* p. 78

APLASIA CUTIS

Presents at birth as an ulcerated red area on the scalp. This heals to leave a permanent scar (*see also* naevus sebaceous, p. 79). It is not due to birth trauma.

MORPHOEA

Linear morphoea on the forehead may extend into the scalp resulting in a linear scar *(en coup de sabre)*. It often involves the underlying subcutaneous fat leaving a depression in the skin. There is no satisfactory treatment for this condition.

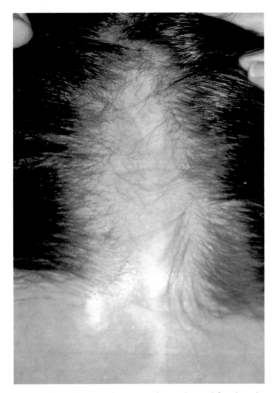

Fig. 3.17 Linear morphoea on the scalp and forehead, also known as 'en coup de sabre'.

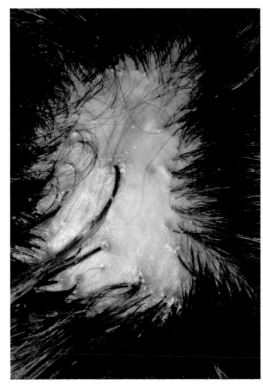

Fig. 3.18 Folliculitis decalvans. Bald area with pustules and crusts around hairs.

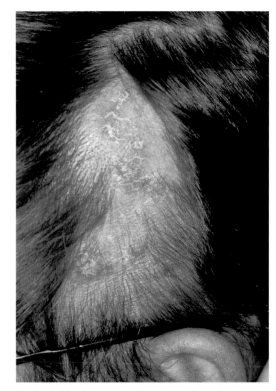

Fig. 3.19 Discoid lupus erythematosus in scalp. Note red scaly plaques in the bald area.

FOLLICULITIS DECALVANS

Folliculitis decalvans is a rare condition in which there is an abnormal host reaction to an infection with *Staphylococcus aureus*. There is a slow progressive scarring alopecia with pustules and crusts around the affected hairs.

TREATMENT FOLLICULITIS DECALVANS

Once scarring has occurred the hair will not regrow. It is important therefore to start treatment as soon as possible to minimise the hair loss. Although due to *Staph. aureus* treatment with flucloxacillin does not work. A combination of rifampicin 600mg/day with doxycycline 100mg/day (or clindamycin 300mg b.i.d.) usually works well. Give it for 10–12 weeks. Septrin 960mg b.i.d. is an alternative for 2–3 years if relapse occurs.

LICHEN PLANUS & DISCOID LUPUS ERYTHEMATOSUS

Lichen planus and discoid lupus erythematosus (DLE) both cause scarring alopecia on the scalp. In lupus the skin over the bald patches is red and scaly and there may be follicular plugging. In lichen planus the skin is mauvish in colour with little scaling.

Sometimes the diagnosis is obvious from the rash elsewhere. If in doubt a biopsy will confirm the diagnosis. Sometimes nothing is seen histologically except the replacement of hair follicles with scar tissue. This is called idiopathic scarring alopecia or **pseudo-pelade of Brocq**.

For treatment for lichen planus *see* p. 171, DLE *see* p. 111.

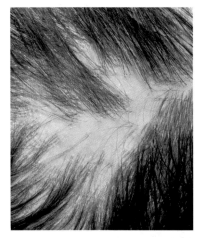

Fig. 3.20 Idiopathic scarring alopecia of the scalp (no cause found on biopsy).

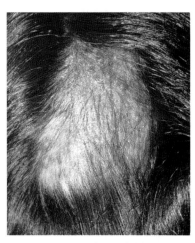

Fig. 3.21 Alopecia due to lichen planus. Note mauve colour of skin.

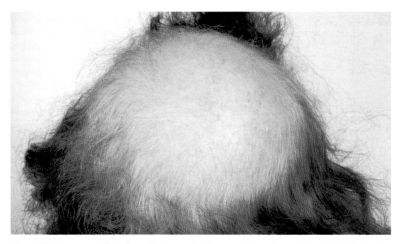

Fig. 3.22 Permanent hair loss due to radiotherapy given during the 1950s to treat ringworm.

POST TRAUMATIC ALOPECIA

Any injury or infection resulting in scarring will result in hair loss. Usually the history will make the cause obvious. Before griseofulvin was introduced in 1958, radiotherapy was the usual treatment for scalp ringworm. It caused the anagen hairs to fall out and resulted in cure. If too big a dose was given the resulting alopecia was permanent. Many of these patients are now developing basal cell and squamous cell carcinomas on their bald scalps.

TUMOURS

Basal cell carcinoma may occur on the hairy scalp as a persistent area of crusting or hair loss. The unusual site may result in a misdiagnosis of eczema or an 'infection' so that the lesion may become quite large before being recognised. (For tumours on the bald scalp *see* Chapter 9.)

ACNE NECROTICA

This condition occurs in adult men and presents as itchy or painful papules and pustules, which crust over and heal leaving scars. The cause is unknown but it is not related to acne.

TREATMENT ACNE NECROTICA

The condition often responds poorly to therapy, but like acne it should improve with oxytetracycline 250mg (or minocycline, lymecycline, doxycycline) given twice daily for 4 months. Once scarring has occurred any hair loss will be permanent.

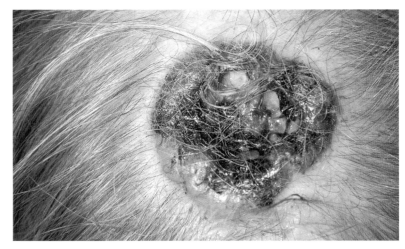

Fig. 3.23 Basal cell carcinoma on the scalp.

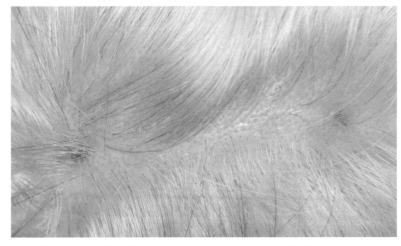

Fig. 3.24 Acne necrotica. Two crusted lesions which may heal with scarring.

Hairy scalp
Diffuse hair loss

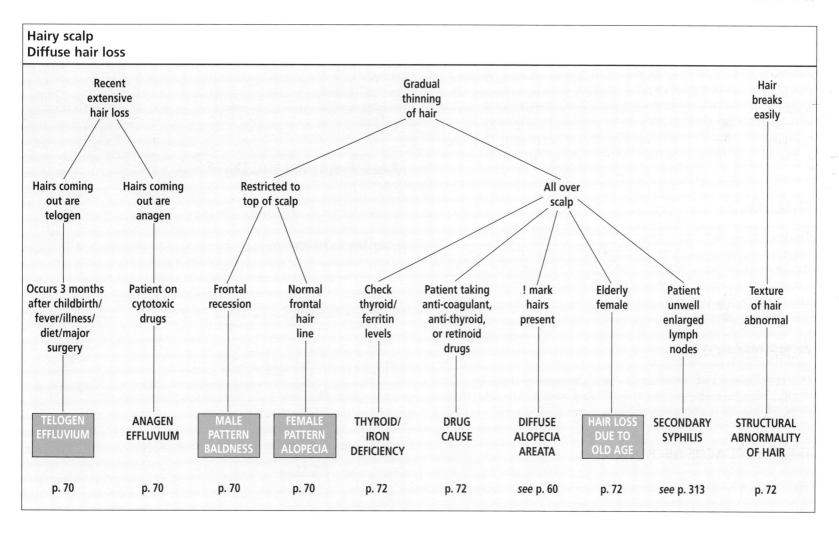

TELOGEN EFFLUVIUM

During pregnancy the hair cycle stops. At the time of delivery all the hairs that should have gone into telogen during the previous 9 months suddenly do so. Three months later these telogen hairs are shed and considerable hair loss occurs. The hair will often come out in handfuls when you pull gently on the hair. Since shedding of telogen hairs is followed by regrowth of anagen hairs, such hair loss is short lived and fully reversible. Similar shedding of telogen hairs can occur three months after any severe illness, major operation or very strict dieting.

TREATMENT ANAGEN & TELOGEN EFFLUVIUM

Both conditions will resolve spontaneously once the precipitating factor has been removed. Reassurance is all that is necessary.

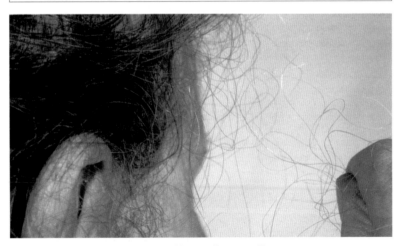

Fig. 3.25 Telogen effluvium. A lot of hair pulls out easily.

ANAGEN EFFLUVIUM

Cytotoxic drugs affect any rapidly dividing cells and the hair matrix is affected as well as the bone marrow and tumour cells. It is the anagen hairs that are shed so 90% of all scalp hair will be lost.

MALE PATTERN BALDNESS

This is hair loss occurring over the temples or on the crown due to androgens (dihydrotestosterone). The hair on the occiput and around the sides of the scalp is never lost. The effect of dihydrotestosterone is a shortening of the anagen growth phase and a corresponding increase in telogen hairs. Gradually the hair follicles get smaller and terminal hairs are replaced by vellus hairs. The amount of hair loss and the age of onset is genetically determined.

FEMALE PATTERN ALOPECIA

This is similar to male pattern baldness but without the frontal recession (Fig. 3.28). Decreased hair density from the crown forward with normal hair density at the back and sides occurs. Minor degrees of this are extremely common.

An androgen secreting tumour should be considered in women with male pattern alopecia if it is very extensive or if there is a change in the menstrual cycle.

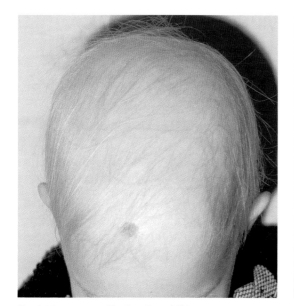

Fig. 3.26 Anagen effluvium in a child on chemotherapy.

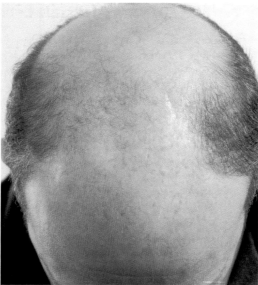

Fig. 3.27 Male pattern baldness. Frontal recession with loss on the crown. The sides and occiput are normal.

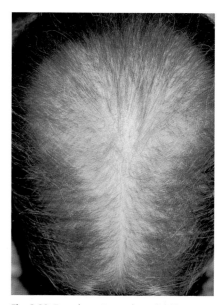

Fig. 3.28 Female pattern alopecia. Note retention of frontal hair line with thinning over vertex of scalp.

TREATMENT MALE PATTERN BALDNESS

For most men, no treatment is needed or sought since this is a normal physiological process. For a few, who cannot come to terms with their baldness, the following are available *(not under the NHS)*:–

1. **5% minoxidil** solution. 1ml is rubbed into the bald scalp twice daily. This does not produce regrowth of normal terminal hair but of long vellus hair in about a third of those who use it. If treatment is stopped, the longer hair will fall out, so once started it will need to be continued indefinitely. A 2% solution is used for maintenance treatment.

2. **Finasteride.** 1mg orally daily (or 5mg weekly, which is much cheaper to buy) inhibits type II 5-α-reductase, the enzyme that converts testosterone to the more active dihydrotestosterone in scalp follicles. One third of men will have marked regrowth of hair, one third moderate regrowth and one third little regrowth. Side effects are uncommon (<2%) and include impotence and loss of libido.

3. **Hair transplants.** Hairs are taken from the occipital area or sides of the scalp by punch biopsy. Follicular units (containing 1–4 follicles) are transplanted into the bald areas.

TREATMENT FEMALE PATTERN ALOPECIA

For minor degrees of this, no treatment is needed, but if it is noticeable consider one of the following options:–

1. **Anti-androgens.** Small doses of cyproterone acetate as in Dianette do not work. To be effective, 50–100mg daily is required. For women of child bearing age, it should be combined with an oestrogen to prevent feminization of a male foetus. The usual regimen is cyproterone acetate 100mg on days 5–14 of the menstrual cycle, together with ethinyl oestradiol 50µg on days 5–25 of the cycle. For post-menopausal women, it can be given alone on a daily basis, either 50mg or 100mg once a day. Side effects include weight gain, nausea, decreased libido, depression and headaches.

2. **Spironolactone.** Start with 50mg/day and increase to 100mg b.i.d depending on side effects. It is worth trying this for 6 months, particularly in older women. In younger women it may cause menstrual irregularities and postural hypotension. Check renal function and electrolytes (potassium).

3. **Topical minoxidil**, as for male pattern baldness.

On stopping treatment with any of these drugs, the hair loss will reoccur.

4. **A wig.**

OTHER CAUSES OF DIFFUSE HAIR LOSS

a. When the hair density is obviously reduced

The hair density gradually decreases with age and the hairs become finer. In younger patients consider:–

- Hypothyroidism.
- Iron deficiency.
- Diffuse alopecia areata. Look for ! mark hairs.
- Secondary syphilis. The patient will be unwell with widespread lymphadenopathy and a rash (*see* p. 193).
- Systemic lupus erythematosus (*see* p. 114).

b. When the hair density looks normal

Many patients complain that they have less hair than they would like, but there is no obvious abnormality or hair loss on examination. Pluck out a group of hairs with a pair of artery forceps and count the proportion of growing/resting (anagen/telogen) hairs. If the percentage of resting (telogen) hairs is greater than 30% check for hypothyroidism or iron deficiency, ask about anti-coagulant or anti-thyroid drugs or whether the patient has had a recent thallium scan.

STRUCTURAL ABNORMALITIES OF HAIR

Some patients notice that their hair breaks easily and will not grow to the desired length. There are numerous structural abnormalities of the hair shaft which cause hair to break off short. All are uncommon (Fig. 3.29).

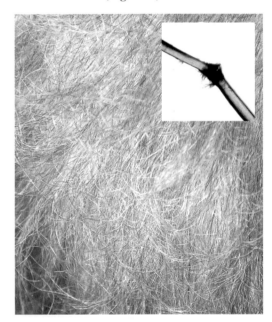

Fig. 3.29a Trichorrhexis nodosa. Hair breaks off easily and is difficult to comb or keep tidy.

Fig. 3.29b (inset) Microscopy showing nodular swelling at which point the hair breaks.

RASHES AND LESIONS IN THE HAIRY SCALP

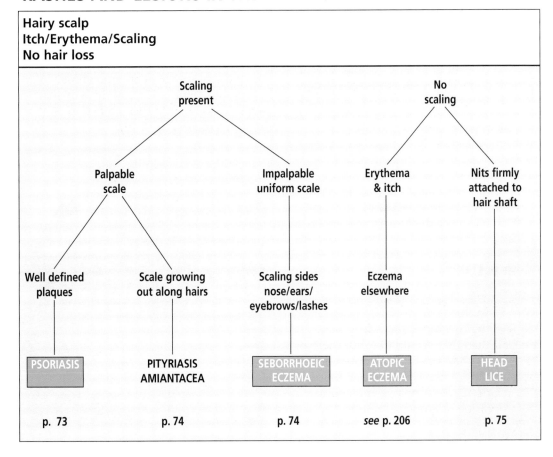

Hairy scalp
Itch/Erythema/Scaling
No hair loss

Scaling present
No scaling

Palpable scale
Impalpable uniform scale
Erythema & itch
Nits firmly attached to hair shaft

Well defined plaques
Scale growing out along hairs
Scaling sides nose/ears/eyebrows/lashes
Eczema elsewhere

PSORIASIS
PITYRIASIS AMIANTACEA
SEBORRHOEIC ECZEMA
ATOPIC ECZEMA
HEAD LICE

p. 73
p. 74
p. 74
see p. 206
p. 75

PSORIASIS

Psoriasis in the scalp is common, and it may first start there. The diagnosis is made by running your hands through the scalp and feeling the thick heaped up scales, which are not shed because the scale binds to the hair. When you look the lesions are identical to those found elsewhere, i.e. discrete, red scaly plaques. Hair loss in scalp psoriasis is very rare but may occur due to persistent rubbing and scratching which causes the hair to break.

The plaques may extend away from the hair line onto the forehead, neck or around the ears.

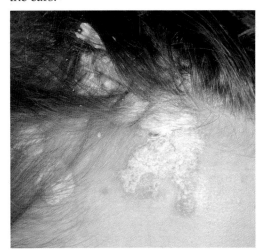

Fig. 3.30 Scalp psoriasis. Thick scale extending from the hairline onto the forehead (compare with seborrhoeic eczema, Fig. 3.32).

PITYRIASIS AMIANTACEA

This term is used to describe thick scales growing out along the hair shaft. It can be due to either psoriasis or eczema. It is seen more commonly in children than in adults.

ECZEMA

Eczema is differentiated from psoriasis on the scalp because it usually covers all the hairy scalp and is more easily seen than felt. Wherever you look it is red and scaly. **Seborrhoeic eczema** typically starts in the scalp causing fine scaling (dandruff). **Atopic eczema** also commonly affects the scalp but typical changes will be seen elsewhere (*see* p. 206).

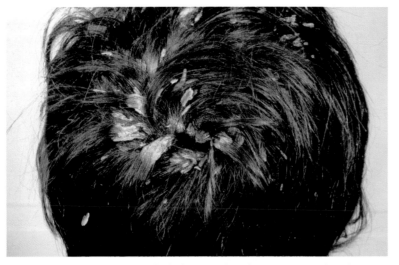

Fig. 3.31 Pityriasis amiantacea. Thick plaque with scale growing out along hairs.

TREATMENT SCALP PSORIASIS/PITYRIASIS AMIANTACEA

Mild scalp psoriasis. Where the scales are not very thick, shampooing the scalp twice weekly with a tar based shampoo such as *Capasal*UK, *Polytar*, *T-gel* etc. may be all that is needed.

If that is not enough, or if the **scalp is very itchy**, a topical steroid lotion or gel can be applied every night until it is clear. Calcipitriol lotion may be tried as an alternative but tends to be less effective. Topical scalp lotions contain alcohol, so warn the patient that it will sting if the skin is broken. Steroid gels are water miscible and will not sting. None of these will work if there is thick scaling.

Thick plaques of psoriasis in the scalp or **pityriasis amiantacea** require something to soften up the scale. The most effective treatment is coconut oil compound ointment (Ung cocois co, [*Cocois*UK] or a keratolytic gel). The hair is parted and the ointment rubbed onto the scalp, it is then parted again a little further along, and more ointment applied; this is continued until the whole scalp has been treated. It is done every night before the patient goes to bed and washed off the following morning with *Polytar* shampoo or whatever shampoo the patient likes. Because it makes a mess, the head should be covered overnight with a scarf or shower cap to keep the ointment off the pillow. The treatment is repeated each night and washed off each morning until the scalp is clear. This usually takes 7–10 days. Once it is clear, the treatment can be done once a week or once a fortnight to keep it clear.

If coconut oil compound ointment does not work (unusual), Ung pyrogallol co, dithranol pomade or oil of Cade ointment can be used instead (*see* p. 75).

TREATMENT SEBORRHOEIC ECZEMA

Ketoconazole (Nizoral) shampoo is used twice weekly for 2 weeks and then once a fortnight to keep it clear.

Coconut oil compound		Dithranol pomade	
Emulsifying wax	65g	Dithranol	2g
Yellow soft paraffin	45g	Salicylic acid	0.8g
Precipitated sulphur	20g	Coconut oil	149.2g
Salicylic acid	10g	(or liquid paraffin)	
Coal tar solution	60ml	Emulsifying wax	45g
Coconut oil	300ml		

Ung pyrogallol co.		Oil of Cade ointment	
Pyrogallol	5g	Cade oil	6g
Salicylic acid	8g	Precipitated sulphur	3g
Phenol	5g	Salicylic acid	2g
White soft paraffin	182g	Emulsifying ointment	89g

HEAD LICE (Pediculosis capitis)

Lice are wingless insects which pierce the skin to feed on human blood. The head louse is about 3mm long. The female lays 7–10 eggs each day during a life span of one month. The eggs are firmly attached to the base of the hair, and hatch in about a week. Head lice are spread by direct contact from head to head, mainly in children. It has nothing to do with poor hygiene. Lice are not transmitted by combs, hats or hair brushes. Infestation is extremely common and usually asymptomatic. If there are large numbers of lice, itching may be intolerable and can cause secondary bacterial infection (impetigo and pustules). Enlarged posterior cervical glands should always make you think of head lice. The diagnosis is made by finding the nits (egg cases), which are white, opalescent oval capsules, firmly attached to hairs (Figs 3.35, 3.36); unlike dandruff where the scale easily comes off.

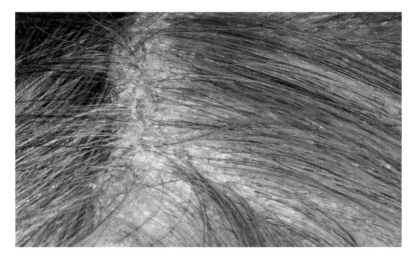

Fig. 3.32 Seborrhoeic eczema in scalp. Note fine uniform scaling.

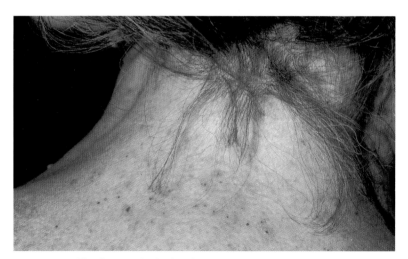

Fig. 3.33 Head lice bites on back of neck.

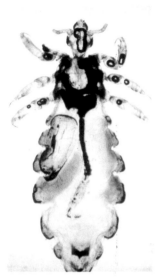

Fig. 3.34 Head louse.
Fertilised female (×20).

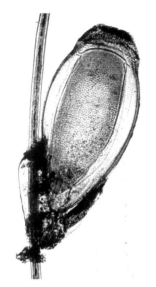

Fig. 3.35 Head louse egg (nit).
Firmly cemented to hair shaft (×30).

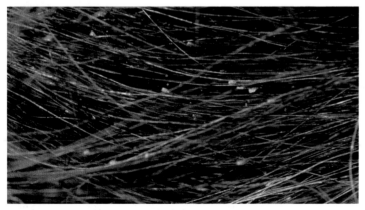

Fig. 3.36 Nits on hair. Looks like 'dandruff' but stuck firmly to hairs.

TREATMENT HEAD LICE

There are a number of insecticides available which kill both adult lice and eggs – malathion, carbaryl[UK] and the pyrethroids (permethrin and *d*-phenothrin) formulated as water or alcohol-based lotions, cream shampoos or cream rinses. All are neurotoxic to the lice. Two treatments should be given, 7 days apart, because young eggs do not possess a nervous system and may survive a single treatment. Lotions are better than shampoo formulations because the latter have too short a contact time to be effective. The lotion is applied all over the scalp, left on for 12 hours, and then washed off with a normal shampoo. The permethrin cream rinse is used like a conditioner. It coats the lice and eggs with a balsam containing the insecticide, so combining a long contact time with a short treatment time. The egg cases can be removed by combing them out with a nit comb.

Problems with treating head lice

1. Resistance to insecticides is now common, and if one treatment fails to cure the infestation, you should try another one. The *Bug Buster* kit consists of a nit comb and a conditioner. The wet hair should be combed for 10 minutes every night for about two weeks. This is useful if you want to avoid excessive use of insecticides.

2. To prevent re-infection, the *whole family* and school friends or contacts should be treated whether or not they are itching. You may need to involve the health visitor, practice nurse or school nurse.

3. People are often worried that some of the lice may be missed in children or adults with very long hair. Since the eggs are laid onto the hairs where they leave the scalp, all the viable eggs will be close to the scalp and will be killed as long as the insecticide has been applied to the scalp (not the hair). In the same way, the adult lice and the immature walking stages have to go to the scalp to feed, so they will be killed by the insecticide then.

4. Only water based insecticide lotions should be used in patients with eczema because the alcoholic ones will sting excoriated skin.

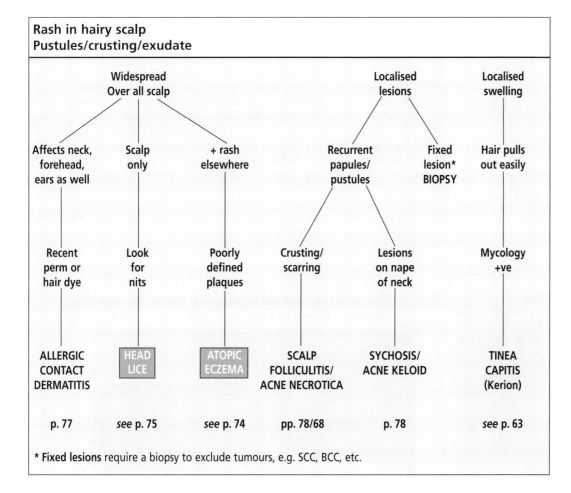

Rash in hairy scalp
Pustules/crusting/exudate

Widespread Over all scalp
- Affects neck, forehead, ears as well → Recent perm or hair dye → **ALLERGIC CONTACT DERMATITIS** — p. 77
- Scalp only → Look for nits → **HEAD LICE** — *see p. 75*
- + rash elsewhere → Poorly defined plaques → **ATOPIC ECZEMA** — *see p. 74*

Localised lesions
- Recurrent papules/pustules
  - Crusting/scarring → **SCALP FOLLICULITIS/ ACNE NECROTICA** — pp. 78/68
  - Lesions on nape of neck → **SYCHOSIS/ ACNE KELOID** — p. 78
- Fixed lesion* BIOPSY

Localised swelling
- Hair pulls out easily → Mycology +ve → **TINEA CAPITIS (Kerion)** — *see p. 63*

* Fixed lesions require a biopsy to exclude tumours, e.g. SCC, BCC, etc.

ALLERGIC CONTACT DERMATITIS

Allergic contact dermatitis on the scalp is not common and is usually due to hair dyes (paraphenylene diamine), or perming solutions (thioglycolates). It usually presents as an acute weeping eczema at the hair margins and on the forehead, face and neck rather than in the scalp itself. The diagnosis is confirmed once the patient is better by patch testing.

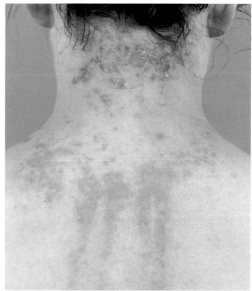

Fig. 3.37 Acute allergic contact dermatitis to hair dye.

TREATMENT ALLERGIC CONTACT DERMATITIS

Stop using hair dyes/perming solutions. If it is very weepy, dry up any exudate by soaking the scalp in a diluted potassium permanganate or aluminium acetate solution (*see* p. 26). Then apply a potent[UK]/group 2–3[USA] steroid ointment. Once it is better refer to a dermatologist for patch testing to establish the cause.

SCALP FOLLICULITIS

Recurrent pustules in the scalp can present diagnostic and therapeutic difficulties. Sometimes the cause is a staphylococcal folliculitis which can be confirmed by taking a swab. Often no bacteria are grown and the condition may be a variant of acne.

Sychosis nuchae refers to a specific pattern of folliculitis primarily affecting the nape of the neck.

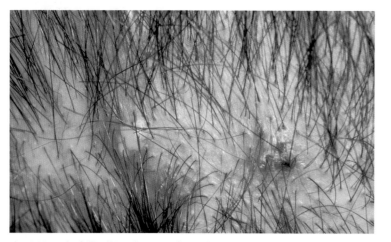

Fig. 3.38 Scalp folliculitis. Close up of pustules and crusted erosions.

TREATMENT SCALP FOLLICULITIS & ACNE KELOID

Take swabs. If *Staph. aureus* is grown treat with flucloxacillin or erythromycin 250mg q.i.d. until clear. If swabs are negative treat with a tetracycline (e.g. lymecycline) or isotretinoin as for acne (*see* p. 101).

ACNE KELOID NUCHALIS

This is a chronic inflammatory condition of the nape of the neck, most commonly seen in Negro men. Itchy follicular pustules develop in the occipital area (sychosis nuchae) which later become keloid scars. In the early stages of the disease (pustules present), long-term, low dose antibiotics as for acne can be used. Once keloid papules, nodules or plaques are present **treatment** is more difficult. Possibilites include intralesional triamcinolone once a month, or wide excision of the affected area down to and including the fat.

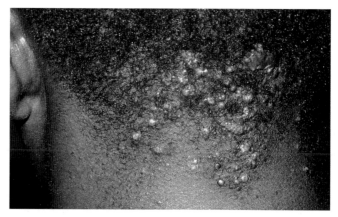

Fig. 3.39 Acne keloid nuchalis. Small keloid papules on nape of neck.

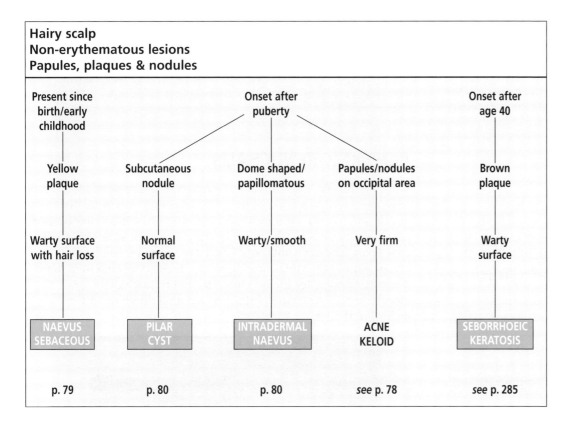

Hairy scalp
Non-erythematous lesions
Papules, plaques & nodules

Present since birth/early childhood	Onset after puberty			Onset after age 40
Yellow plaque	Subcutaneous nodule	Dome shaped/ papillomatous	Papules/nodules on occipital area	Brown plaque
Warty surface with hair loss	Normal surface	Warty/smooth	Very firm	Warty surface
NAEVUS SEBACEOUS	**PILAR CYST**	**INTRADERMAL NAEVUS**	ACNE KELOID	**SEBORRHOEIC KERATOSIS**
p. 79	p. 80	p. 80	*see p. 78*	*see p. 285*

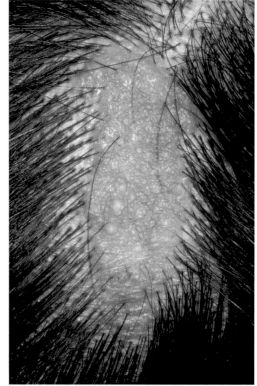

Fig. 3.40 Naevus sebaceous present since birth.

NAEVUS SEBACEOUS

This is present from birth or early childhood. It differs from a congential melanocytic naevus in being yellowish with a flat warty surface and hair loss. A basal cell carcinoma or an adnexal tumour may develop within it in middle age. When this happens it is obvious because there will be a lump within the naevus or a discharge from it.

TREATMENT NAEVUS SEBACEOUS

Excise if they are a nuisance. Otherwise only remove if a tumour develops.

PILAR (Trichilemmal) CYST

Pilar (or trichilemmal) cysts are derived from the external root sheath of hair follicles and occur predominantly on the scalp. They are inherited as an autosomal dominant trait, appear between the ages of 15 and 30, and present to the doctor because the patient notices a lump when brushing or combing the hair. One or several subcutaneous nodules are present. They do not have a punctum and do not usually become inflamed (compare with epidermoid cysts, p. 238).

TREATMENT PILAR CYST

These cysts shell out very easily under local anaesthetic once you are in the right plane since they have a connective tissue sheath around them. An alternative method of removal is to cut straight into them with a scalpel, squeeze out the contents and then remove the cyst lining with a pair of artery forceps. It should come out intact and very easily.

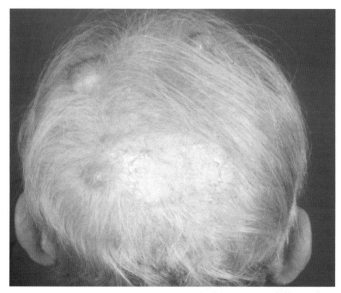

Fig. 3.41 Pilar cysts on the scalp.

INTRADERMAL NAEVUS

Flat pigmented naevi are not usually recognised on the hairy scalp. Once they become raised they are likely to be caught in combs. Most skin coloured or light brown papules in the scalp will be intradermal naevi. They may have a smooth or papillomatous surface (*see* p. 233).

TREATMENT INTRADERMAL NAEVUS

Reassure the patient that they are harmless. They can be easily removed by shave and cautery if they become a problem.

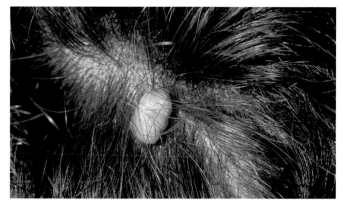

Fig. 3.42 Intradermal naevus on the scalp.

Acute erythematous rash on the face

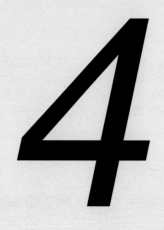

4

Normal surface

Crust or exudate on surface

Face
Acute erythematous rash
Surface normal/smooth
Widespread patches/papules/plaques/swelling

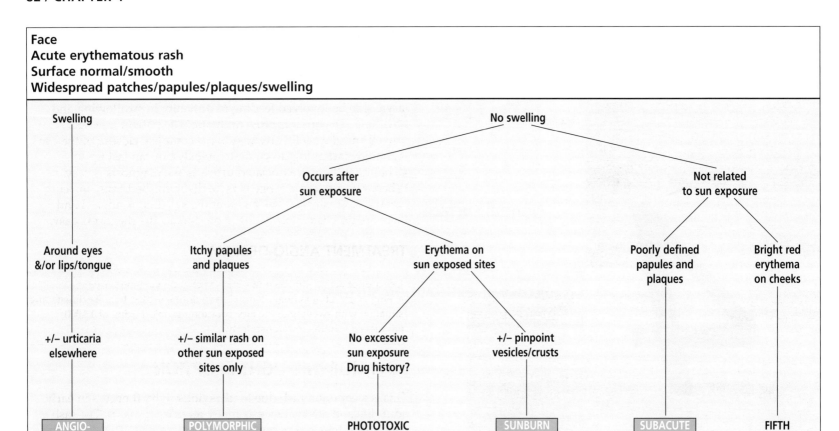

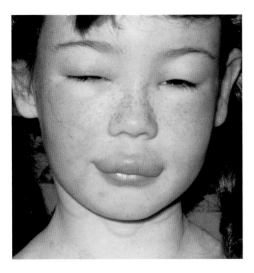

Fig. 4.01 Angio-oedema involving the upper lip and eyelids. There is oedema without exudate or scaling. Note associated urticaria on face and neck.

Compare with Fig. 4.02.

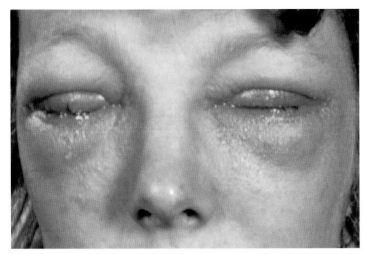

Fig. 4.02 Acute eczema: swelling associated with exudate and crusting.

ANGIO-OEDEMA

Angio-oedema is oedema in the dermis due to increased vascular permeability (*see* urticaria, p. 150). On the face the swelling involves the eyelids and lips. Less commonly the tongue and larynx can be involved leading to difficulty in swallowing and breathing. The onset is often dramatic. The patient may feel unwell and the eyelid swelling cause complete closure of the eyes. It should start going down quite quickly but can last up to 48 hours. If there is associated urticaria the diagnosis is easy. When it occurs alone it needs to be distinguished from an acute eczema or erysipelas. The fact that the swelling is not red and there are no blisters or scaling should make the diagnosis easy.

TREATMENT ANGIO-OEDEMA

Use a short-acting antihistamine such as chlorphenamine (*Piriton*), 4–8mg every 4 hours (max. 24mg/24hrs) until it settles. In a life-threatening situation with swelling of the larynx or tongue, inject 0.5ml of 1:1000 adrenaline solution intramuscularly.

POLYMORPHIC LIGHT ERUPTION

This is a common rash due to ultraviolet light. It occurs in early adult life and affects twice as many females as males. The rash consists of itchy red papules, vesicles or plaques. The size of the papules varies in different patients from pin point up to 5mm. The plaques may be urticarial (i.e. non-scaly dermal oedema) or eczematous (scaly & poorly defined). Vesicles are less common. It occurs only on sun-exposed parts, especially the back of the hands, forearms, 'V' of neck and below the ears, as well as the face, but not all sun-exposed sites need to be involved, and quite often the face may be clear.

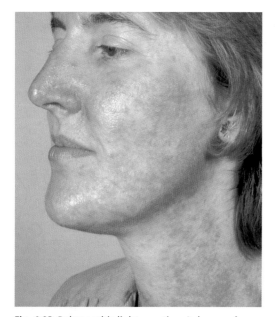

Fig. 4.03 Polymorphic light eruption. Itchy papules and vesicles on the face and neck, sparing under chin.

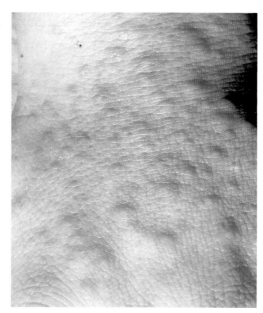

Fig. 4.04 Polymorphic light eruption. Itchy papules on dorsum of the hand.

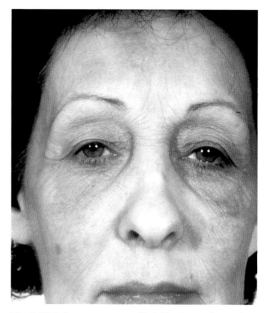

Fig. 4.05 Subacute eczema. Ill defined papules and patches with no exudate or scaling.

Most patients are aware of the connection with the sun. The rash typically occurs several hours after sun exposure and, if there is no further exposure, lasts for 2–5 days. It usually occurs in spring and early summer and tends to improve as the summer progresses due to some form of tolerance. In some patients it only occurs when they are away from home (on holiday) in more intense sunlight.

TREATMENT POLYMORPHIC LIGHT ERUPTION

1. Keep out of strong sunlight, wear protective clothing and use a high factor sun block with both UVB & UVA protection.
2. Refer to dermatology department for PUVA therapy. This can be given in early summer to prevent the rash developing, or as a treatment to induce tolerance. It is given twice a week for 6 weeks.
3. Systemic steroids (prednisolone 20mg/day) may suppress the eruption for the duration of a short two-week holiday.
4. Hydroxychloroquine 400mg daily may provide partial protection.

SUBACUTE ECZEMA

Subacute eczema occurs without obvious vesicles and exudate. There will be erythematous patches and plaques where the border of the rash is ill defined merging imperceptibly into normal skin. It can be due to an allergic contact dermatitis (to cosmetics, perfumes, medicaments), or to an exacerbation of existing eczema (atopic or seborrhoeic).

PHOTOTOXIC RASHES

A phototoxic rash looks like sunburn but occurs in a patient who has not been exposed to excessive sunlight. It is caused by sunlight plus:–

a. Chemicals applied to the skin, e.g. psoralens in suncreams.

b. Accidental contamination of the skin by wood tars in creosote.

c. Drugs taken by mouth, e.g.:–

- amiodarone (30–50% of patients on this drug)
- furosemide
- nalidixic acid
- psoralens
- sulphonamides
- tetracyclines – especially demethylchlortetracycline
- thiazide diuretics.

The diagnosis is suggested by the distribution of the rash with shaded sites (upper eyelids, behind ears, under chin) spared. It can be confused with a contact allergic eczema but there should not be any scaling. The history of drug ingestion or creams applied to the face should enable the cause to be identified.

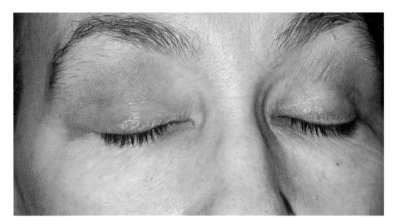

Fig. 4.06 Subacute eczema involving the eyelids. The surface is scaly, and involvement of the upper eyelids (shaded from sunlight) distinguish it from a phototoxic rash.

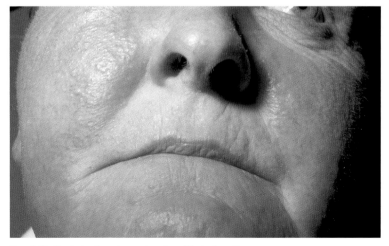

Fig. 4.07 Phototoxic rash sparing the skin below the nose.

TREATMENT PHOTOTOXIC RASHES

Stop the drug responsible. If this is not possible, use an opaque sun screen (*see* p. 33) containing titanium dioxide or zinc oxide to screen out all UVA (almost all drug sensitivity rashes are due to UVA). Note that UVA penetrates glass so protection is needed even indoors or inside a car.

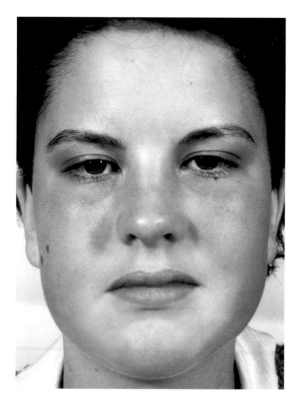

Fig. 4.08 Fifth disease. Typical 'slapped cheek' appearance.

FIFTH DISEASE (Erythema infectiosum)

This is a viral infection due to parvovirus B19. It is characterised by the appearance of red papules on the cheeks which coalesce within hours to form symmetrical, red, oedematous plaques sparing the nasolabial folds and eyelids, the so called 'slapped cheek' appearance. Other symptoms are mild (sore throat, pruritis, fever) or even absent. The rash on the face fades after 4 days, but within 48 hours of the onset of the facial erythema, a lace-like pattern of erythema appears on the proximal limbs extending to the trunk and extremities. This fades within 6–14 days.

TREATMENT FIFTH DISEASE

It gets better on its own after about a week; no treatment is needed.

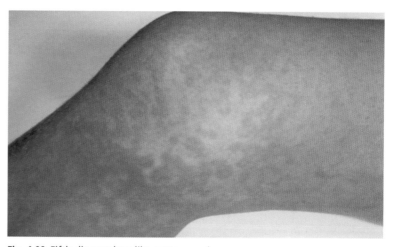

Fig. 4.09 Fifth disease: lace-like pattern on leg.

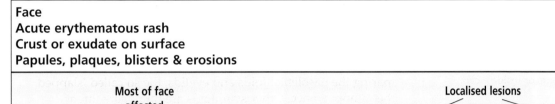

Face
Acute erythematous rash
Crust or exudate on surface
Papules, plaques, blisters & erosions

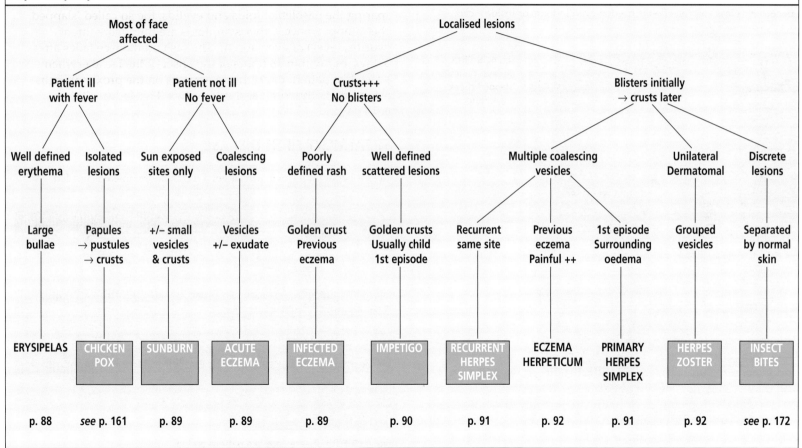

Most of face affected

Localised lesions

Patient ill with fever — **Patient not ill No fever**

Crusts+++ No blisters — **Blisters initially → crusts later**

Well defined erythema | **Isolated lesions** | **Sun exposed sites only** | **Coalescing lesions** | **Poorly defined rash** | **Well defined scattered lesions** | **Multiple coalescing vesicles** | **Unilateral Dermatomal** | **Discrete lesions**

Large bullae | Papules → pustules → crusts | +/– small vesicles & crusts | Vesicles +/– exudate | Golden crust Previous eczema | Golden crusts Usually child 1st episode | Recurrent same site | Previous eczema Painful ++ | 1st episode Surrounding oedema | Grouped vesicles | Separated by normal skin

ERYSIPELAS | **CHICKEN POX** | **SUNBURN** | **ACUTE ECZEMA** | **INFECTED ECZEMA** | **IMPETIGO** | **RECURRENT HERPES SIMPLEX** | **ECZEMA HERPETICUM** | **PRIMARY HERPES SIMPLEX** | **HERPES ZOSTER** | **INSECT BITES**

p. 88 | *see* p. 161 | p. 89 | p. 89 | p. 89 | p. 90 | p. 91 | p. 92 | p. 91 | p. 92 | *see* p. 172

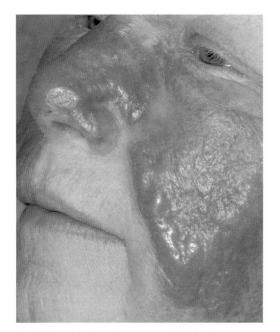

Fig. 4.10 Erysipelas. Blisters on well defined erythema.

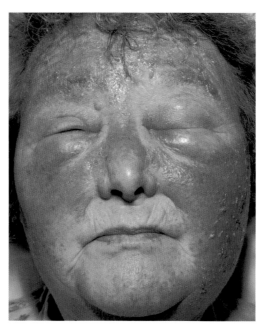

Fig. 4.11 Acute contact allergic dermatitis due to lanolin in a moisturising cream – exudate and crusting.

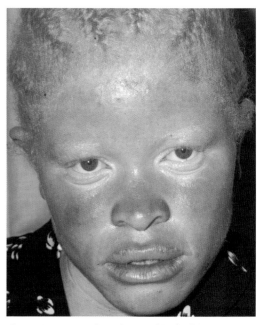

Fig. 4.12 Acute sunburn in an African albino.

ERYSIPELAS

This is an acute, rapidly spreading rash caused by a Group A beta-haemolytic streptococcus. The patient is unwell with fever, rigors and general malaise. The rash itself is bright red, well demarcated and may or may not contain large blisters in the centre. There is no associated lymphangitis or lymphadenopathy. It is not usually possible to culture the organism and measurement of the ASO titre is not helpful. Diagnosis is made on the characteristic clinical picture.

TREATMENT ERYSIPELAS

Intravenous benzyl penicillin 600mg six hourly for 5 days. If the patient is allergic to penicillin use oral erythromycin 500mg six hourly, but this is not as good as benzyl penicillin. The patient should be dramatically better within 24 hours.

ACUTE SUNBURN

Acute sunburn presents as painful erythema with or without blisters, between a few hours to 2 days after sun exposure. Usually the cause will be obvious as the patient will have been exposed to strong sunlight, although a delay in symptoms can lead to misdiagnosis. Any exposed areas will be burnt.

TREATMENT ACUTE SUNBURN

> Topical calamine lotion will produce symptomatic relief. If severe, a single application of a very potent[UK]/group 1[USA] topical steroid (0.05% clobetasol propionate) ointment will reduce redness and bring instant relief.

ACUTE ECZEMA

Acute eczema presents as tiny vesicles, weeping and crusting, and is usually due to an allergic contact dermatitis. The onset of the rash is sudden with erythema followed by vesicles, profuse exudate and crusting. If the eyelids are involved there may be marked oedema and the patient may not be able to open the eyes (Fig. 4.11). The rash is usually symmetrical and uncomfortable and itchy rather than painful as in herpes zoster. Angio-oedema causes swelling only with no weeping and there is no associated fever as in erysipelas.

Acute allergic contact dermatitis of the face can be due to medicaments applied to the face or airborne allergens such as sawdust, cement dust or phosphorus sesquisulphide from the smoke of 'strike anywhere' matches. Common applied allergens include lanolin (in ointment bases), parabens (a preservative in creams), topical antihistamines or antibiotics, cosmetics and perfumes. The exact pattern of the rash depends on the allergen responsible. Airborne allergens cause a symmetrical eczema especially affecting the eyelids and cheeks while allergens in medicaments and cosmetics only involve areas where they have been applied. Linear streaking can be due to nail varnish. A rash around the hair margins and ears can be due to hair dyes or perming solutions (*see* p. 77).

A **photoallergic dermatitis** is identical in appearance to an allergic contact dermatitis but it needs a combination of long wave ultraviolet light (UVA) and a drug to cause it. The commonest drugs are:-

- chlorpromazine
- sulphonamides
- promethazine
- alimemazine (trimeprazine).

TREATMENT ALLERGIC CONTACT DERMATITIS

> Remove the patient from all possible allergens. Dry up any exudate with wet dressings of potassium permanganate (1:10,000) or Burow's solution (*see* p. 26) twice a day. Dry the skin and then apply 1% hydrocortisone ointment b.i.d. Always use a steroid ointment rather than a cream which may contain potential allergens. Once the rash is better refer the patient to a dermatologist for patch testing.

IMPETIGINIZED ECZEMA

Any itchy rash may become secondarily infected with *Staphylococcus aureus* once the skin has been broken by scratching. Weeping occurs and golden yellow crusts form on the surface. The diagnosis is made by the history of a preceding rash (usually atopic eczema or scabies). Individual lesions may be difficult to distinguish from impetigo.

TREATMENT IMPETIGINIZED ECZEMA

It is best to give a systemic antibiotic, either flucloxacillin or erythromycin four times a day (125mg dose for children, 250mg for adults). At the same time treat the atopic eczema (*see* p. 208) or scabies (*see* p. 218), or the infection will reoccur.

IMPETIGO

This is a very superficial infection of the epidermis due to *Staphylococcus aureus*, a group A beta-haemolytic streptococcus or a mixture of both. Children are mainly affected since the organisms gain entrance through broken skin (cuts and grazes). It is very contagious. Typically it starts as vesicles, which rapidly break down to form honey-coloured crusts; less commonly there may be just a glazed erythema.

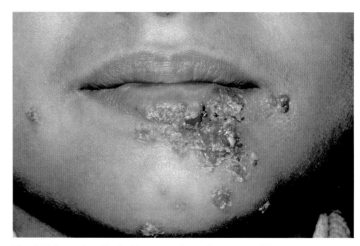

Fig. 4.14 Impetigo. Typical honey-coloured crusts on chin.

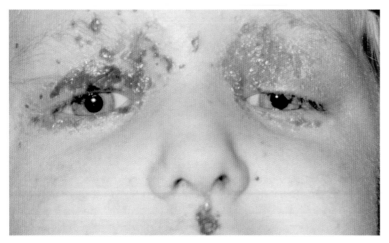

Fig. 4.13 Impetiginized eczema. Exudate and golden crusts in a patient with atopic eczema.

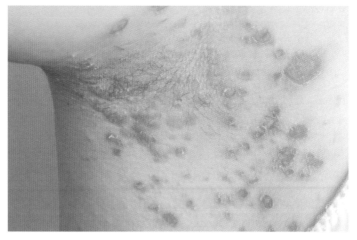

Fig. 4.15 Impetigo. Superficial erosions around the axilla in a teenage girl.

TREATMENT IMPETIGO

Because the infection is very superficial, topical antibiotics are more effective than systemic. If thick crust is present, remove it by applying arachis oil (or olive/sunflower oil) for 15–20 minutes. This will soften it so that it can be wiped off. Once the crust has been removed apply 2% mupirocin (*Bactroban*), 2% fusidic acid (*Fucidin*) or 0.3% neomycin ointment four times a day for 3 days. Apply the antibiotic ointment to the anterior nares at the same time.

In parts of the world where impetigo is commonly due to a group A beta-haemolytic streptococcus, the child will need to be treated with oral penicillin V four times a day for 7 days to prevent acute glomerulonephritis from occurring.

PRIMARY HERPES SIMPLEX

Infection with the *Herpes hominis virus type 1* most commonly affects the buccal mucosa (*see* p. 125) and occurs in the first five years of life. It is usually asymptomatic but may cause an acute gingivo-stomatitis. A primary infection on the skin causes painful blistering on an oedematous background.

RECURRENT HERPES SIMPLEX

If the primary infection of herpes simplex was in the mouth, recurrent episodes affect the lips or the skin around the lips. Primary infections elsewhere on the skin produce recurrences at the same site (e.g. finger, buttock). Most patients know that a recurrence is beginning because of the prodromal sensation of itching, burning or tingling. A few hours later, small grouped vesicles appear (*see* Fig. 1.29, p. 9), burst, crust and then heal in

7–10 days. These episodes can be precipitated by fever (hence the name 'cold sores'), sunlight, menstruation and stress and can continue throughout life. Herpes simplex is differentiated from impetigo by the history of recurrent episodes, prodromal pain and initial vesicles containing clear fluid and in adults is the more likely diagnosis. If in doubt, a Tzanck smear from the base of a blister will show multinucleate giant cells in herpes simplex.

TREATMENT HERPES SIMPLEX

Most patients need no treatment. Topical aciclovir or penciclovir cream applied 2 hourly for 2 days, beginning as soon as the prodromal symptoms occur, will shorten the attack but will not prevent further episodes. If recurrent episodes occur frequently or result in erythema multiforme, these can be suppressed by giving oral aciclovir 400mg b.i.d. or famciclovir 250mg daily for at least 6 months.

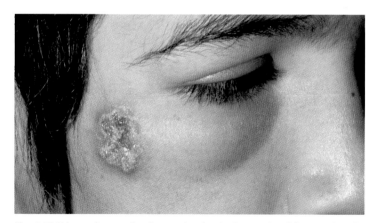

Fig. 4.16 Primary herpes simplex on the cheek. Grouped vesicles associated with marked surrounding oedema.

ECZEMA HERPETICUM

Atopic eczema may become secondarily infected by herpes simplex. The characteristic feature is small umbilicated vesicles which are painful rather than itchy. The patient will be ill and more miserable than might be expected from normal eczema. Swabs from the vesicles will confirm the presence of the herpes simplex virus. Pemphigus, pemphigoid and Darier's disease may all become similarly infected with the herpes simplex virus. Treat the same as herpes zoster (*see* p. 158).

HERPES ZOSTER

Herpes zoster on the face is the result of involvement of the trigeminal nerve. It presents as groups of small vesicles on a red background, followed by weeping and crusting. The rash is unilateral. Healing takes 3–4 weeks. With ophthalmic zoster the rash extends from the upper eyelid to the vertex of the skull, but if vesicles occur on the side of the nose (nasociliary branch), the eye is likely to be involved (Fig. 4.19). These patients should be referred to an ophthalmologist. (*See also* p. 158.)

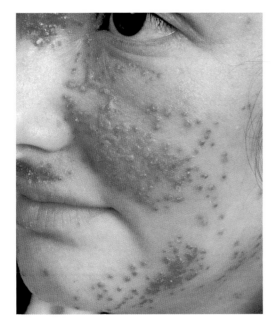

Fig. 4.17 Eczema herpeticum: umbilicated vesicles becoming pustules and rupturing to leave painful erosions.

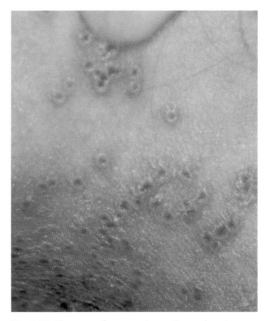

Fig. 4.18 Close up of eczema herpeticum showing umbilicated vesicles.

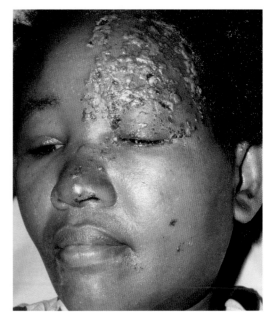

Fig. 4.19 Herpes zoster affecting ophthalmic branch of the Vth cranial nerve.

Chronic erythematous rash on the face

5

Normal surface

Scaly surface

Crust, exudate or excoriated surface

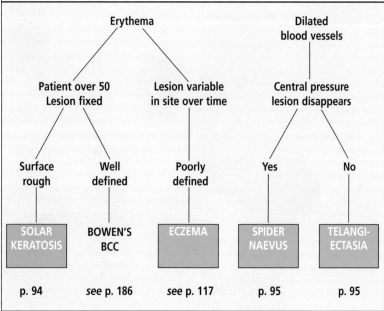

Face
Chronic erythematous lesions
Surface normal
Macules

Erythema

Dilated
blood vessels

Patient over 50
Lesion fixed

Lesion variable
in site over time

Central pressure
lesion disappears

Surface
rough

Well
defined

Poorly
defined

Yes

No

SOLAR KERATOSIS	BOWEN'S BCC	ECZEMA	SPIDER NAEVUS	TELANGI-ECTASIA
p. 94	*see* p. 186	*see* p. 117	p. 95	p. 95

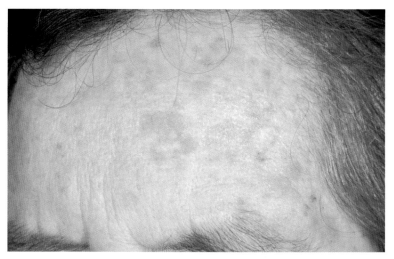

Fig. 5.01 (above) Multiple solar keratoses on the forehead – often misdiagnosed as eczema.

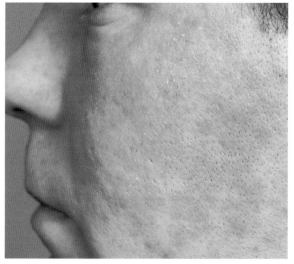

Fig. 5.02 Eczema on the face. The lesions are not always in the same place.

SOLAR KERATOSIS

These may present as an area of fixed erythema on the face of a middle aged or elderly fair-skinned individual who has had a lot of sun exposure in the past. They are often misdiagnosed (as eczema), but the key to the diagnosis is to feel the surface, which is rough. The individual lesions remain fixed over a period of time.

SPIDER NAEVUS

A red papule with a central arteriole and peripheral radiating arms is a common normal finding in children. Pressure (use a paper clip) on the central vessel results in obliteration of the lesion. Large numbers occur in pregnancy and in association with chronic liver disease.

TREATMENT SPIDER NAEVUS

The central feeding vessel can be cauterised with a 'cold point' or fine looped wire cautery. This takes about 1 second so local anaesthetic is not necessary unless the lesion is very large. The pulse dye laser is also effective – a single shot is all that is necessary, and if available may be preferable in children.

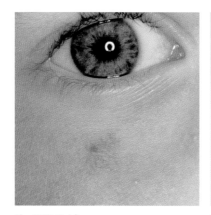

Fig. 5.03 Spider naevus.

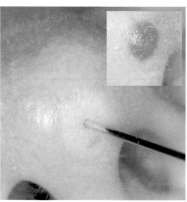

Fig. 5.04 Spider naevus: central arteriole compressed (inset before compression).

TELANGIECTASIA

Small areas of visibly dilated blood vessels where there is no central vessel feeding it is called telangiectasia. It is very common on the face due to weathering and may be associated with rosacea, scleroderma, and the application of potent topical steroids.

TREATMENT TELANGIECTASIA

Any vascular laser such as the pulse dye or KTP laser will remove visible telangiectasia on the face (*see* p. 53). The KTP laser does not cause bruising so patients can continue to work. Several treatments may be needed at 6-weekly intervals. The patient should not have a suntan otherwise post-inflammatory hyperpigmentation can occur.

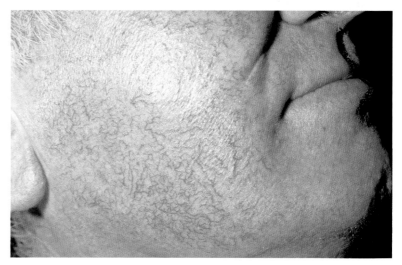

Fig. 5.05 Telangiectasia.

Face
Chronic erythematous rash
Surface normal
Multiple papules & pustules (Single/few lesions *see* p. 230)

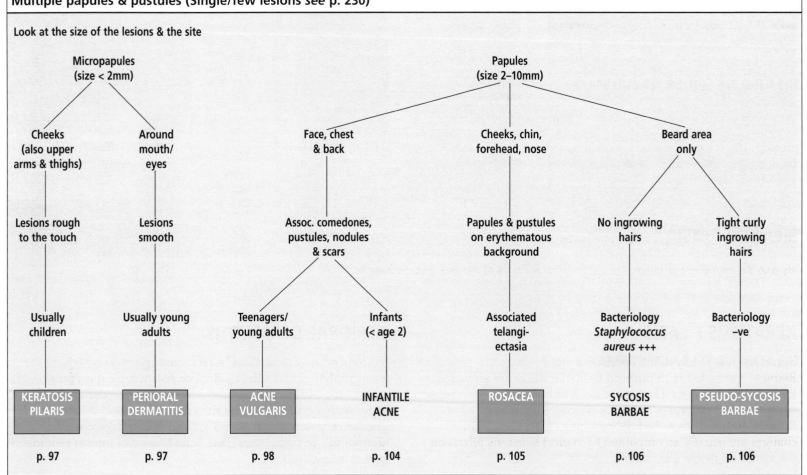

Look at the size of the lesions & the site

Micropapules
(size < 2mm)

Papules
(size 2–10mm)

Cheeks
(also upper
arms & thighs)

Around
mouth/
eyes

Face, chest
& back

Cheeks, chin,
forehead, nose

Beard area
only

Lesions rough
to the touch

Lesions
smooth

Assoc. comedones,
pustules, nodules
& scars

Papules & pustules
on erythematous
background

No ingrowing
hairs

Tight curly
ingrowing
hairs

Usually
children

Usually young
adults

Teenagers/
young adults

Infants
(< age 2)

Associated
telangi-
ectasia

Bacteriology
*Staphylococcus
aureus* +++

Bacteriology
–ve

KERATOSIS
PILARIS

PERIORAL
DERMATITIS

ACNE
VULGARIS

INFANTILE
ACNE

ROSACEA

SYCOSIS
BARBAE

PSEUDO-SYCOSIS
BARBAE

p. 97

p. 97

p. 98

p. 104

p. 105

p. 106

p. 106

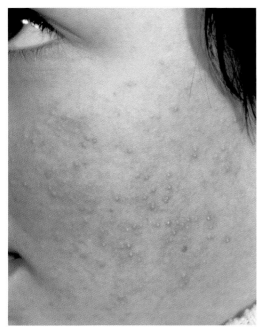

Fig. 5.06 Keratosis pilaris on the cheek.

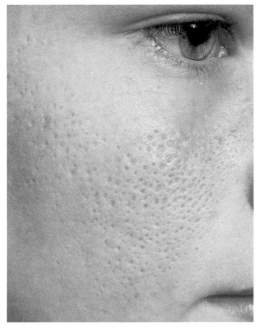

Fig. 5.07 Atrophoderma vermiculata.

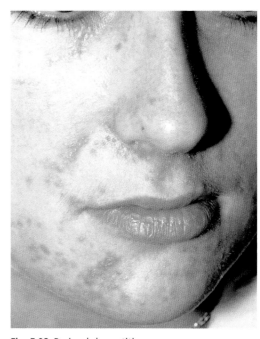

Fig. 5.08 Perioral dermatitis.

KERATOSIS PILARIS

Keratosis pilaris may affect the cheeks and eyebrows in children. Redness associated with pinhead follicular plugs are seen, and as the plugs are shed atrophy can occur (atrophoderma vermiculata). On the (outer) eyebrows this is associated with loss of hair follicles. In some cases the forehead may be involved. These changes are usually accompanied by typical keratosis pilaris on the arms and thighs (*see* p. 294).

PERIORAL DERMATITIS

Perioral dermatitis is a condition of young adults who have been applying moderately potent or potent topical corticosteroids to the face. Minute red papules and pustules appear around the mouth, typically sparing the skin immediately adjacent to the lips. Occasionally it occurs around the eyes (periocular dermatitis). In some cases there is no history of topical steroid use.

TREATMENT PERIORAL DERMATITIS

Stop any topical steroid use. This may lead to worsening of the rash initially; warn the patient about this and tell him on no account to use the topical steroid again. Oxytetracycline 250mg b.d. taken on an empty stomach for 6 weeks usually speeds up its resolution.

ACNE VULGARIS

Acne is a disease of the pilosebaceous unit. The hallmark of the disease is the comedo, a single blocked follicle. Everyone gets some acne. In girls it may appear before menstruation commences, sometimes as early as 9 years of age. In both sexes the peak incidence is 13–16 years, although it may continue into the 20s, 30s and occasionally later. Acne occurs on the face, chest and back depending on the distribution of the sebaceous follicles in that individual.

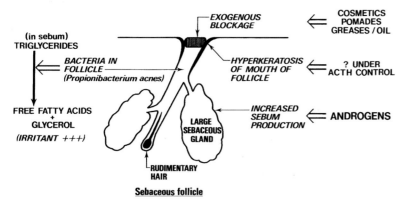

Fig. 5.09 Aetiology of acne.

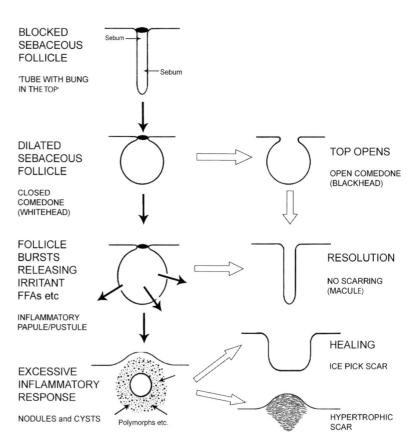

Fig. 5.10 Diagram to show evolution of acne lesions.

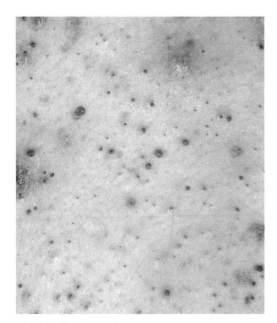

Fig. 5.11 Acne vulgaris – open comedones (blackheads) and a few inflammatory papules.

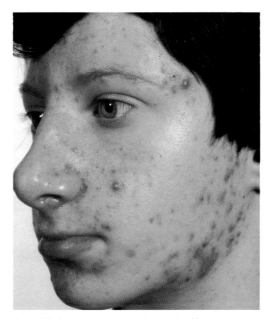

Fig. 5.12 Acne – papules and pustules (few comedones).

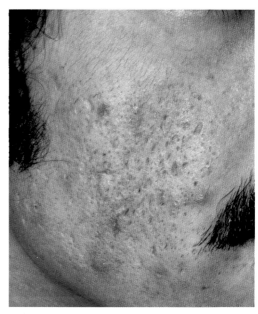

Fig. 5.13 Acne – ice pick scars.

The factors involved in the aetiology are shown in Fig. 5.09. Genetic factors are important in determining the severity, duration and clinical pattern. There is no evidence that diet influences acne, and it is certainly not a result of over indulgence in chocolates, fatty or 'junk' food. The evolution of acne lesions from a blocked sebaceous follicle is shown in Fig. 5.10. The black colour of open comedones is due to melanin not dirt.

The diagnosis of acne is usually easy, but comedones must be present before it is made. Comedones, papules, pustules, nodules, cysts and scars on the face or trunk of a young person is unique to acne, but occasionally folliculitis or even a papular form of eczema can mimic acne. Multiple epidermoid cysts may be confused with severe nodulo-cystic acne. Rosacea looks similar but affects an older population. There are no comedones, and the papules and pustules occur over a general erythematous background (*see* Fig. 5.22). In perioral dermatitis there are no comedones, and tiny papules and pustules occur around the mouth (*see* Fig. 5.08).

TREATMENT OF ACNE VULGARIS

1. COMEDONES

Keratolytic agents remove the surface keratin and unplug the follicular openings. Retinoids are the most effective e.g.:–

- Adapalene 0.1% cream or gel (*Differin*)
- Isotretinoin 0.05% gel (*Isotrex*^{UK})
- Tretinoin (0.01%, 0.025%) gel, (0.025%*, 0.05%**) cream or (0.025%) lotion (*Acticin*^{UK}, *Avita*^{USA}, *Retin-A**, *Retinova***)

If inflammatory lesions are present as well as the comedones use:–

- Benzoyl peroxide (2.5%, 5%, 10%) as a cream, lotion or gel (*Acnecide*^{UK}, *Benzagel*^{USA}, *Benzac*^{USA}, *Brevoxyl*, *Desquam*^{USA}, *PanOxyl*, *Persa-Gel*^{USA}, *Triaz*^{USA}), or combined (5%) with clindamycin 1% (*Duac*^{UK}, *Clindoxyl*^{USA}) or erythromycin 3% (*Benzamycin*). Note that benzoyl peroxide can bleach bed linen and clothing
- Adapalene 0.1% cream or gel (*Differin*)
- Azelaic acid 20% cream (*Azelex*^{USA}, *Skinoren*^{UK})

Instructions for the use of keratolytic agents

Before going to bed the patient should wash the skin with soap and water (medicated washes are not any better) and then apply the weakest strength of retinoid cream or benzoyl peroxide. If the skin becomes too sore, stop the treatment for a few days and then restart on alternate nights. In the morning if the skin becomes dry apply a non-greasy moisturiser. Increase the strength of the keratolytic if side effects are tolerated.

Ultraviolet light has a similar effect and a suntan tends to hide acne spots.

Squeezing with the fingers should be avoided, since this can convert a comedone into an inflammatory papule. Female patients can use makeup to cover their spots during the daytime, but they must wash it off at night so that the follicles do not become blocked causing more comedones.

2. INFLAMMATORY LESIONS

Systemic antibiotics

Oxytetracycline 500mg b.i.d. is cheap and effective. It must be given on an empty stomach (half an hour before a meal or 2 hours after) as it chelates with calcium in milk and food and also with iron and antacids. Improvement of the acne is slow and usually not apparent for at least 2–3 months with gradual improvement thereafter. Maintenance treatment must be continued until the acne gets better spontaneously, however long that is. Don't use tetracyclines in those under the age of 12, in females who are pregnant or breast feeding (it causes staining of teeth in the foetus and in children) or if renal function is impaired. Side effects are few – diarrhoea and vaginal candidiasis. At this dose they do not interfere with the absorption of the contraceptive pill although extra precautions are needed for the first month of treatment as the gut flora changes.

If no improvement occurs and *compliance has been good*, change to doxycycline 100mg daily, lymecycline 408mg daily or minocycline 100mg daily. Treatment with antibiotics should be given for at least 6 months, but if response is poor or relapse occurs after stopping treatment consider referral to a dermatologist for oral isotretinoin.

Topical antibiotics

Erythromycin (*Acne-mycin*^{USA}, *Emgel*^{USA}, *Erycette*^{USA}, *EryDerm*^{USA}, *Eryacne*^{USA}, *Stiemycin*^{UK})

Tetracycline (*Topicycline*)

Clindamycin (*Cleocin T*^{USA}, *Clindets*^{USA}, *Clinda-Derm*^{USA}, *Dalacin T*^{UK}, *Zindaclin*^{UK})

These all work nearly as well as systemic antibiotics but have the disadvantage of causing resistant bacteria on the skin surface. This can be reduced by using a combination such as *Duac* (clindamycin and benzoyl peroxide) or *Zineryt* (erythromycin and zinc). They are useful in pregnancy as there is negligible systemic absorption. There is no evidence that combining topical and systemic antibiotics is beneficial.

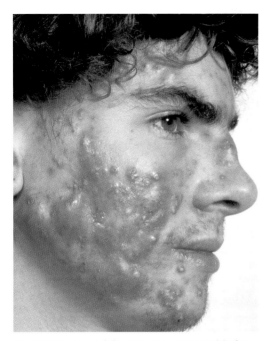

Fig. 5.14 Severe nodulo-cystic acne cyst suitable for treatment with isotretinoin.

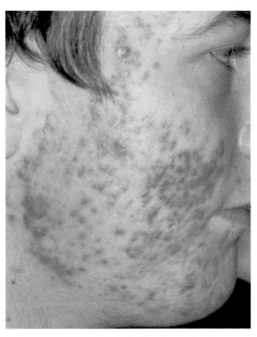

Fig. 5.15 Acne in teenager before isotretinoin therapy.

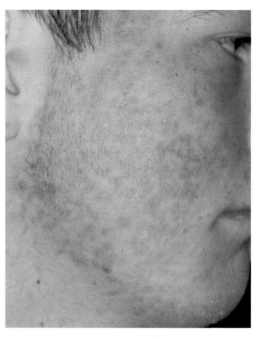

Fig. 5.16 Same patient as 5.15 after 4 months on isotretinoin.

Anti-androgens

Anti-androgens are useful in female patients if antibiotics have not worked and they are already on a contraceptive pill. They should be avoided in women who smoke, who are over 35 years of age, or who are hypertensive, because of the increased risk of cardiovascular and thromboembolic disease. Dianette contains 2mg of cyproterone acetate plus 35µg of oestrogen. It will act as a contraceptive pill as well as an anti-acne agent. The maximum effect does not occur for 2–3 months and treatment needs to be continued long term.

3. NODULES, CYSTS & SCARS

These patients should be referred immediately to a dermatologist for treatment with isotretinoin. It is given with food as a single daily dose (0.5–1mg/kg body weight/day) for 4 months. Although it is expensive early use can prevent scarring. A single course of treatment gives long-term remission (permanent in over 70% of individuals). Recurrence is more likely with lower doses. For the side effects of isotretinoin *see* pp. 41, 42 and for indications for oral isotretinoin *see* p. 102.

Isolated acne cysts can be injected with 10mg/ml triamcinolone.

Indications for oral isotretinoin treatment

1. Severe acne that is leading to permanent scarring.
2. Acne that has not responded to 6 months or more of oral antibiotics or anti-androgens.
3. Patients who are depressed by the state of their skin.
4. Persistent low grade acne especially in patients over the age of 30.
5. Patients with acne excoriée.

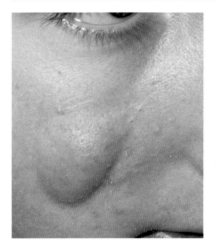

Fig. 5.17 (left) Acne cyst suitable for injection with triamcinolone.

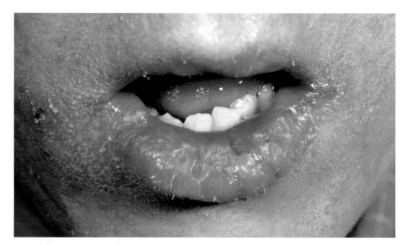

Fig. 5.18 Dry lips and dryness of the skin around the lips due to isotretinoin.

DRUG AND CHEMICAL INDUCED ACNE

A rash that looks like acne occurring in the wrong place or in the wrong age group may be due to drugs or chemicals. Systemic steroids, isoniazid and ACTH may worsen or precipitate acne. Chlorinated aromatic hydrocarbons used in insecticides, fungicides and wood preservatives cause severe acne which may continue after exposure has ceased. Insoluble cutting oils, coal tars, corticosteroids and cosmetics may induce acne when applied topically to the skin.

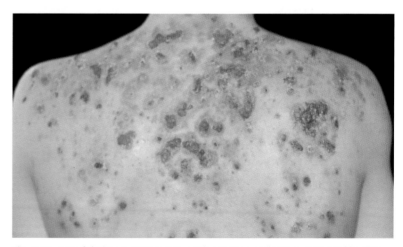

Fig. 5.19 Acne fulminans. Severe acne with erosions and ulcers. Patients like this should be referred urgently to a dermatologist. This patient needed treatment with corticosteroids as well as isotretinoin.

SUMMARY OF TREATMENT OF ACNE VULGARIS

	COMEDONAL ACNE	INFLAMMATORY ACNE		
		Mild	Moderate	Severe
Lesions	Comedones only	Comedones, papules & pustules	Papules & pustules	Nodules & cysts
First Choice	Topical retinoid e.g. adapalene isotretinoin tretinoin	Topical retinoid plus topical antibiotic	Long-term tetracycline plus topical retinoid	Oral isotretinoin
Alternatives	Azelaic acid Benzoyl peroxide	Benzoyl peroxide plus topical antibiotic Azelaic acid	Other antibiotic e.g. doxycycline, erythromycin lymecycline, minocycline	High-dose oral antibiotic plus topical retinoid
Female alternative	As above	As above	Oral anti-androgen plus topical retinoid	Oral isotretinoin plus oral contraceptive
Maintenance	Topical retinoid or benzoyl peroxide			

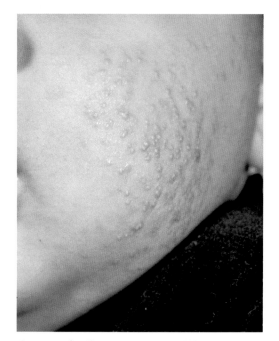

Fig. 5.20 Infantile acne in a 1-year-old boy.

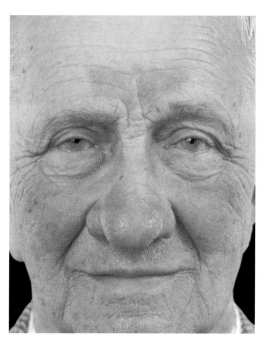

Fig. 5.21 Rosacea. Red patches on cheeks, nose and forehead.

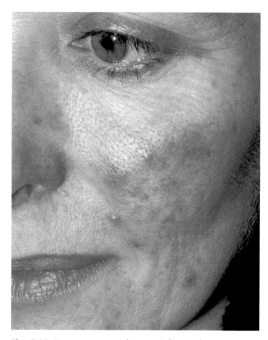

Fig. 5.22 Rosacea – papules, pustules and telangiectasia.

INFANTILE ACNE

Acne is occasionally seen in boys in the first 2 years of life. It is confined to the face, with comedones, papules, pustules and nodules. It gets better spontaneously and is presumably due to maternal androgens. It is not seen in girls.

TREATMENT INFANTILE ACNE

Systemic antibiotics for 4–6 months are usually needed. All forms of tetracycline are contraindicated because they stain developing teeth. Co-trimoxazole paediatric suspension 240mg b.i.d. or erythromycin 125mg b.d. can be used, although the latter needs replacing weekly. If there are only comedones present a keratolytic agent can be used instead (*see* p. 100).

ROSACEA

This is a rash which looks like acne but on a red background. Red patches (erythema and telangiectasia) occur on the cheeks, chin, forehead, and tip of the nose. On top of this there are papules and pustules but no comedones. If the patient is undressed papules and pustules may be seen on the upper trunk as well. Rosacea affects women more commonly than men, and the main incidence is over the age of 40 (although it can occur at any age). Complications, such as sore red eyes (blepharitis, conjunctivitis and keratitis), chronic lymphoedema of the face and rhinophyma occur more commonly in men.

Rosacea needs to be distinguished from acne, seborrhoeic eczema and perioral dermatitis. Acne occurs at a younger age and there should be comedones present. Seborrhoeic eczema is scaly, there are no pustules and the naso-labial folds rather than cheeks are affected; scaling will also be present in the scalp and possibly elsewhere (*see* p. 118). Perioral dermatitis occurs in young adults, is around the mouth only and the individual papules and pustules are very small. Systemic lupus erythematosus may be confused with rosacea because of the redness of the face but there are no papules or pustules and the patient is usually unwell.

TREATMENT ROSACEA

Broad spectrum antibiotics are the mainstay of treatment but how they work is not understood. Oxytetracycline 250mg b.i.d. (on an empty stomach) for 2 months is the cheapest option. One course clears up a third of patients. Another third respond to a second course, while a third may need more long-term therapy. There is no harm in giving oxytetracycline indefinitely if necessary.

Other options include doxycycline 100mg/day, erythromycin 250mg b.i.d., lymecycline 408mg/day, minocycline 100mg/day or metronidazole 200mg t.d.s. If you do not want to use a systemic antibiotic, 0.75% metronidazole gel or cream (*Rozex*UK/*Metrogel*) applied b.i.d. is effective in some instances.

If the main problem is telangiectasia, treatment with a vascular laser is the treatment of choice (*see* p. 54). If flushing is the main problem, try clonidine 25–50µg b.i.d.

RHINOPHYMA

Enlargement of the skin of the nose due to hyperplasia of the sebaceous glands (Fig. 5.24) can occur in individuals with rosacea. Contrary to popular belief it is not associated with excessive alcohol intake.

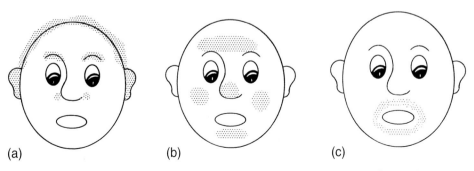

(a)   (b)   (c)

Fig. 5.23 Distribution of rash in (a) seborrhoeic eczema, (b) rosacea, (c) perioral dermatitis.

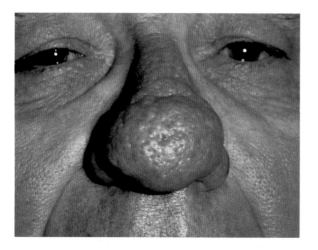

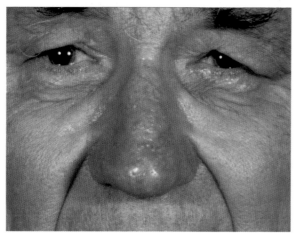

Fig. 5.24 & 5.25 Rhinophyma in a 68-year-old man before (above) and after (below) the excess tissue had been shaved off.

TREATMENT RHINOPHYMA

First treat any active rosacea. The excess sebaceous tissue can then be shaved off under a local or general anaesthetic using a suitable electrocautery machine or a carbon dioxide laser. Provided the shave is no deeper than the base of the sebaceous glands, complete healing without scarring occurs in 4 weeks.

TREATMENT STEROID ROSACEA

The topical steroids must be stopped or the rash will not get better. Usually when the steroids are stopped the rash gets very much worse. You will need to warn the patient about this and it is a good idea to see her 3 days later for reassurance or she may be tempted to restart the topical steroid.

The resolution of the rash can be speeded up by taking oxytetracycline 250mg twice a day for 6 weeks. If the patient wants to use a topical preparation for dry skin or itching prescribe a moisturiser such as Aqueous cream which can be used as often as she likes.

STEROID ROSACEA

Application of potent topical fluorinated steroids to the face can result in a rosacea-like rash. Telangiectasia is the most obvious feature although small papules and pustules may also be present.

SYCOSIS BARBAE

This is folliculitis of the beard area caused by infection with *Staph. aureus*. Shaving results in spread and innoculation of the bacteria over the beard area. The organism is often cultured from the nose as well as the infected follicles. It occurs only in men who shave, and presents with follicular papules and pustules in the beard area.

PSEUDO-SYCOSIS BARBAE

This is a condition due to ingrowing hairs in the beard area. It occurs in men with tight curly hair. The inflammatory papules and pustules are due to a foreign body reaction to the ingrowing hairs.

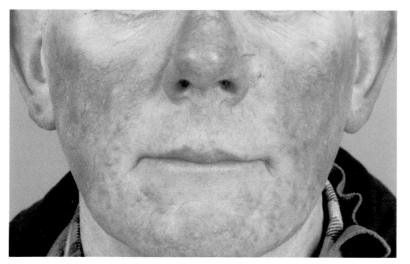

Fig. 5.26 Steroid rosacea with telangiectasia and papules involving cheeks and chin.

TREATMENT SYCOSIS BARBAE

Take swabs for bacteriology culture from a pustule and from the anterior nares before starting treatment. Start with flucloxacillin 250mg q.d.s. orally for 7 days. If staphylococci are grown from the nose apply topical mupirocin (*Bactroban*) q.d.s. for 2 weeks. Recurrent infection may require long-term antibiotics for 6 months or more with erythromycin 250mg b.i.d. or co-trimoxazole 480–960mg b.i.d.

TREATMENT PSEUDO-SYCOSIS BARBAE

This is not an infection, so antibiotics are not needed. If the patient will grow a beard or put up with a short stubble by shaving less closely, the hairs will uncurl as they get longer and the problem will be solved. The only other alternative is to persuade a partner to uncurl the in-growing hairs with a needle each day which is both time consuming and tedious.

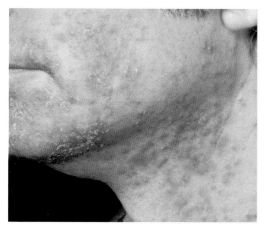

Fig. 5.27 Sycosis barbae. Follicular papules involving neck, cheeks and chin.

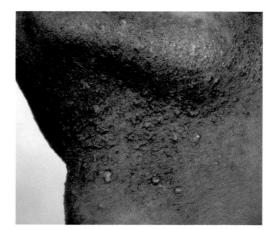

Fig. 5.28 Pseudo-sycosis barbae.

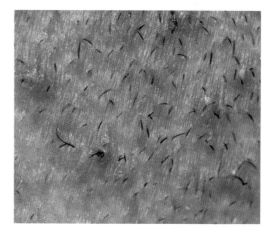

Fig. 5.29 Pseudo-sycosis barbae. Close up showing tight hairs curling back into the skin.

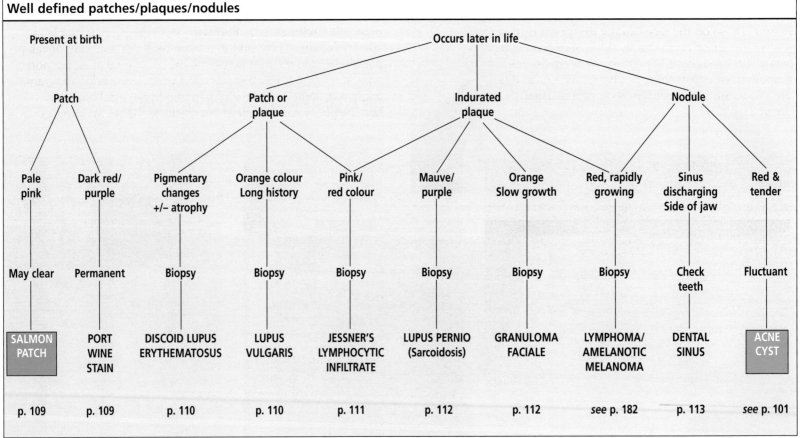

Face
Chronic erythematous rash
Normal surface
Well defined patches/plaques/nodules

Present at birth

Occurs later in life

Patch

Patch or plaque

Indurated plaque

Nodule

Pale pink	Dark red/ purple	Pigmentary changes +/– atrophy	Orange colour Long history	Pink/ red colour	Mauve/ purple	Orange Slow growth	Red, rapidly growing	Sinus discharging Side of jaw	Red & tender
May clear	Permanent	Biopsy	Biopsy	Biopsy	Biopsy	Biopsy	Biopsy	Check teeth	Fluctuant
SALMON PATCH	PORT WINE STAIN	DISCOID LUPUS ERYTHEMATOSUS	LUPUS VULGARIS	JESSNER'S LYMPHOCYTIC INFILTRATE	LUPUS PERNIO (Sarcoidosis)	GRANULOMA FACIALE	LYMPHOMA/ AMELANOTIC MELANOMA	DENTAL SINUS	ACNE CYST
p. 109	p. 109	p. 110	p. 110	p. 111	p. 112	p. 112	*see* p. 182	p. 113	*see* p. 101

SALMON PATCH (Naevus flammeus)

This is a pale pink patch present from birth, situated on the nape of the neck, forehead or eyelid. Pressure over the area will cause blanching, showing that it is due to dilated blood vessels. Those on the face usually disappear during the first year of life; those on the nape of the neck do not, usually persisting throughout life. Often the occipital patch is not noticed unless there has been hair loss at this site. No treatment is needed because it is usually covered by hair.

PORT WINE STAIN

A permanent, more obvious and cosmetically disfiguring birth mark, being darker in colour than a salmon patch. It is present at birth and is usually unilateral. It increases in size only in proportion with growth. Port wine stains are very variable in size and colour. They tend to darken with age and may develop papules within them. If involving the trigeminal area, the port wine stain may rarely be associated with ocular and intracranial angiomas, sometimes resulting in blindness, focal epilepsy, hemiplegia or mental retardation (Sturge–Weber syndrome).

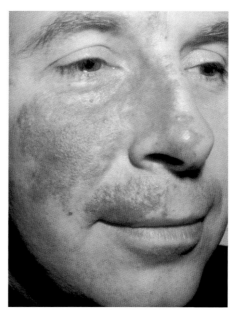

Fig. 5.31 Port wine stain before pulse dye laser treatment.

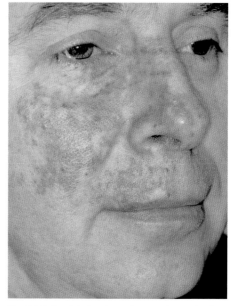

Fig. 5.32 Partial clearing of port wine stain after 15 pulse dye laser treatments.

Fig. 5.30 Salmon patch on occiput – visible due to alopecia.

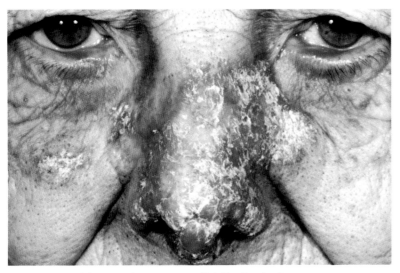

Fig. 5.33 Discoid lupus erythematosus. Well defined scaly plaques.

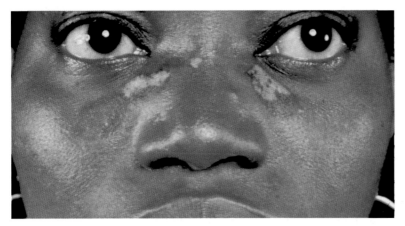

Fig. 5.34 Discoid lupus erythematosus with both hypo- and hyper-pigmentation.

TREATMENT PORT WINE STAIN

The pulse dye laser is the treatment of choice although results are variable. Only 10% of patients get complete clearance. The majority respond but do not totally clear (*see* Figs 5.31 & 5.32). Recurrence can occur later. Treatment is painful so children will need a general anaesthetic. If laser treatment is not successful or possible, then cosmetic camouflage can be used to hide the mark.

DISCOID LUPUS ERYTHEMATOSUS (DLE)

This is a benign form of lupus erythematosus where the skin is involved usually without any systemic involvement (although 5% of patients have autoantibodies). Females are more commonly affected than males and it usually starts between the ages of 25 and 40 years. Well defined red scaly plaques occur on the face and scalp. The scale is quite different from that occurring in psoriasis or eczema. Scratching with the fingernail does not produce silver scaling as in psoriasis and the scale is rougher and more adherent than that of eczema. There may also be follicular plugging, atrophy and a change in pigment (both hypo- and hyper-pigmentation). It is exacerbated by sunlight, so often starts or worsens in the summer. The diagnosis should only be considered when more common causes of scaling on the face are excluded. On occasions indurated non-scaly plaques are seen and the diagnosis will need to be confirmed by skin biopsy.

LUPUS VULGARIS

This is a chronic tuberculous infection of the skin. A slowly enlarging orangy-pink plaque is typical. Nowadays it is exceedingly rare but is a diagnosis that still needs to be considered. Confirm the diagnosis by biopsy.

TREATMENT LUPUS ERYTHEMATOSUS

This is the only condition where a very potent[UK]/group 1[USA] topical steroid can be used on the face. 0.05% clobetasol propionate (*Dermovate*[UK], *Temovate*[USA]) ointment should be applied carefully to the plaques twice daily until they disappear. Only use while there are active lesions present (the plaques are red and scaly). It will not help atrophy or pigment change.

DLE is also made worse by sunlight, so use a sunscreen (SPF 30+) in the summer.

If topical steroids do not help or if there are extensive lesions, use an antimalarial by mouth instead. Try hydroxychloroquine 200mg b.d. or mepacrine 100mg b.i.d. for at least 3 months. Mepacrine makes the patient's skin and urine yellow and can also cause vomiting or diarrhoea. The patient should be warned about these.

Hydroxychloroquine can affect the retina so check the visual acuity and fields yearly. The nails may be stained a greyish-blue colour.

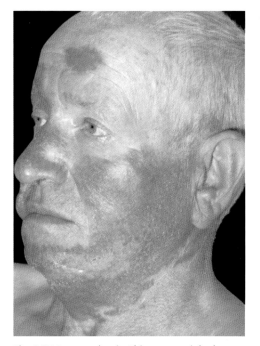

Fig. 5.35 Lupus vulgaris. This orangy-pink plaque had been present for 50 years, gradually extending. It had been assumed to be a birth mark.

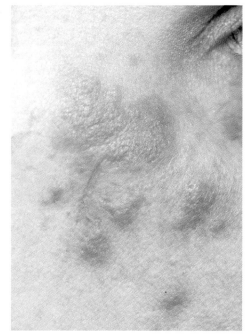

Fig. 5.36 Jessner's lymphocytic infiltrate. Fixed plaques on the cheek.

TREATMENT LUPUS VULGARIS

Triple therapy as for pulmonary tuberculosis: isoniazid 300mg/day single dose, rifampicin 600mg/day single dose and pyrazinamide 20mg/kg body weight 3–4 times a day or ethambutol 15mg/kg weight as single dose. After two months two drugs can be used for the next 4 months, usually isoniazid and rifampicin.

JESSNER'S LYMPHOCYTIC INFILTRATE

Fixed red indurated plaque(s) with a smooth non-scaly surface is scattered over the face or trunk. Individual lesions are round, oval or serpiginous in outline. The diagnosis can be confirmed by taking a skin biopsy which shows a dense perivascular lymphocytic infiltrate in the dermis. A biopsy will distinguish this condition from discoid lupus erythematosus and a lymphoma. It tends to be unresponsive to treatment but antimalarials (*see* DLE) can be tried.

SARCOIDOSIS (Lupus pernio)

Around a quarter of patients with sarcoid have skin involvement. Sarcoid of the skin can present with macules, papules, patches and plaques. They can be red, orange or purple in colour. On the face the commonest appearance is of a mauve/purple plaque (lupus pernio) on the nose or cheek. Sarcoid seems to be commoner in Negroes.

TREATMENT SARCOIDOSIS

Refer the patient to a dermatologist to confirm the diagnosis and to look for sarcoid elsewhere. For multi-system disease the patient will need systemic steroids; this will also improve the skin lesions. Alternatives are methotrexate (10–25mg/week), azathioprine (100–150mg/day), hydroxychloroquine (200mg b.i.d.) or acetretin (25mg/day). If there is only lupus pernio, inject triamcinalone (5 mg/ml) intradermally every 4–6 weeks. Err on the side of caution because steroid-induced atrophy of the skin may be unsightly and permanent.

GRANULOMA FACIALE

A nodule or indurated plaque with an orange colour and prominent follicular openings. Histologically both a granuloma and a vasculitis are present. The lesion tends to be chronic.

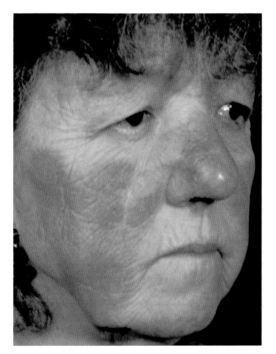

Fig. 5.37 Lupus pernio. Purple plaques on the cheek.

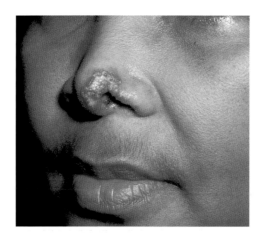

Fig. 5.38 Lupus pernio in black skin.

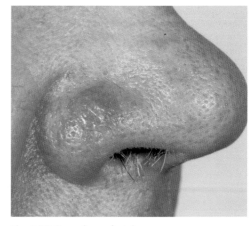

Fig. 5.39 Granuloma faciale.

DENTAL SINUS

This is due to a tooth abscess which discharges through the the skin on the cheek, chin or under the jaw. It presents as a nodule or a discharging sinus. The diagnosis can be confirmed by looking in the mouth where a rotten tooth is usually seen. The offending tooth should be removed.

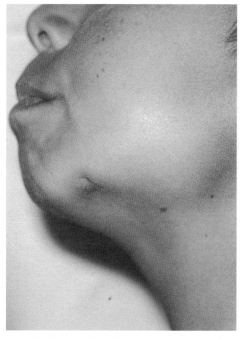

Fig. 5.40 Dental sinus discharging through skin.

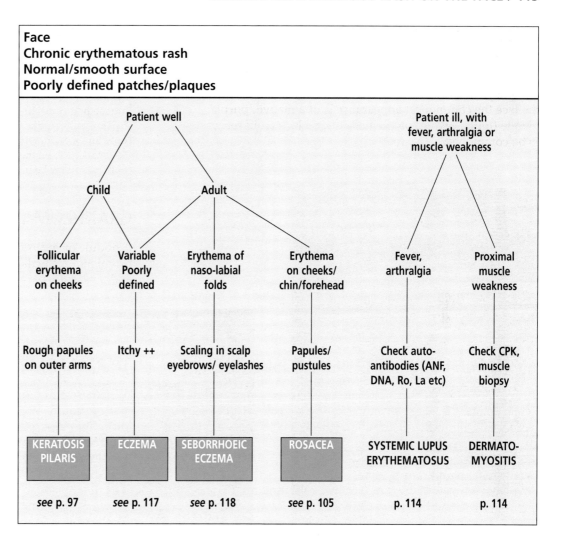

Face
Chronic erythematous rash
Normal/smooth surface
Poorly defined patches/plaques

Patient well

Patient ill, with fever, arthralgia or muscle weakness

Child — Adult

Follicular erythema on cheeks → Rough papules on outer arms → **KERATOSIS PILARIS** — *see p. 97*

Variable Poorly defined → Itchy ++ → **ECZEMA** — *see p. 117*

Erythema of naso-labial folds → Scaling in scalp eyebrows/ eyelashes → **SEBORRHOEIC ECZEMA** — *see p. 118*

Erythema on cheeks/ chin/forehead → Papules/ pustules → **ROSACEA** — *see p. 105*

Fever, arthralgia → Check auto-antibodies (ANF, DNA, Ro, La etc) → **SYSTEMIC LUPUS ERYTHEMATOSUS** — p. 114

Proximal muscle weakness → Check CPK, muscle biopsy → **DERMATO-MYOSITIS** — p. 114

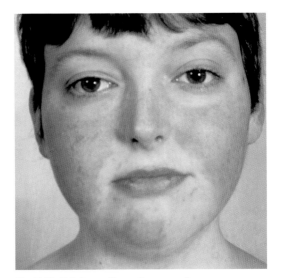

Fig. 5.41 SLE. Butterfly erythema on face.

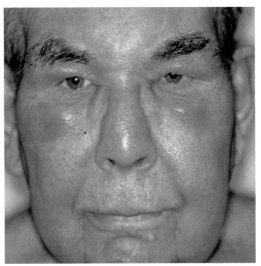

Fig. 5.42 Dermatomyositis. Marked oedema around the eyes.

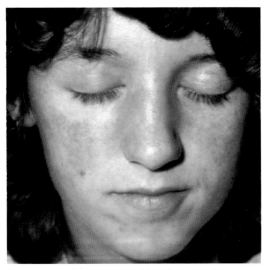

Fig. 5.43 Dermatomyositis. Note involvement of the upper eyelids.

SYSTEMIC LUPUS ERYTHEMATOSUS (SLE)

An erythema on the face associated with fever and arthralgia in a female patient is suggestive of SLE. The rash characteristically occurs in a 'butterfly' distribution (cheeks and bridge of nose), but does not always do so. There is also nail fold telangiectasia with ragged cuticles. Although the site may be similar to rosacea, there are no papules or pustules. The patient may have renal involvement, psychiatric or neurological symptoms, pericarditis, pleurisy or abdominal pain. Chilblains and Raynaud's phenomenon are likely. A positive anti-nuclear factor will confirm the diagnosis. An illness identical to SLE can be caused by procainamide, hydralazine and minocycline.

DERMATOMYOSITIS

Weakness and tenderness of proximal muscles associated with a mauve or pink rash on the face, 'V' of the neck or in lines along the backs of the fingers and over the metacarpal bones (Fig. 5.45) is typical. There may be considerable oedema on the face and arms (Fig. 5.42) and dilatation of the nail fold capillaries (Fig. 5.44). The diagnosis can be confirmed by measuring muscle enzymes (creatine phosphokinase), muscle biopsy or electromyography. In patients over the age of 40 there may be an associated internal malignancy.

TREATMENT SYSTEMIC LUPUS ERYTHEMATOSUS

Referral to a specialist (rheumatologist, physician or dermatologist) with an interest in this condition is necessary. Treatment depends on which organs are involved. Severe disease involving the kidneys, pleura, pericardium, CNS, or blood require high doses of systemic steroids, e.g. prednisolone 60mg/day.

The skin should be protected from the sun by using a high factor sunscreen (SPF 15 or above). A very potent[UK]/group 1[USA] topical steroid ointment or cream applied twice a day can be very helpful in getting rid of the rash.

If the joints are the main problem, non-steroidal anti-inflammatory drugs will be the treatment of choice. If it is only the skin and joints involved, hydroxychloroquine 200mg b.i.d. or mepacrine 100mg b.i.d. can be used.

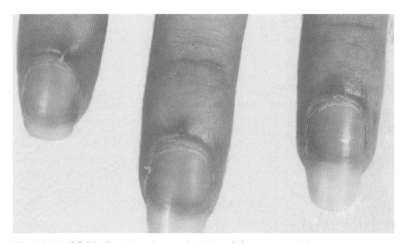

Fig. 5.44 Nail fold telangiectasia seen in SLE and dermatomyositis.

TREATMENT DERMATOMYOSITIS

Refer urgently to a dermatologist for diagnosis and treatment. A search for an internal malignancy is essential (especially Ca lung, stomach, ovary or breast); if found and treated successfully, the dermatomyositis will disappear. If the cancer is not curable it may be very difficult to control the dermatomyositis.

Initial treatment is with prednisolone 60mg/day. This is gradually reduced as the disease comes under control. Steroid sparing agents such as azathioprine or methotrexate may also be needed. Patients not responding to these may require high dose intravenous immunoglobulin as well.

Muscle enzyme levels can be used to monitor disease activity. In the acute phase rest is important; later passive muscle exercises and physiotherapy will be needed.

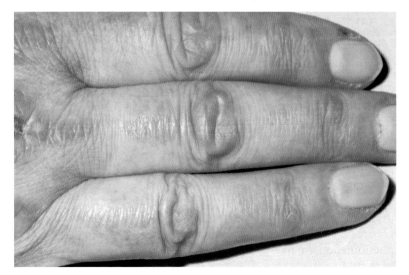

Fig. 5.45 Dermatomyositis. Linear mauve plaques along the back of the fingers.

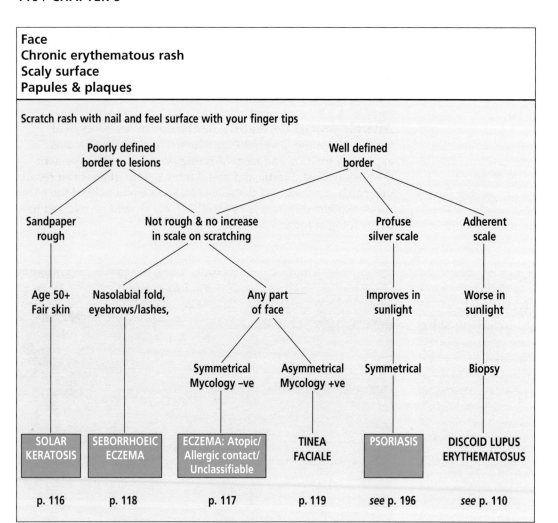

Face
Chronic erythematous rash
Scaly surface
Papules & plaques

Scratch rash with nail and feel surface with your finger tips

Poorly defined
border to lesions

Well defined
border

Sandpaper
rough

Not rough & no increase
in scale on scratching

Profuse
silver scale

Adherent
scale

Age 50+
Fair skin

Nasolabial fold,
eyebrows/lashes,

Any part
of face

Improves in
sunlight

Worse in
sunlight

Symmetrical
Mycology –ve

Asymmetrical
Mycology +ve

Symmetrical

Biopsy

SOLAR KERATOSIS	SEBORRHOEIC ECZEMA	ECZEMA: Atopic/ Allergic contact/ Unclassifiable	TINEA FACIALE	PSORIASIS	DISCOID LUPUS ERYTHEMATOSUS
p. 116	p. 118	p. 117	p. 119	*see* p. 196	*see* p. 110

SOLAR KERATOSES

Widespread solar keratoses may be confused with eczema on the face, but will feel rough to the touch. The patient will probably be over 50, have fair skin (burn rather than tan on sun exposure) and blue eyes.

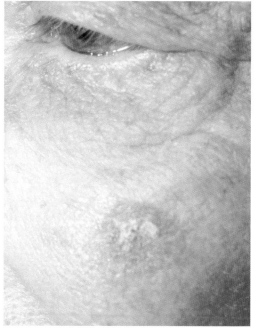

Fig. 5.46 Solar keratosis on the cheek.

Often there will be a history of working out of doors or living abroad (20+ years ago). Solar elastosis (*see* p. 251) will be present. This is a yellowish discolouration of the skin with increased skin markings and follicular openings on the face, neck and back of the neck. These 'wrinkles' are not due to ageing *per se* but to prolonged sun damage.

ECZEMA ON THE FACE

The most likely cause of poorly defined scaly plaques on the face is chronic eczema. The distribution of the plaques and age of the patient determine the type of eczema.

Atopic eczema Eczema on the face in infants and children is likely to be due to atopic eczema. In infants it often starts on the cheeks and scalp before affecting the rest of the body especially the antecubital and popliteal fossae. Atopic eczema persisting into adult life is often lichenified.

Allergic contact dermatitis may be due to cosmetics, nail varnish (from the fingernails touching the face skin), creams applied to the face and from airborne allergens such as cement dust or sawdust. Plastic and metal frames from glasses can result in a patch of eczema on the sides of the nose and behind the ears. All unexplained instances of facial eczema should be referred to a dermatologist for patch testing.

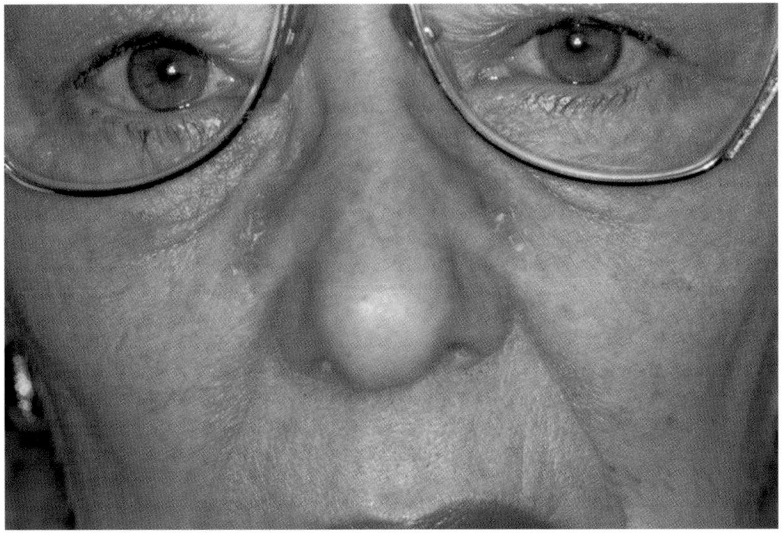

Fig. 5.47 Allergic contact dermatitis on the side of the nose from spectacle frames.

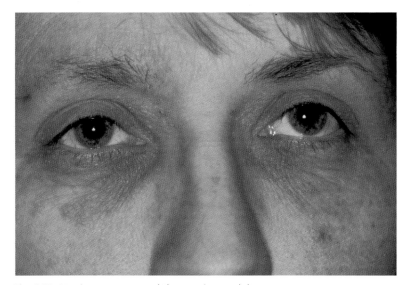

Fig. 5.48 Atopic eczema around the eyes in an adult.

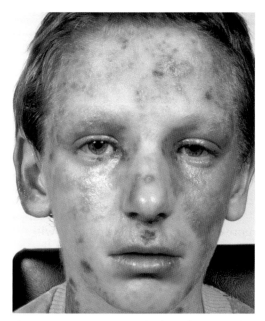

Fig. 5.49 Atopic eczema on the face of a 9-year-old boy.

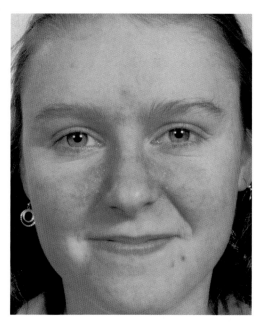

Fig. 5.50 Seborrhoeic eczema affecting the nasolabial folds.

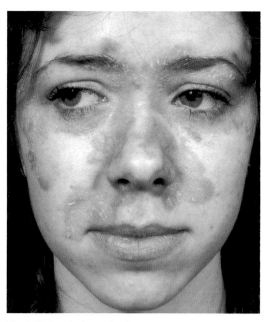

Fig. 5.51 Psoriasis on the face.

TREATMENT ECZEMA ON FACE

On the face use only a weak[UK]/group 7[USA] topical steroid such as 1% hydrocortisone. Use an ointment if the skin is particularly dry or an allergic contact dermatitis is suspected (creams can contain preservatives which are potential sensitizers). In addition instead of soap use a light moisturiser such as Aqueous cream[UK] or hydrophilic ointment[USA]. Tacrolimus 0.1% ointment is an alternative in atopic eczema (*see* p. 29).

SEBORRHOEIC ECZEMA

In adults this common type of eczema is due to an overgrowth of the yeast *Pityrosporum ovale*. It is diagnosed by its distribution on the skin – scalp, eyebrows, eyelashes, nasolabial folds, external ear, centre of chest and centre of back (*see also* p. 211).

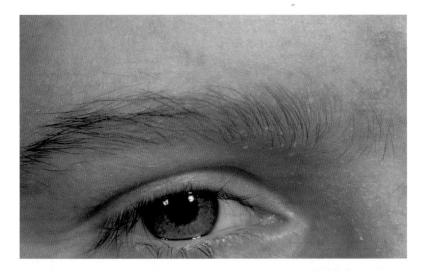

TREATMENT SEBORRHOEIC ECZEMA

Only treat it when it is present. Start with 2% ketoconazole (*Nizoral*) cream twice a day until it is clear. This will reduce the pityrosporum yeasts.

If it does not work use 1% hydrocortisone cream b.i.d. or 2% miconazole plus 1% hydrocortisone cream (*Daktacort*). Treat the scalp with ketoconazole shampoo (*see* p. 74).

TINEA

Although frequently diagnosed in general practice, ringworm is uncommon on the face. It should be suspected if a red scaly rash is unilateral or very much more on one side than the other. It will have a well demarcated edge with relatively normal skin in the centre. It is often itchy and slowly gets bigger. The border needs to be scraped and the scale sent off for mycology (*see* p. 19).

TREATMENT TINEA

Apply either terbinafine (*Lamasil*) cream once daily for 7–10 days or an imidazole cream twice a day for 2 weeks. All the imidazoles work equally well (<u>clotrimazole</u>, <u>econazole</u>, <u>ketoconazole</u>, <u>miconazole</u> and <u>sulconazole</u>*).

Whitfield's ointment is a cheaper alternative. Apply twice a day until the rash has gone and then for a further 2 weeks. Systemic antifungals are not needed.

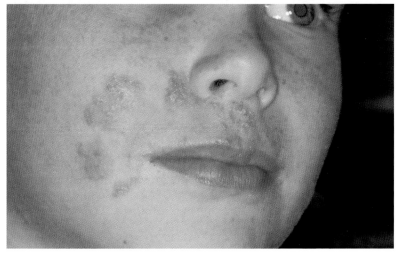

Fig. 5.52 (above left) Seborrhoeic eczema involving the eyebrows and eyelashes.

Fig. 5.53 (below left) Tinea around the mouth in a young boy.

*<u>*Drug names</u> which are underlined are those prescribable in the UK by specialist nurse practitioners.

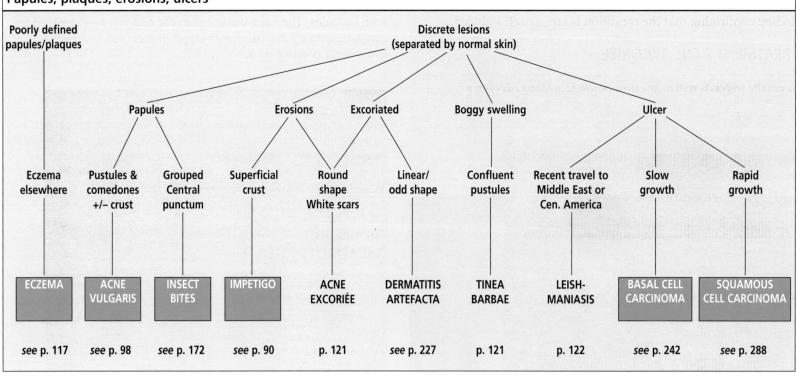

Face
Chronic erythematous rash
Crust, excoriated or eroded surface
Papules, plaques, erosions, ulcers

Poorly defined papules/plaques

Discrete lesions (separated by normal skin)

Papules — Erosions — Excoriated — Boggy swelling — Ulcer

Eczema elsewhere — Pustules & comedones +/– crust — Grouped Central punctum — Superficial crust — Round shape White scars — Linear/ odd shape — Confluent pustules — Recent travel to Middle East or Cen. America — Slow growth — Rapid growth

ECZEMA — ACNE VULGARIS — INSECT BITES — IMPETIGO — ACNE EXCORIÉE — DERMATITIS ARTEFACTA — TINEA BARBAE — LEISH-MANIASIS — BASAL CELL CARCINOMA — SQUAMOUS CELL CARCINOMA

see p. 117 — see p. 98 — see p. 172 — see p. 90 — p. 121 — see p. 227 — p. 121 — p. 122 — see p. 242 — see p. 288

ACNE EXCORIÉE

This variety of acne occurs predominantly in women over the age of 30. The acne is usually mild but most of the lesions are excoriated. Round or oval white scars are the most obvious finding confirming that the condition is largely self induced.

TREATMENT ACNE EXCORIÉE

It usually responds well to low dose isotretinoin (20mg/day) on a long-term basis (*see* p. 41). Adequate contraception is essential if this is going to be used.

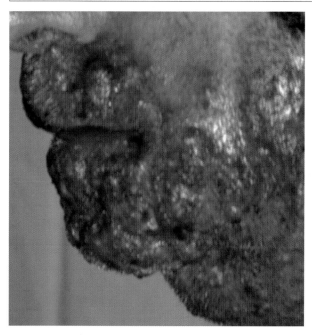

Fig. 5.54 Tinea barbae.

TINEA BARBAE

An uncommon infection of the beard area due to an animal ringworm (usually *Trichophyton verrucosum* from calves). It usually occurs in farm workers. A confluent boggy swelling is studded with pustules. The hairs come out easily and can be examined for fungi. Secondary infection with staphylococci can produce a misleading positive bacterial culture.

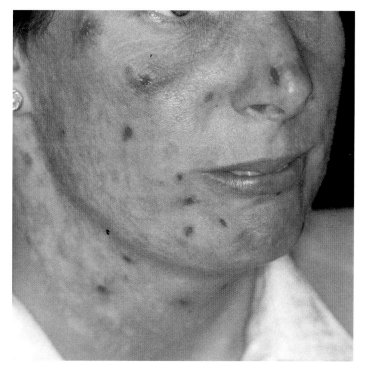

Fig. 5.55 Acne excoriée showing all the lesions excoriated, no comedones and white circular scars.

TREATMENT TINEA BARBAE

Griseofulvin 0.5–1g daily is given as a single oral dose with food for
4–6 weeks. *See* p. 39 for side effects.

LEISHMANIASIS

Leishmaniasis results from the bite of an infected sandfly. It
is a common disease around the Mediterranean, in the Middle
East, North Africa, India and Pakistan. A few weeks after the
sandfly bite, a boil-like nodule appears at the site of the bite. It
gradually flattens off to form a plaque which may or may not
ulcerate. One or more lesions appear on exposed sites – face,
arms and legs. They are painless and heal spontaneously after
about 1 year to leave a cribriform scar. In Central and South
America a much more destructive picture is seen with
ulcerated nodules, and later systemic spread to mucous
membranes (muco-cutaneous leishmaniasis).

TREATMENT LEISHMANIASIS

1. Leave alone to heal spontaneously.
2. Weekly intralesional injection with sodium stibogluconate (*Pentostam*)
   or n-methylglucamine antimonate (*Glucantime*) until healed.
3. Intravenous (through a peripherally inserted central catheter –
   PICC line) sodium stibogluconate at a daily dose of 20mg/kg
   body weight for 20 days. This is particularly recommended for
   New World leishmaniasis.

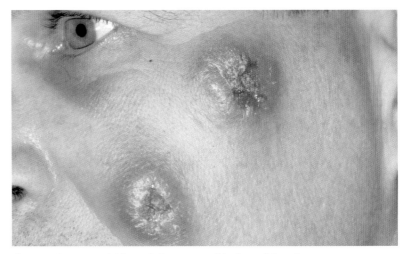

Fig. 5.56 Cutaneous leishmaniasis contracted in Central America.

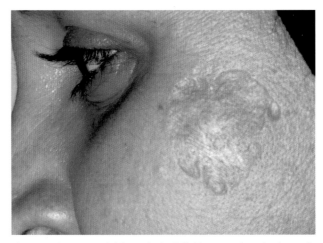

Fig. 5.57 Cutaneous leishmaniasis. Cribriform scar on the face of
an Iranian lady.

Mouth, tongue, lips and ears

6

Mouth

Tongue

Lips

Ears

LESIONS AFFECTING THE MOUTH & TONGUE

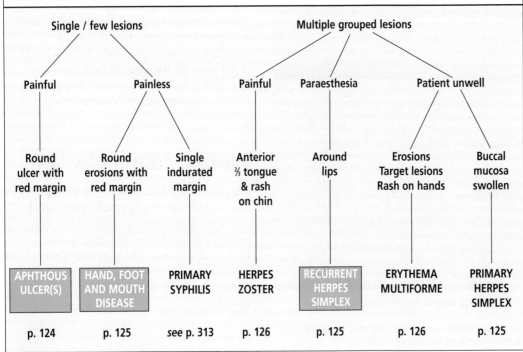

Mouth, tongue, lips
Acute lesions (<2 weeks duration)
Ulcers and erosions

APHTHOUS ULCERS

These are the commonest cause of recurrent mouth ulcers. Single or multiple small round ulcers with a red margin last 7–10 days before healing spontaneously. They begin in teenagers and may continue throughout life. Rarely they are associated with Crohn's disease, ulcerative colitis or coeliac disease.

TREATMENT APHTHOUS ULCERS

This is a self limiting condition which often needs no treatment. Most patients will use things like *Bonjela* (choline salicylate & cetalkonium chloride) for symptomatic relief. For more troublesome ulcers consider one of the following:–

1. 2% sodium cromoglycate spray (*Rynacrom*) sprayed directly onto the ulcers three times a day. About 50% of patients find this extremely helpful. It is not known how it works.

2. Tetracycline mouthwash, 250mg/5ml, held in the mouth and swished around for about five minutes 4–5 times a day. Do not use in children under 12 since it stains teeth.

3. 0.1% triamcinolone acetonide (*Adcortyl*) in orobase applied to the ulcers t.d.s.

4. Beclomethasone dipropionate, 50μg/puff (*Becotide 50*), can be sprayed on the ulcers several times a day until they heal.

5. 10% hydrocortisone in equal parts of glycerine and water as a mouthwash three times a day. The patient must spit it out after use rather than swallow it, to make sure that not too much steroid is absorbed.

6. 2.5% hydrocortisone sodium succinate (*Corlan*) pellet, held against the ulcer(s) until the pellet dissolves, twice daily.

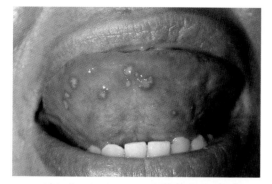

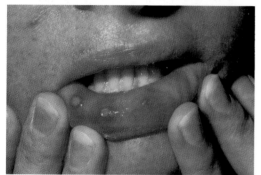

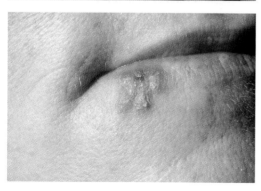

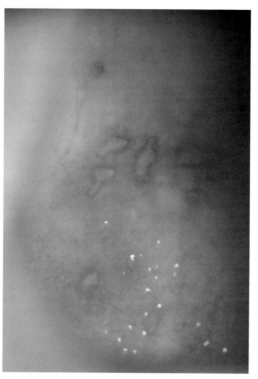

Fig. 6.01 (top left) Aphthous ulcers on tongue.

Fig. 6.02 (middle left) Hand, foot and mouth disease. Blisters and erosions on the lower lip.

Fig. 6.03 (bottom left) Recurrent herpes simplex.

Fig. 6.04 (above) Primary herpes simplex. Erosions on the hard palate.

HAND, FOOT & MOUTH DISEASE

This mild infection is due to a Coxsackie A16 virus. Round erosions with a red margin are seen in the mouth. They look like small aphthous ulcers but are associated with small grey blisters with a red halo on the fingers and toes (*see* Fig. 13.02, p. 361). The condition gets better spontaneously in a few days.

PRIMARY HERPES SIMPLEX

Most primary infections with the herpes simplex virus occur in early childhood and are asymptomatic with only a few vesicles/erosions on the hard palate or buccal mucosa. Occasionally they may cause an acute gingivostomatitis associated with fever and general malaise.

RECURRENT HERPES SIMPLEX

Recurrent herpes simplex is usually preceded by prodromal itching, burning or tingling on the lips. Small grouped vesicles appear, burst, crust and then heal in 7–10 days (*see also* p. 91).

HERPES ZOSTER

Herpes zoster involving the mandibular branch of the 5th cranial nerve is uncommon, but presents with unilateral vesicles and ulceration on the anterior two-thirds of the tongue as well as the characteristic vesicles on the same side of the chin (*see also* p. 157).

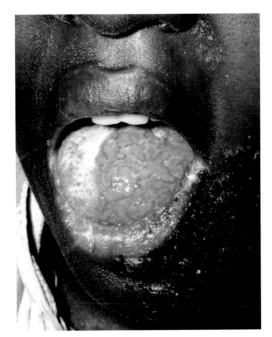

Fig. 6.05 Herpes zoster affecting the mandibular branch of 5th cranial nerve. Blisters and ulceration on anterior ⅔ of the tongue and a rash on the side of the chin.

STEVENS–JOHNSON SYNDROME

Erythema multiforme involving the mouth presents with multiple irregular erosions on the buccal mucosa. Extensive involvement of the mouth, lips, conjunctiva and genitalia is called Stevens–Johnson syndrome. The causes of this are the same as for erythema multiforme (*see* p. 153) but usually drugs (often co-trimoxazole) rather than infections are the cause.

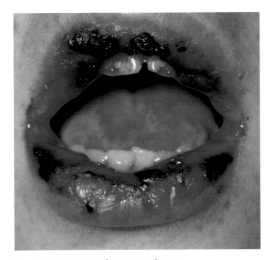

Fig. 6.06 Stevens–Johnson syndrome.

TREATMENT STEVENS–JOHNSON

Many of these patients will need to be admitted to hospital because they are unable to eat or drink. Frequent mouth washes with glycerine and thymol (made up by dissolving a glycerine and thymol tablet in a tumbler of water) should be swished around the mouth for several minutes every hour, or applied on a cotton wool swab by a nurse if the patient cannot manage a mouth wash by himself. This will keep the buccal mucosa relatively comfortable. If this is not done, the lips can stick together, which initially will make eating and drinking even more difficult, and will at some stage necessitate surgical separation. Benzydamine hydrochloride (*Difflam*) or chlorhexidine gluconate (*Corsodyl*) are alternative mouthwashes.

Frequent bathing of the eyes with normal saline and insertion of hypromellose eye drops (artificial tears) will be needed to keep them comfortable. If there are extensive skin lesions as well as extensive mucosal involvement, the patient may need nursing in a burns unit where there are facilities to prevent ulceration of the skin.

There is no evidence that systemic steroids are helpful.

Mouth ulcers and erosions
Chronic lesions (> 2 weeks duration)

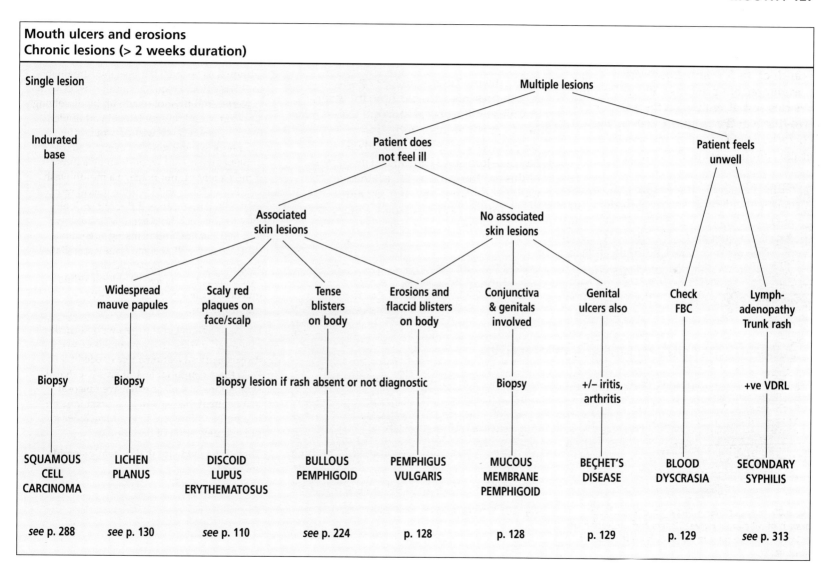

PEMPHIGUS VULGARIS

Blisters and erosions in the mouth are usually the first sign of pemphigus vulgaris; the rash often comes later (*see* p. 225).

MUCOUS MEMBRANE PEMPHIGOID

This is a rare auto-immune disease in which there are antibodies against the epidermal basement membrane. Mucous membranes (mouth, eyes and genitalia) are predominantly involved with blisters, erosions and scarring. Blisters can also occur on the skin adjacent to orifices. The diagnosis is usually made by looking in the eyes. Scarring and adhesions between the palpebral conjuctivae are characteristic, and can lead to blindness if not treated. **Bullous pemphigoid** less commonly involves the mucous membranes. The diagnosis is made by the characteristic skin rash (*see* p. 224).

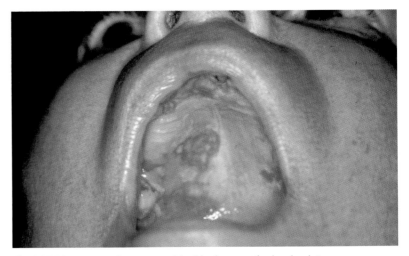

Fig. 6.07 Mucous membrane pemphigoid: ulcers on the hard palate.

TREATMENT MUCOUS MEMBRANE PEMPHIGOID

Unlike bullous pemphigoid mucous membrane pemphigoid does not respond well to systemic steroids. There is no single treatment that always works and it is a question of finding the right drug for any individual patient. Start with dapsone 50mg t.d.s. as this is the safest alterenative. It can cause haemolytic anaemia and/or methaemoglobinaemia so check the FBC after 1 week and every 2–3 months. If this fails to work cyclophosphamide 50mg b.i.d. is more effective but you will need to check the FBC regularly (monthly). A third alternative is azathioprine 50mg t.d.s. If there is scarring of the conjunctivae, it may sometimes be necessary to inject steroids intralesionally to inactivate the disease. All patients with this rare disorder should be under the care of a dermatologist or ophthalmologist.

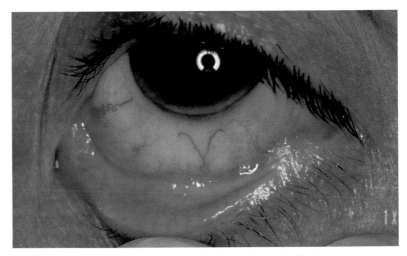

Fig. 6.08 Mucous membrane pemphigoid with conjunctival adhesions.

BEÇHET'S SYNDROME

A rare condition mainly affecting young men. You should think of it in any patient with recurrent oral and genital ulceration. The ulcers tend to be larger, deeper and last longer than aphthous ulcers. There will also be one or more of the following: iritis, arthritis, thrombophlebitis, sterile pustules on the skin, erythema nodosum and meningo-encephalitis. Such patients should be referred to hospital for treatment.

TREATMENT BEÇHET'S SYNDROME

Since the cause is unknown treatment is empirical and often unsatisfactory. The drugs used are:-

- Colchicine 500µg b.i.d.
- Azathioprine 2mg/kg body weight/day (average = 50mg t.d.s.)
- Thalidomide 100mg nocte given 'on a named patient basis'

For the mouth ulcers it is worth the patient trying:–

1. 10% hydrocortisone in equal parts of glycerine and water used as a mouthwash after each meal. The patient should be warned that it has a very bitter taste. It should be spat out so that the steroid is not absorbed.

2. Steroid inhaler. Beclomethasone dipropionate, 50µg/puff (*Becotide 50*), is usually used for asthma, but instead of inhaling it, the patient sprays it on the ulcers several times a day until the ulcers heal.

BLOOD DYSCRASIA

Agranulocytosis and neutropenia can cause mouth ulcers. They may be the first manifestation of leukaemia, or be a side effect of cytotoxic drugs such as methotrexate.

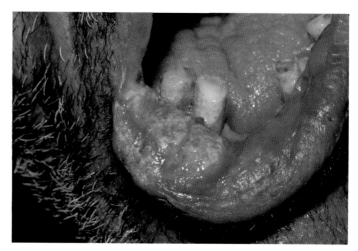

Fig. 6.09 Squamous cell carcinoma of the lower lip.

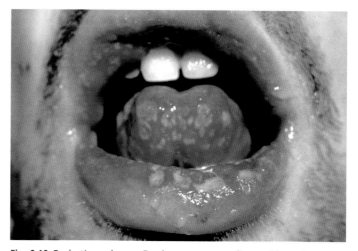

Fig. 6.10 Beçhet's syndrome. Erosions on tongue, lips and buccal mucosa.

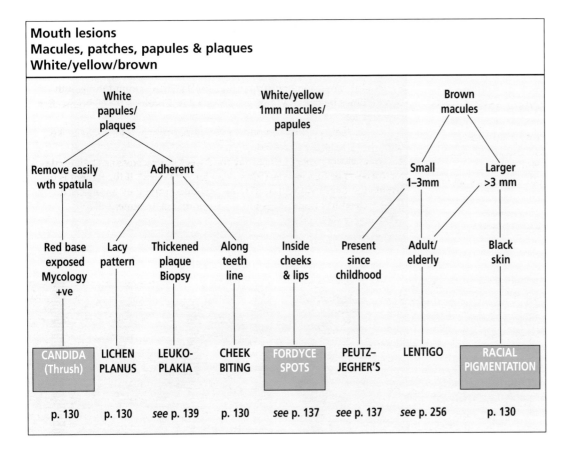

Mouth lesions
Macules, patches, papules & plaques
White/yellow/brown

White papules/ plaques
- Remove easily wth spatula
  - Red base exposed Mycology +ve → **CANDIDA (Thrush)** — p. 130
  - Lacy pattern → **LICHEN PLANUS** — p. 130
- Adherent
  - Thickened plaque Biopsy → **LEUKO-PLAKIA** — see p. 139
  - Along teeth line → **CHEEK BITING** — p. 130

White/yellow 1mm macules/ papules
- Inside cheeks & lips → **FORDYCE SPOTS** — see p. 137
- Present since childhood → **PEUTZ–JEGHER'S** — see p. 137

Brown macules
- Small 1–3mm
  - Adult/ elderly → **LENTIGO** — see p. 256
- Larger >3 mm
  - Black skin → **RACIAL PIGMENTATION** — p. 130

PIGMENTATION IN THE MOUTH

Melanin pigmentation in the mouth is a normal finding in blacks. If present from childhood multiple small brown macules may be due to Peutz–Jegher's syndrome (*see* p. 137). In later life pigmented macules are likely to be lentigines (*see* p. 256).

LICHEN PLANUS

Lichen planus in the mouth is usually asymptomatic. The diagnosis is made in a patient with the typical rash (*see* p. 171). In the mouth there is a lacy pattern on the buccal mucosa. Rarely there may be erosions and ulceration and the patient will have a sore mouth and find eating painful. The edge of the ulcer is usually white. At the start there may have been the characteristic rash of lichen planus, but ulceration can go on for years, and continue long after the rash is gone. It needs to be distinguished from **cheek biting** where a fold of mucous membrane is seen heaped up along the teeth line.

ORAL CANDIDIASIS

Thrush occurs in the very young, the very old and in patients who are immunosuppressed or who are taking antibiotics or cytotoxic drugs. Small white papules scrape off easily with a spatula to leave a red surface. If these are mixed with potassium hydroxide, the spores and hyphae are easily seen on direct microscopy (*see* p. 305) or can be cultured on Sabouraud's dextrose agar.

TREATMENT ORAL LICHEN PLANUS

Most oral lichen planus is asymptomatic and needs no treatment. Treatment of erosive lichen planus is unsatisfactory. The following can be tried:–

1. Ordinary mouth washes as used for aphthous ulcers (*see* p. 124). If these fail to work some kind of systemic therapy is necessary.
2. Prednisone 15–30mg/day may occasionally be needed for the most severe forms of ulceration. The dose is reduced as soon as the ulceration is healed down to a maintenance dose of 5–10mg/day. You want to get the patient off steroids as soon as possible because otherwise they will end up taking them for years.
3. Rarely one of the oral retinoids may be needed as an alternative to systemic steroids (acetretin, 0.5–1mg/kg body weight/day, *see* p. 41).

TREATMENT ORAL CANDIDIASIS

1. In infancy, miconazole gel applied directly to the plaques by an adult's finger 4 times daily.
2. In adults, nystatin oral suspension (1ml) swirled around the mouth several times before swallowing 4 times a day. Continue for 48 hours after clinical cure.
3. Alternatives are nystatin pastilles or amphoteracin B lozenges sucked until they dissolve 4 times a day.
4. Oral ketoconazole (200mg/day for 2 weeks), itraconazole (100mg/day for 2 weeks) or fluconazole (50mg/day for 7–14 days). If the patient is on antibiotics, treatment will need to be continued until they are finished. If the patient has cancer or is immunosuppressed, treatment may need to be prolonged.

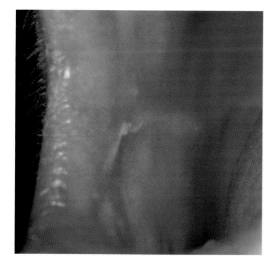

Fig. 6.11 Bite line along the buccal mucosa.

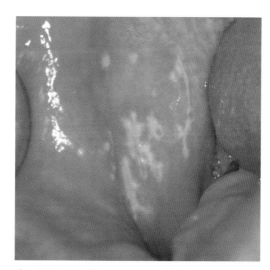

Fig. 6.12 Buccal lichen planus: white lacy pattern.

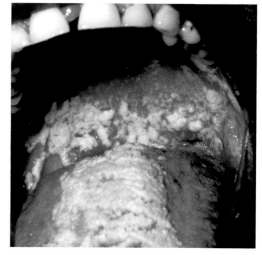

Fig. 6.13 Oral candidiasis.

ABNORMALITIES OF THE TONGUE

ORAL HAIRY LEUKOPLAKIA

A white plaque consisting of multiple papules (looking like hairs) is found along the side of the tongue. It is due to the *Epstein–Barr* virus and is found in patients with HIV infection. It is usually asymptomatic.

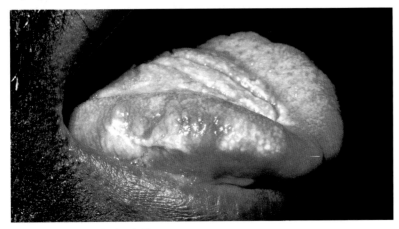

Fig. 6.14 Oral hairy leukoplakia.

LARGE TONGUE (MACROGLOSSIA)

The tongue may be large from birth or from early childhood in individuals with Down's syndrome or with a lymphangioma, haemangioma or neurofibroma of the tongue. Intermittent enlargement of the tongue (lasting <24 hours) is usually due to angio-oedema (*see* p. 83) which is usually associated with urticaria. After middle age, enlargement of the tongue should make you think of systemic amyloid.

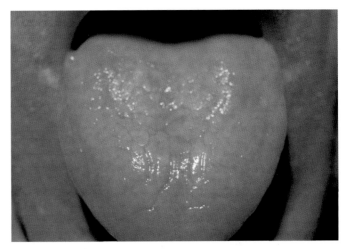

Fig. 6.15 Smooth tongue.

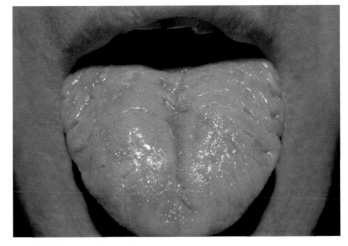

Fig. 6.16 Fissured (scrotal) tongue.

GEOGRAPHIC TONGUE

A very common benign condition where smooth red patches appear on the dorsum of the tongue giving a map-like appearance. These move about from day to day. The condition is generally asymptomatic although its appearance can cause alarm.

FURRED & BLACK HAIRY TONGUE

These common conditions are due to hypertrophy of the filiform papillae, and are completely harmless. They are asymptomatic and not indicative of any internal disease.

TREATMENT GEOGRAPHIC TONGUE

Any soreness can be treated with glycerine and thymol mouthwash. Tell the patient to avoid acidic foods such as vinegar or citrus fruits.

TREATMENT BLACK HAIRY TONGUE

Apply 0.025% tretinoin gel (*Retin-A*) and brush it off with a soft toothbrush 5 minutes later. This is repeated daily until it clears (about 2 weeks).

SMOOTH TONGUE

A smooth tongue may be associated with iron deficiency, malabsorption or pernicious anaemia.

FISSURED TONGUE (SCROTAL TONGUE)

Deep groves in the tongue may be a congenital abnormality or seen together with facial nerve palsy and swelling of the lips in the **Melkersson–Rosenthal syndrome**.

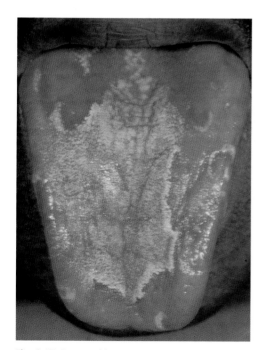

Fig. 6.17 Geographic tongue.

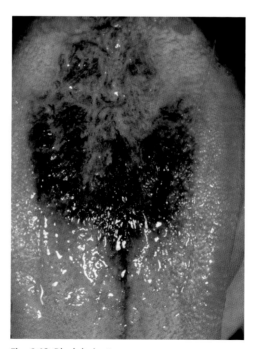

Fig. 6.18 Black hairy tongue.

LIPS

Lips
Surface normal

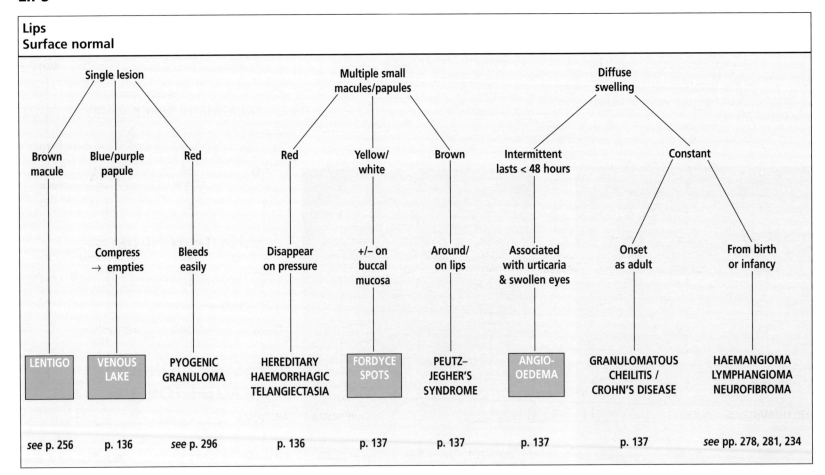

Single lesion → Brown macule → **LENTIGO** — *see p. 256*

Single lesion → Blue/purple papule → Compress → empties → **VENOUS LAKE** — p. 136

Single lesion → Red → Bleeds easily → **PYOGENIC GRANULOMA** — *see p. 296*

Multiple small macules/papules → Red → Disappear on pressure → **HEREDITARY HAEMORRHAGIC TELANGIECTASIA** — p. 136

Multiple small macules/papules → Yellow/white → +/− on buccal mucosa → **FORDYCE SPOTS** — p. 137

Multiple small macules/papules → Brown → Around/on lips → **PEUTZ–JEGHER'S SYNDROME** — p. 137

Diffuse swelling → Intermittent lasts < 48 hours → Associated with urticaria & swollen eyes → **ANGIO-OEDEMA** — p. 137

Diffuse swelling → Constant → Onset as adult → **GRANULOMATOUS CHEILITIS / CROHN'S DISEASE** — p. 137

Diffuse swelling → Constant → From birth or infancy → **HAEMANGIOMA LYMPHANGIOMA NEUROFIBROMA** — *see pp. 278, 281, 234*

Lips
Scale/fissures/hyperkeratotic/crust/warty surface
Chronic papules/plaques/ulcers (Acute ulcers & erosions, *see* Mouth p. 124)

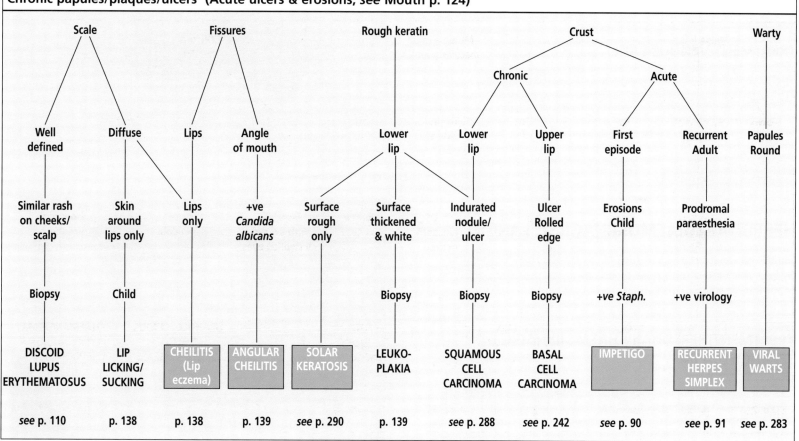

Scale		**Fissures**		**Rough keratin**			**Crust**			**Warty**
							Chronic	Acute		
Well defined	Diffuse	Lips	Angle of mouth		Lower lip	Lower lip	Upper lip	First episode	Recurrent Adult	Papules Round
Similar rash on cheeks/scalp	Skin around lips only	Lips only	+ve *Candida albicans*	Surface rough only	Surface thickened & white	Indurated nodule/ulcer	Ulcer Rolled edge	Erosions Child	Prodromal paraesthesia	
Biopsy	Child				Biopsy	Biopsy	Biopsy	+ve *Staph.*	+ve virology	
DISCOID LUPUS ERYTHEMATOSUS	LIP LICKING/ SUCKING	CHEILITIS (Lip eczema)	ANGULAR CHEILITIS	SOLAR KERATOSIS	LEUKO-PLAKIA	SQUAMOUS CELL CARCINOMA	BASAL CELL CARCINOMA	IMPETIGO	RECURRENT HERPES SIMPLEX	VIRAL WARTS
see p. 110	p. 138	p. 138	p. 139	*see* p. 290	p. 139	*see* p. 288	*see* p. 242	*see* p. 90	*see* p. 91	*see* p. 283

VENOUS LAKE

A solitary soft purple papule on the upper or lower lip is common in the middle aged or elderly.

TREATMENT VENOUS LAKE

Most patients do not seem to mind having these lesions on their lips. If they want them removed there are various ways of doing it.

1. Surgical excision under a local anaesthetic. The lip will heal well if the excision line is sited perpendicularly across the lip.
2. The pulse dye laser can be used without any anaesthetic and gives excellent cosmetic results. This is the treatment of choice if there is one in use near where the patient lives.

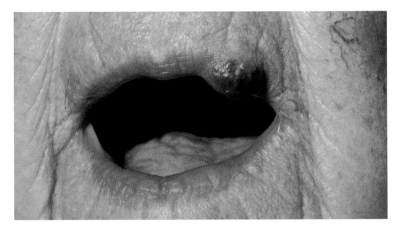

Fig. 6.19 Venous lake on the upper lip.

HEREDITARY HAEMORRHAGIC TELANGIECTASIA

Small red macules and papules occur on the lips, tongue and fingers associated with nose bleeds and gastro-intestinal bleeding. It is inherited as an autosomal dominant trait.

TREATMENT HEREDITARY HAEMORRHAGIC TELANGIECTASIA

The skin lesions do not need any treatment although the pulse dye laser is very effective at removing them. Nose bleeds may need cauterising if they will not stop with ordinary pressure. Anaemia due to recurrent bleeding from the nose or gastrointestinal tract will need treating with oral iron. The familial nature of the disorder should be explained to the patient and his family.

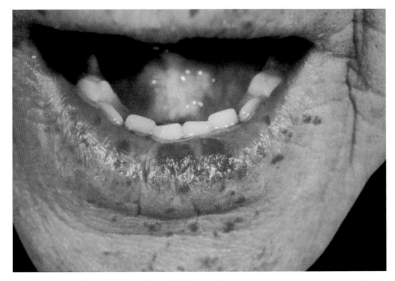

Fig. 6.20 Hereditary haemorrhagic telangiectasia.

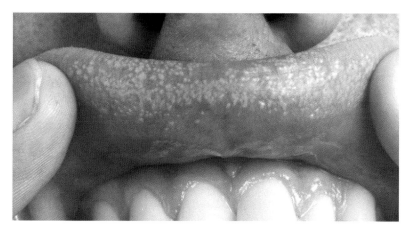

Fig. 6.21 Fordyce spots inside the upper lip.

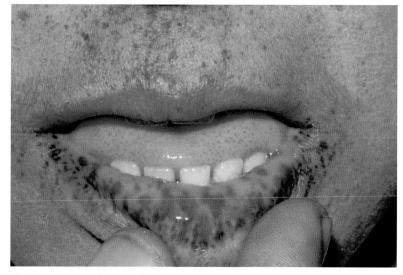

Fig. 6.22 Peutz–Jegher's syndrome.

FORDYCE SPOTS

These are small discrete white or yellow papules on the lips or buccal mucosa due to sebaceous gland hyperplasia. They are very common and completely harmless.

PEUTZ–JEGHER'S SYNDROME

A rare genetically determined condition, transmitted as an autosomal dominant trait. Brown macules on the lips, the skin around the mouth and on the fingers and toes occur in early childhood. They may be associated with small bowel polyps which can cause intussusception.

ANGIO-OEDEMA

Intermittent swelling of the lips lasting less than 24 hours before starting to go down is usually associated with urticaria and swelling around the eyes (*see* p. 83).

GRANULOMATOUS CHEILITIS

In granulomatous cheilitis the whole lip (upper or lower) is swollen. Initially this may fluctuate quite a lot, but eventually the swelling becomes permanent. The cause is unknown. If the buccal mucosa is also thickened consider Crohn's disease. Ask about abdominal symptoms and look inside the mouth for the characteristic cobblestone appearance of the buccal mucosa. If necessary do a barium follow through and a biopsy. If there is an associated facial nerve palsy and/or a fissured tongue (*see* p. 133) consider the **Melkersson–Rosenthal syndrome**.

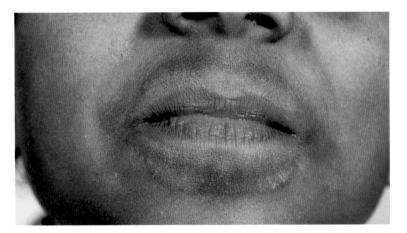

Fig. 6.23 Lip licking.

TREATMENT GRANULOMATOUS CHEILITIS

Injection of triamcinolone 5mg/ml into the swollen lip is often helpful.

ECZEMA ON THE LIPS (CHEILITIS)

Allergic contact dermatitis can occur on the lips from lipstick, lip salves, toothpaste or mouth washes. The diagnosis is confirmed by patch testing (*see* p. 20). Atopic eczema may affect the lips as well as the rest of the skin of the face (*see* p. 206). Many children suck or lick their lips causing a red scaly rash around the mouth which only extends as far as the tongue can reach.

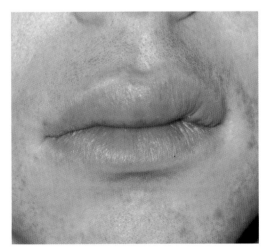

Fig. 6.24 Granulomatous cheilitis. Swollen upper lip.

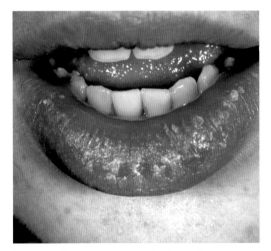

Fig. 6.25 Cheilitis. Eczema on the lower lip.

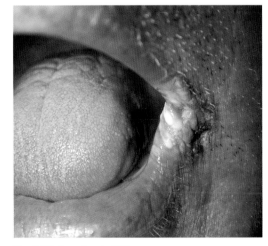

Fig. 6.26 Angular cheilitis.

TREATMENT LIP ECZEMA

It is important to use white soft paraffin[UK]/petrolatum[USA] as a regular moisturiser. A weak[UK]/group 7[USA] topical steroid such as 1% hydrocortisone ointment will be effective if applied twice a day.

Lip licking/sucking in children can usually be stopped once the parents realise what is happening. Applying a thick paste (e.g. Lassar's paste) will discourage the habit.

ANGULAR CHEILITIS

Cheilitis means inflammation of the lips, and in angular cheilitis only the corners of the lips are involved. It occurs in individuals who wear dentures, and is usually due to infection with *Candida albicans* from under the top denture. Poorly fitting dentures may also lead to overlap of the lower by the upper lip resulting in angular cheilitis.

TREATMENT ANGULAR CHEILITIS

First scrape the underside of the denture and examine for the spores and hyphae of *Candida albicans* or send for culture. Tell the patient to clean his dentures after every meal with a hard tooth brush and soap. Specific anti-candida treatment is not usually necessary.

LEUKOPLAKIA

This is a persistent white, hyperkeratotic plaque in the mouth, on the tongue or lips due to epithelial dysplasia or carcinoma-in-situ.

TREATMENT OF LEUKOPLAKIA

Since leukoplakia is usually caused by smoking, the first thing for the patient to do is to stop smoking. This may result in the lesion(s) disappearing. If it does not, consider one of the following:–

- If the area involved is small, excise it.
- If it is too large for excision, it can be frozen with liquid nitrogen (two freeze-thaw cycles, *see* p. 46).
- Widespread involvement can be treated by removing the lip epidermis with the carbon dioxide laser and allowing the epidermis to regenerate.

Such patients are probably best cared for by an oral surgeon.

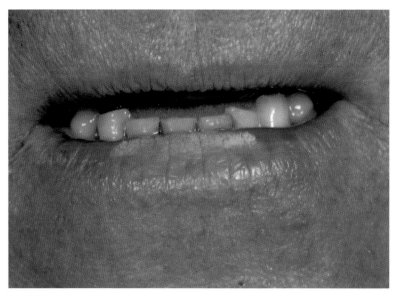

Fig. 6.27 Leukoplakia on the lower lip.

LESIONS AFFECTING THE EARS

Ears
Patches and plaques

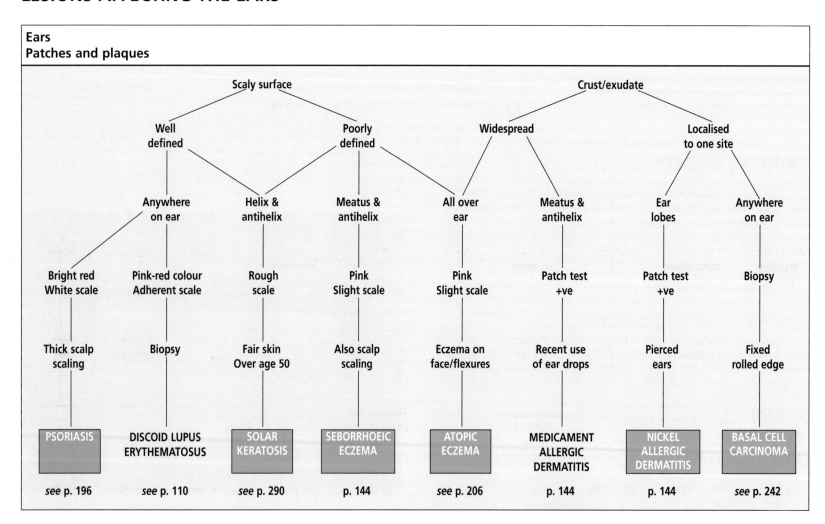

Ears
Papules and nodules

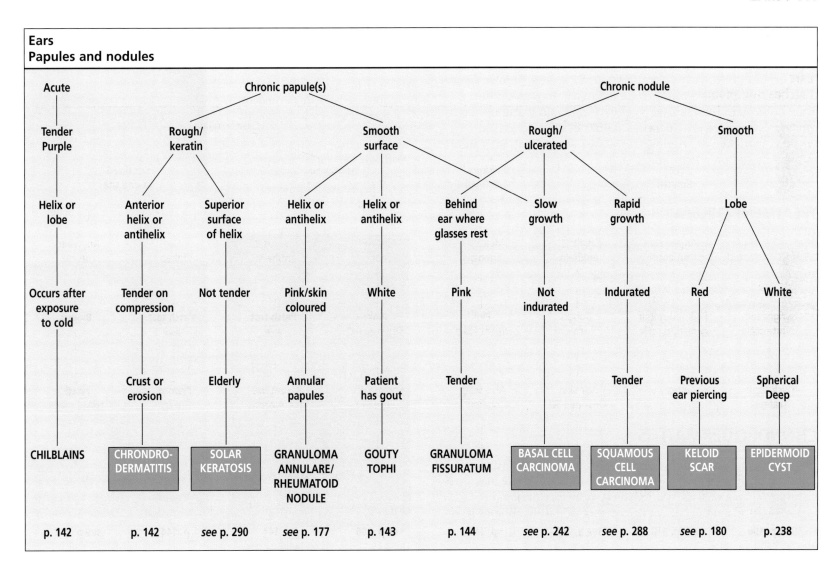

CHILBLAINS

Tender, itchy, mauve papules and nodules on the earlobes and helix occur in cold weather and last up to 2 weeks. Similar lesions can occur on other exposed sites, e.g. fingers, toes and nose. They occur in individuals who get very cold and warm up too quickly. The lesions are due to an abnormal reaction to cold where constriction of arterioles is followed by exudation of fluid into the tissues on rewarming.

TREATMENT CHILBLAINS

Prevention is better than cure, i.e. do not allow the skin to get too cold. Those at risk, particularly individuals who work out of doors and the elderly who live in unheated accommodation, should wear warm gloves, boots and hats in the winter. When they come in from the cold they should warm up slowly.

Nifedipine retard 20mg three times a day can reduce the pain, soreness and irritation of chilblains. For patients who get severe recurrent chilblains it is worth considering continuing the drug for several weeks if the weather is particularly cold.

CHONDRODERMATITIS

Chondrodermatitis nodularis helicis chronicus is a painful skin coloured or pink papule on the helix or antihelix. There may be a central area of scaling or crusting. A history of pain in bed at night when the patient lies on that side differentiates it from solar keratoses and skin tumours, which if painful, hurt all the time.

TREATMENT CHONDRODERMATITIS

Excision biopsy of the painful papule together with the underlying cartilage is usually curative. Removing the cartilage is more important than removing the skin. It is sometimes necessary to take the adjoining cartilage away to prevent the problem returning.

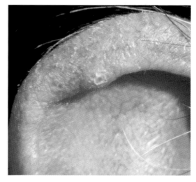

Fig. 6.29 Chondrodermatitis nodularis helicis chronicus.

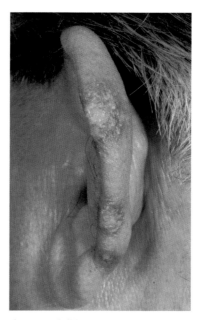

Fig. 6.28 Chilblains on helix.

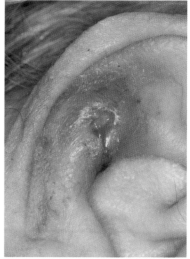

Fig. 6.30 Chondrodermatitis on antihelix. This may be difficult to differentiate from a BCC.

GOUTY TOPHI

These are hard white or cream coloured papules or plaques due to deposition of sodium urate crystals in the dermis. Classically they occur on the helix or antihelix of the ear, but occasionally are found on the dorsum of the hands and feet. Patients with tophi are likely to suffer from gout.

TREATMENT GOUTY TOPHI

Allopurinol competitively inhibits the enzyme xanthine oxidase, which oxidises xanthine to uric acid. It causes a rapid fall in serum uric acid. Start with 100mg daily as a single oral dose, and gradually increase to 300–400mg a day which will need to be continued indefinitely. By gradually increasing the dose you will hope to avoid precipitating acute attacks of gout at the beginning of treatment. With this treatment the tophi gradually become smaller and disappear.

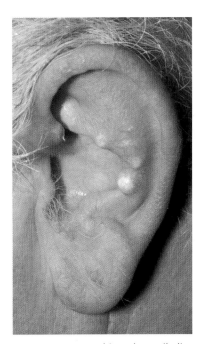

Fig. 6.31 Gouty tophi on the antihelix.

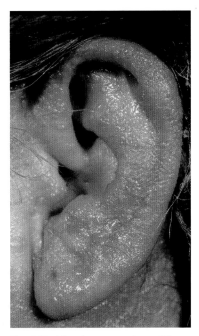

Fig. 6.32 Allergic contact dermatitis due to neomycin ear drops.

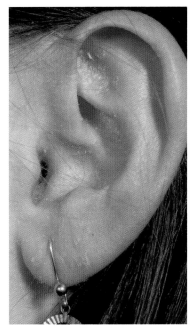

Fig. 6.33 Seborrhoeic eczema in the external meatus and on the antihelix.

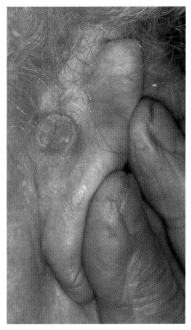

Fig. 6.34 Granuloma fissuratum behind the ear where the glasses rest.

ECZEMA ON THE EAR

Eczema on the ear usually occurs in association with eczema elsewhere. **Otitis externa**, i.e. eczema of the external auditary canal and meatus, is usually due to seborrhoeic eczema (Fig. 6.33), and there will be other evidence of this, e.g. scaling in the scalp (*see* p. 74). **Psoriasis** is red rather than pink and there will be typical plaques elsewhere +/– thick scaly plaques in the scalp (*see* p. 73). **Discoid lupus erythematosus** (*see* p. 110) usually involves the antihelix but not the external auditory canal. A biopsy will be needed to confirm this diagnosis.

Because of the narrow ear canal, eczema here can cause problems:–

- Scale tends to accumulate blocking the ear and causing pain.
- Secondary infection (with *Staphylococcus aureus*, Gram-negative organisms, *Candida albicans* and aspergillus) is common especially in wet conditions (e.g. after swimming).
- The itching encourages the patient to poke things down the ear canal.

Allergic contact dermatitis on the ears presents with an acute eczema (vesicles, exudate and crusting, Fig. 6.32). On the ear lobes this is usually due to nickel in cheap earrings. In the external auditory meatus and on the rest of the ear it is usually due to antibiotic or antihistamine ear drops, creams or ointments.

KELOID SCAR

A round pink/purple papule or nodule may develop on the ear lobe following ear piercing. It may gradually increase in size and become unsightly. It is differentiated from an inclusion epidermoid cyst (due to epidermis being implanted into the dermis at the time of ear piercing) by its colour, an epidermoid cyst being white.

TREATMENT OTITIS EXTERNA

If the eczema is dry and scaly, the treatment is the same as for seborrhoeic eczema elsewhere, i.e. 1% hydrocortisone cream or 2% ketoconazole cream used twice a day until it is better.

If there is a lot of scale and/or pain, the patient should see an ENT surgeon. A perforated ear drum and a co-existant otitis media must be excluded. Aural toilet, with removal of the excess scale can be done in the ENT clinic and will help the pain.

If there is an acute weeping eczema, do not be tempted to use one of the topical steroid/antibiotic (+/– antifungal) ear drops or sprays. You will only make things worse by exposing the patient to the risk of developing an acute allergic contact dermatitis on top of what he already has. Take a swab for bacteriology and mycology culture. If there is a bacterial infection present, use a systemic antibiotic depending on the sensitivities (probably flucloxacillin or erythromycin 250mg four times a day for 7 days). If there is a fungal infection, ketoconazole will be required rather than a topical steroid. First dry up the exudate with an astringent such as 13% aluminium acetate ear drops. When it is dry, use 1% hydrocortisone cream or ointment twice a day until it is better. Send the patient for patch testing when the rash has settled to exclude allergic contact dermatitis.

An ichthammol wick inserted into the ear canal is useful in patients with recurrent otitis externa.

GRANULOMA FISSURATUM

This occurs from the pressure of spectacles and occurs at the side of the bridge of the nose or behind the ear (Fig. 6.34). It looks like a basal cell carcinoma, and is distinguished by skin biopsy. Changing from heavy to light-framed glasses usually resolves the problem.

Acute erythematous rash on the trunk

7

Surface normal: no blisters or exudate

Crusting on surface

Generalised rash (>50% body surface)

Trunk & limbs
Acute progressive erythematous rash
Surface normal
Macules and papules
Erythematous maculo-papular rashes consist of small red macules and papules which coalesce to become confluent.

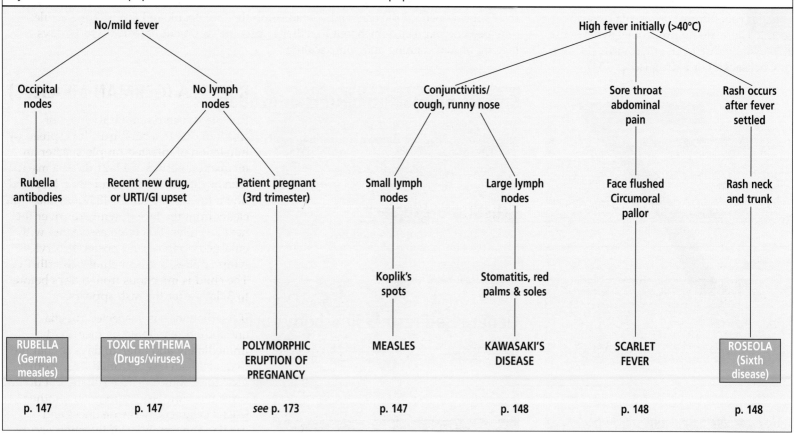

TOXIC ERYTHEMA

This is a rash in which pink/red macules and papules appear and then coalesce to become a widespread erythema. The rash may look like measles (morbilliform), rubella (rubelliform) or roseola (roseoliform). There are no prodromal symptoms. It is usually due to an enterovirus (ECHO or Cocksackie) or a drug (*see* p. 154).

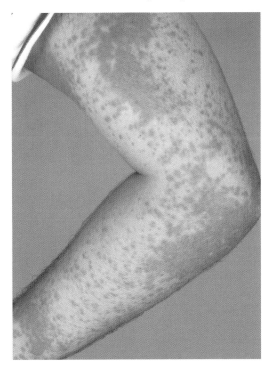

Fig. 7.01 Toxic erythema on the arm.

MEASLES

Measles is caused by the RNA morbillivirus. After an incubation period of about 10 days, the child becomes miserable with a high fever, runny nose, conjunctivitis, photophobia, brassy cough, and inflamed tonsils. Koplik spots on the buccal mucosa are diagnostic at this stage (look like grains of salt on a red base). On day 4 of the illness a red macular rash appears behind the ears and spreads onto the face, trunk and limbs. The macules may become papules, which join together to become confluent. It lasts up to 10 days leaving brown staining and some scaling.

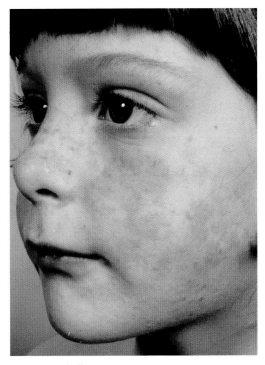

Fig. 7.02 Rubella.

RUBELLA (GERMAN MEASLES)

Rubella is a common viral illness of children due to a rubivirus. It is spread by inhalation of infected droplets. After an incubation period of 14–21 days, a macular rash begins on the face and neck. It spreads down the body over 24–48 hours and then clears from the face downwards over the next 2–3 days. It is often associated with enlarged occipital and posterior cervical lymph nodes, and sometimes an arthritis. The child is infectious from 5 days before to 3 days after the rash appears.

If the diagnosis is suspected rubella antibody titres should be measured immediately and after 10 days so that the diagnosis can be confirmed. Many other viral infections look like rubella but do not carry the same risk to pregnant mothers (foetal cataracts, nerve deafness and cardiac abnormalities) if infection occurs in the first trimester.

ROSEOLA INFANTUM (Sixth disease)

This is the commonest rash of this kind in children under the age of 2, and is due to the human herpes virus-6. The rash is preceded by a high fever but the child remains well. After 3–5 days the fever goes and the rash, which looks like rubella, appears on the trunk. It lasts only 1–2 days and then disappears.

TREATMENT MEASLES & OTHER VIRAL EXANTHEMS

Treatment is symptomatic since they get better spontaneously. Bed rest is necessary if the child is sick and pyrexia can be treated with cool sponging and paracetamol elixir.

Measles and rubella can be prevented by immunisation, but with reduced uptake of vaccines, these diseases are becoming more common.

KAWASAKI'S DISEASE

(MUCOCUTANEOUS LYMPH NODE SYNDROME)

This disease may be confused with measles, but must be recognised because of the potentially serious association with myocarditis. It occurs in young children under the age of 5 (50% under 2 years of age). The onset is acute with fever, red eyes, dry lips and prominent papillae on the tongue. The most characteristic signs are the large glands in the neck, the rash on the trunk and limbs, and the red palms and soles which later peel.

TREATMENT KAWASAKI'S DISEASE

If given immediately, a high dose of i.v. gammaglobulin (2g/kg body weight) as a single infusion over 10 hours will reduce the overall morbidity.

SCARLET FEVER

Scarlet fever is due to an infection with a group A β-haemolytic streptococcus which produces an erythrogenic toxin. The condition seems to be less common than it used to be. After an incubation period of 2–5 days there is a sudden fever with anorexia and sore throat. The tonsils are swollen with a white exudate and there is a painful lymphadenopathy in the neck. The tongue is furred initially, but later becomes red with prominent papillae (strawberry tongue). The rash appears on the 2nd day as a widespread punctate erythema which rapidly becomes confluent. The face is flushed except for circumoral pallor. After about a week the rash fades followed by skin peeling. *Streptococcus pyogenes* can be grown from the throat and the ASOT is raised.

TREATMENT SCARLET FEVER

Give oral phenoxymethylpenicillin (Penicillin V) 62.5–125mg every 6 hours for ten days depending on the child's age. The sore throat may be helped by gargling with paracetamol suspension (120mg/5ml) every 4 hours and then swallowing it.

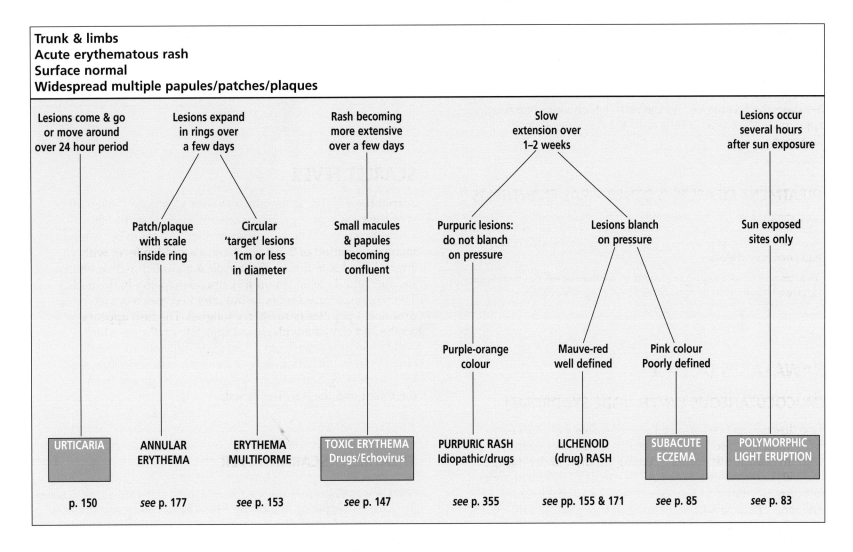

Trunk & limbs
Acute erythematous rash
Surface normal
Widespread multiple papules/patches/plaques

Lesions come & go or move around over 24 hour period

Lesions expand in rings over a few days

Rash becoming more extensive over a few days

Slow extension over 1–2 weeks

Lesions occur several hours after sun exposure

Patch/plaque with scale inside ring

Circular 'target' lesions 1cm or less in diameter

Small macules & papules becoming confluent

Purpuric lesions: do not blanch on pressure

Lesions blanch on pressure

Sun exposed sites only

Purple-orange colour

Mauve-red well defined

Pink colour Poorly defined

URTICARIA

ANNULAR ERYTHEMA

ERYTHEMA MULTIFORME

TOXIC ERYTHEMA Drugs/Echovirus

PURPURIC RASH Idiopathic/drugs

LICHENOID (drug) RASH

SUBACUTE ECZEMA

POLYMORPHIC LIGHT ERUPTION

p. 150   see p. 177   see p. 153   see p. 147   see p. 355   see pp. 155 & 171   see p. 85   see p. 83

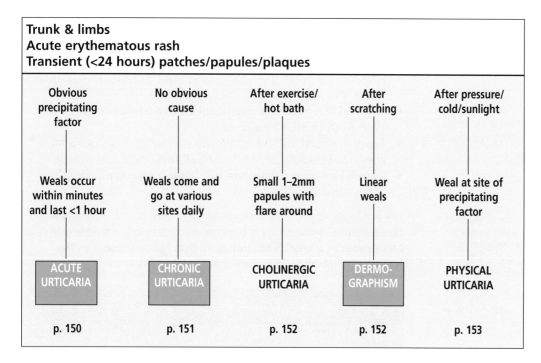

Trunk & limbs Acute erythematous rash Transient (<24 hours) patches/papules/plaques				
Obvious precipitating factor	No obvious cause	After exercise/ hot bath	After scratching	After pressure/ cold/sunlight
Weals occur within minutes and last <1 hour	Weals come and go at various sites daily	Small 1–2mm papules with flare around	Linear weals	Weal at site of precipitating factor
ACUTE URTICARIA	CHRONIC URTICARIA	CHOLINERGIC URTICARIA	DERMO-GRAPHISM	PHYSICAL URTICARIA
p. 150	p. 151	p. 152	p. 152	p. 153

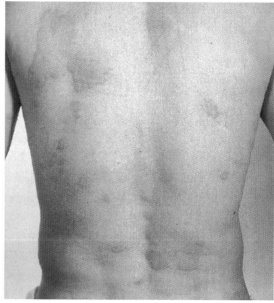

Fig. 7.03 Urticaria. Large weals.

ACUTE URTICARIA

Acute urticaria is defined as urticaria which has been present for less than 6 weeks. Individual lesions come and go within a few hours. A central itchy white papule or plaque due to dermal oedema (weal) is surrounded by an erythematous flare. The lesions are variable in size and shape, and may be associated with swelling of the soft tissues of the eyelids, lips and tongue (angio-oedema, *see* p. 83). Urticaria is due to release of histamine and other mediators from mast cells in the skin; why this occurs is not always understood.

Acute urticaria may be caused by:–

1. **Type 1 allergic response** which occurs within a few minutes of contact with an allergen either on the skin (e.g. nettle rash, latex allergy, *see* p. 364) or ingested (e.g. strawberries or penicillin). The rash disappears spontaneously within an hour. Contact with the same allergen again will result in a further episode.
2. **Direct release of histamine** from mast cells by aspirin, codeine or opiates. IgE is not involved. This is the commonest cause of infrequent acute episodes of urticaria, occurring when a patient takes aspirin for a cold or headache.

3. **Drugs** which cause serum sickness (an immune complex reaction). Urticaria, arthralgia, fever and lymphadenopathy are the hallmarks of this. It may be caused by the following drugs:–

- penicillin
- nitrofurantoin
- phenothiazines
- thiazide diuretics
- thiouracils.

TREATMENT ACUTE URTICARIA

Use a short-acting antihistamine such as chlorphenamine, 4–8mg every 4 hours (max 24mg/24 hours) until it settles. If life-threatening swelling of the larynx or tongue occurs, inject 0.5ml of 1:1000 adrenaline/ epinephrine solution intramuscularly.

Serum sickness may be severe and need treatment with systemic steroids. This is the only reason to give systemic steroids for urticaria.

CHRONIC URTICARIA

Here the weals come and go over a period of months or years. Individual lesions always last less than 24 hours, new lesions appearing daily or every few days. It can occur at any time of the day or night and is not a type 1 allergic response.

Possible causes of chronic urticaria can be identified by a good history so extensive investigation unless supported by this is not indicated.

Most cases will be idiopathic – no cause can be found, but exclude:–

- Psychological factors – ongoing stress; very hectic lifestyle.
- Regular ingestion of drugs such as aspirin, codeine and opiates (*see* p. 150).
- Food additives such as tartrazines, benzoates etc., which are chemically similar to aspirin.
- Chronic infections and infestations – bacterial (sinus, dental, chest, gall bladder), fungal (candidiasis), intestinal worms.
- General medical conditions, e.g. hyperthyroidism, chronic active hepatitis, SLE.

Around 40% of patients show a positive autologuous skin test. The patient's own serum is injected intradermally into the forearm and produces a weal. This indicates that IgE is present in the serum which will degranulate mast cells in the skin.

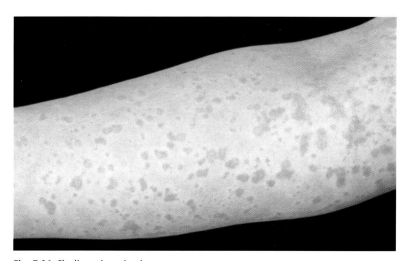

Fig. 7.04 Cholinergic urticaria.

TREATMENT CHRONIC URTICARIA

Ask the patient to avoid aspirin (and proprietary cold and 'flu remedies), codeine, and foods containing azo dyes (tartrazine – orange-yellow) and benzoic acid (used as a preservative in peas and bananas).

Long-acting non-sedative antihistamines need to be given regularly and in sufficient dosage to prevent the urticaria. Try one of the following:–

- Cetirizine 10mg daily (*Zirtek*UK/*Zyrtec*USA) or levocetirizine 5mg daily (*Xyzal*)
- Fexofenadine 180mg daily (*Telfast*UK/*Allegra*USA)
- Loratadine 10mg (*Clarityn*) or desloratadine 5mg daily (*Neoclarityn*)

Sometimes larger doses need to be used to control the urticaria. Once the patient has been free of the rash for 4 weeks, the antihistamine can be stopped. If it reoccurs then further long-term treatment is needed, and in some cases this can last for months.

If non-sedative antihistamines do not work try adding:–

- A sedative antihistamine such as hydroxyzine (*Atarax*) at night 10–50 mg (dose depending on effect and degree of sedation produced).
- An H_2 blocker such as cimetidine 200–400mg four times a day.
- Oral ciclosporin is useful in patients with a positive autologous skin test (inject the patients own serum into dermis to produce a weal at site of injection) not responding to antihistamines.

Do not use systemic steroids in urticaria. They do work but generally the problem reoccurs on stopping and there is a risk of long-term dependence.

CHOLINERGIC URTICARIA

Small red papules (1–3mm diameter) surrounded by an area of vasoconstriction (*see* Fig. 7.04) occur after exercise or hot baths, mainly in young adults. The diagnosis can be confirmed by making the patient exercise vigorously for a few minutes.

DERMOGRAPHISM

Weals occur only after scratching or rubbing the skin. Obviously the more the skin is scatched in response to itch, the worse the lesions can become. Dermographism is not usually associated with urticaria.

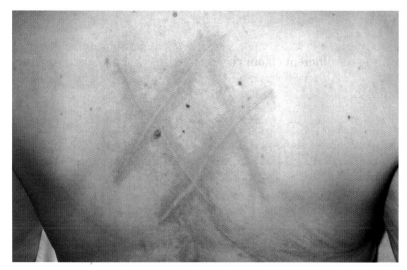

Fig. 7.05 Dermographism.

PHYSICAL URTICARIA

Cold, pressure, water and sunlight can all induce an immediate urticarial reaction.

TREATMENT CHOLINERGIC & PHYSICAL URTICARIAS

The options are to take a long-acting antihistamine on a regular basis to prevent the attacks, or take a short-acting one (such as chlorphenamine 4–8mg) before exercise or the precipitating cause.

Avoidance of exercise or the physical cause should be an obvious priority.

ERYTHEMA MULTIFORME

Multiple small (< 1cm diameter) round circular blisters, made up of rings of different colours ('target' or 'iris' lesions), occur on the palms, dorsum of hands and forearms, knees and dorsum of the feet. They may be very itchy.

The rash occurs 10–14 days after some precipitating cause, e.g.:–

- Viral infections, especially herpes simplex. This is the commonest cause of recurrent episodes of erythema multiforme.
- Immunisations.
- Bacterial infections, especially streptococcal sore throats.
- *Mycoplasma pneumoniae* infection.
- Drugs – sulphonamides, phenylbutazone and other non-steroidal anti-inflammatory drugs.

Occasionally the skin lesions may be widespread and associated with blisters or erosions in the mouth. **Stevens–Johnson syndrome** is erythema multiforme with extensive mucous membrane involvement (*see* p. 126).

TREATMENT ERYTHEMA MULTIFORME

Erythema multiforme gets better on its own after 2 weeks and does not require treatment. Even in severe episodes the case for systemic steroids is controversial. Treatment is symptomatic. Causes of erythema multiforme should be sought and treated if necessary.

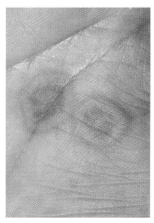

Fig. 7.07 (above) Close up of 'target' lesions.

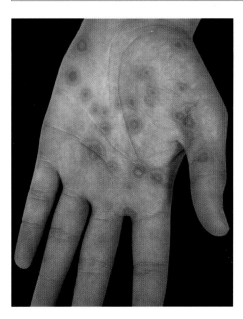

Fig. 7.06 (left) Erythema multiforme on the palm.

DRUG RASHES

Some drug rashes are life threatening and it is essential that the offending drug is stopped. Others are no problem at all; they are asymptomatic and get better whether or not the drug is stopped. Unfortunately there is no simple test to identify the cause of a drug rash and if patients are taking numerous drugs it is often not possible to be sure of the exact cause or even whether a drug is responsible (a viral exanthem may look identical). This leaves the doctor with a problem, not only during the current episode, but also in the future because he needs to know whether it is safe to prescribe the drug again.

If you think the patient has a drug rash find out:–

- What drug(s) has recently been started.
- The exact date each one was started and stopped. It is more likely that a rash is from a recently started drug than one that has been taken for years. A drug rash is unlikely to have developed in less than 4 days if the drug has not been taken before. Most drug rashes take 7–10 days to occur, but they sometimes do not appear for 28 days.
- Has the suspected drug or any chemically related drug been taken before?
- Has there ever been an adverse reaction to a drug before and to which one?

Avoid drug rashes by remembering the following:–

- Only prescribe drugs that are actually necessary.
- Always ask the patient if he has had any previous drug allergies.
- Make sure you know what is in a tablet or injection when you prescribe it.
- Do not give ampicillin for sore throats.

EXANTHEMATOUS DRUG RASH

This is the most common kind of drug rash. In the UK, antibiotics, sleeping tablets and tranquillisers are the most frequent causative agents. The rash mimics the common viral exanthems and is made up of symmetrical red or pink macules or papules mainly on the trunk; on the legs it may be purpuric. Almost any drug can cause this kind of reaction but the commonest are:–

- ampicillin
- benzodiazepines
- carbamazepine
- phenothiazines
- thiazide diruetics
- other penicillins
- captopril
- NSAIDS
- sulphonamides
- thiouracils.

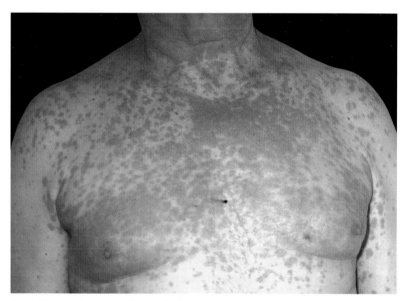

Fig. 7.08 Exanthematous drug rash due to a sulphonamide.

LICHENOID DRUG REACTION

A rash which looks like lichen planus (although usually atypical) can rarely be due to a drug. The rash has the typical mauve hue of lichen planus but the lesions are larger and more confluent. Drugs which can cause it include:–

- beta blockers
- chlorpropamide
- gold
- methyl dopa
- quinine
- chloroquine
- ethambutol
- mepacrine
- penicillamine
- thiazides.

OTHER DRUG RASHES covered elsewhere:–

Acne, *see p. 102*
Bullous, *see p.160*
Erythema multiforme, *see p. 153*
Erythema nodosum, *see p. 335*
Erythrodermic, *see p. 168*
Fixed drug eruption, *see p. 160*
Hair loss, *see p. 72*
Hyperpigmentation, *see p. 265*
Hypertrichosis, *see p. 58*
Lupus erythematosus, *see p. 114*
Photoallergic, *see p. 89*
Phototoxic, *see p. 85*
Purpuric/vasculitic, *see p. 355*
Serum sickness, *see p.151*
Toxic epidermal necrolysis, *see p. 166*
Urticarial drug rashes, *see p. 150*

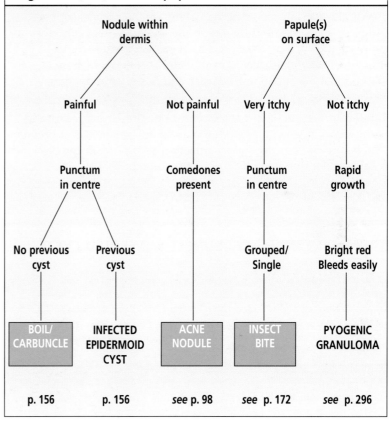

BOIL AND CARBUNCLE

A boil is an abscess of a single hair follicle (*see* Fig. 7.19, p. 164) caused by *Staphylococcus aureus* which may also be isolated from the nose or perineum. Single or multiple tender red nodules with a central punctum can occur anywhere on the body except the palms or soles. Without treatment the abscess will eventually point on the surface, discharge and heal leaving a scar. An abscess of several adjacent hair follicles is called a **carbuncle**. It looks just like a boil but is larger and has several openings to the surface.

Epidermoid cysts have a microscopic opening and through this staphylococci can enter. Sudden painful enlargement of a previous cyst is indicative of secondary infection or rupture of the cyst and a subsequent foreign body reaction (*see also* p. 238).

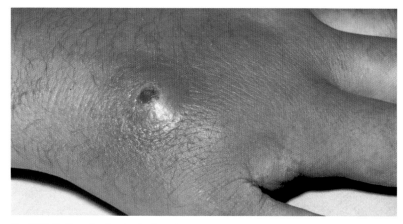

Fig. 7.09 Boil on the back of a hand.

TREATMENT BOILS, CARBUNCLE & INFECTED CYSTS

Check the patient's urine for sugar to exclude diabetes. If the boil is already pointing, it can be lanced to let out the pus. Otherwise treat with oral flucloxacillin (or erythromycin) 500mg four times a day for 7 days. Take swabs for bacteriology from the boil, the nose, perianal skin and any rash. The infection usually comes from the patient himself so carriage sites should be treated with topical mupirocin, fucidic acid or neomycin ointment twice daily for two weeks. If recurrent boils occur, even if carriage sites have been treated, take swabs from other members of the family and treat them if infected. Long-term oral low-dose antibiotics (flucloxacillin or erythromycin 250mg twice a day) may be necessary if the boils reoccur or persist. For cysts, excise after the infection has settled down, not at the time the cyst is red and painful.

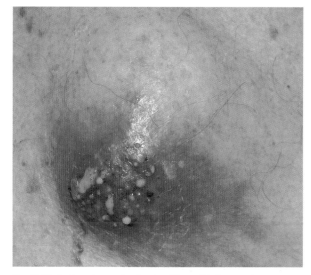

Fig. 7.10 Carbuncle on the back with multiple openings.

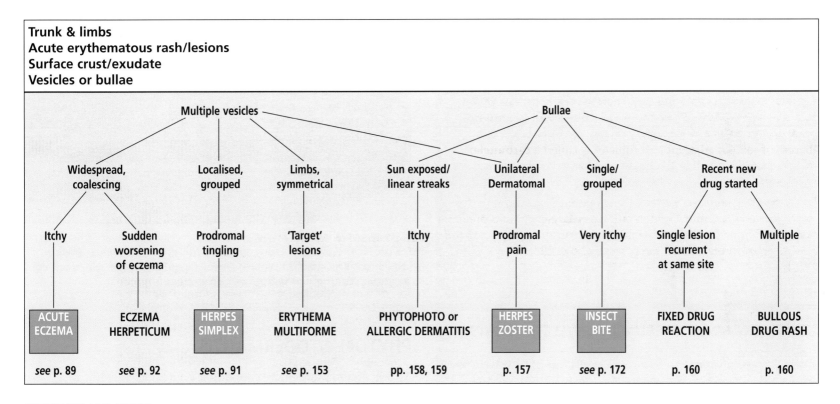

Trunk & limbs
Acute erythematous rash/lesions
Surface crust/exudate
Vesicles or bullae

Multiple vesicles — Bullae

Widespread, coalescing | Localised, grouped | Limbs, symmetrical | Sun exposed/ linear streaks | Unilateral Dermatomal | Single/ grouped | Recent new drug started

Itchy | Sudden worsening of eczema | Prodromal tingling | 'Target' lesions | Itchy | Prodromal pain | Very itchy | Single lesion recurrent at same site | Multiple

| ACUTE ECZEMA | ECZEMA HERPETICUM | HERPES SIMPLEX | ERYTHEMA MULTIFORME | PHYTOPHOTO or ALLERGIC DERMATITIS | HERPES ZOSTER | INSECT BITE | FIXED DRUG REACTION | BULLOUS DRUG RASH |

see p. 89 | see p. 92 | see p. 91 | see p. 153 | pp. 158, 159 | p. 157 | see p. 172 | p. 160 | p. 160

HERPES ZOSTER

Herpes zoster occurs in people who have previously had chickenpox. The virus *Herpes varicella-zoster* lies dormant in the dorsal root ganglion following chickenpox, and later travels down the cutaneous nerves to infect the epidermal cells. Destruction of these cells results in the formation of intra-epidermal vesicles. For several days before the rash appears there is pain or an abnormal sensation in the skin. Then comes the rash – groups of small vesicles on a red background, followed by weeping and crusting. Healing takes 3–4 weeks. The rash is unilateral and confined to one or two adjacent dermatomes with a sharp cut off at or near the midline. This feature and the associated pain makes any other diagnosis unlikely. The pain may continue until healing occurs, but in the elderly may go on for months or even years.

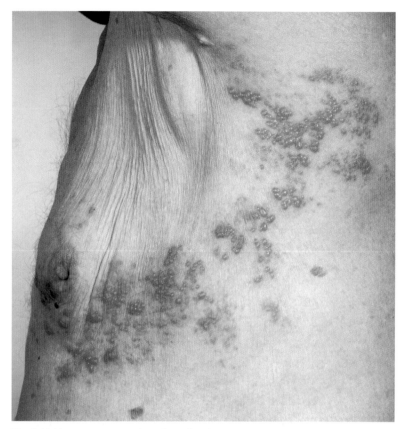

Fig. 7.11 Herpes zoster on chest (*see also* Fig. 1.07, p. 5 & Fig. 4.19, p. 92).

TREATMENT HERPES ZOSTER

If the patient is seen during the *prodromal phase* of pain or paraesthesia, or *within 48 hours of the development of blisters*, treat with a 7-day course of an oral antiviral agent such as:–

- Aciclovir 800mg 5 times/day
- Famciclovir 250mg t.d.s.
- Valaciclovir 1gram t.d.s.

These drugs are competitive inhibitors of guanosine and because they are converted to the triphosphate by viral thymidine kinase, they are effective only in the presence of actively replicating virus. They are all very expensive so should only be given in the early phase of the disease (within 48 hours of the rash appearing).

Give regular analgesics for the pain, e.g. paracetamol 1g every 4 hours, or co-proxamol 2 tablets 4 hourly. In the elderly, prophylactic amitriptyline 10–25mg taken at night, gradually increasing to 75mg, may help to prevent post-herpetic neuralgia if given as soon as the rash appears.

PHYTOPHOTODERMATITIS

This is due to plant juices containing photoactive chemicals (usually psoralens) being accidentally brushed onto the skin. In the presence of sunlight this causes an irritant or toxic dermatitis. Giant hogweed, rue, mustard and St. John's wort are often responsible. The patient gives a history of having been in the garden clearing weeds, often using a strimmer, or walking in the countryside on a sunny day. The rash is characteristically linear made up of blisters where the plants have touched the skin.

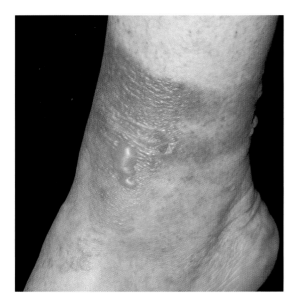

Fig. 7.12 Phytophotodermatitis or 'strimmer rash'. Sun exposed skin affected around ankles where plant juices containing psoralens have triggered a phototoxic reaction.

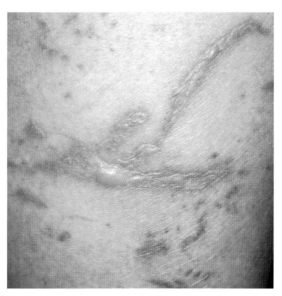

Fig. 7.13 Allergic contact dermatitis on the forearm due to *Primula obconica*.

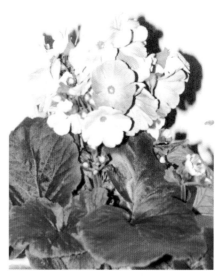

Fig. 7.14 *Primula obconica* plant (the indoor primula).

ALLERGIC CONTACT DERMATITIS

Linear blisters on the front of the wrist are characteristically due to the indoor primula (*Primula obconica*) where the leaves have brushed against the skin when dead heading the flowers. Linear acute eczema can sometimes be due to some medicament which contains a psoralen (e.g. suntan lotion) which has run down the skin (Berloque dermatitis).

TREATMENT PHYTOPHOTO and ALLERGIC DERMATITIS

Ideally the plant involved should be identified, so that it can be avoided in the future, but this is often not possible. If the rash is due to strimming the patient should wear trousers tucked inside his socks or boots in future. If the rash is very acute with blistering and weeping, dry it with potassium permanganate[UK] or aluminium acetate[USA] soaks (*see* p. 26). Once dry apply a potent[UK]/group 2–3[USA] topical steroid ointment until better.

FIXED DRUG ERUPTION

This is a curious reaction, whereby each time a drug is given, a well demarcated round or oval red plaque with/without blistering occurs at the same site, usually within 2 hours, and certainly within 24 hours. The only differential diagnosis is a recurrent herpes simplex infection. Any drug can cause it but in the UK/USA the common ones are:–

- sulphonamides
- phenophthalein (in *over-the-counter* laxatives)
- non-steroidal anti-inflammatory drugs
- tetracycline
- barbiturates
- quinine (tablets & in tonic water or bitter lemon drinks)
- tranquillisers.

The redness and swelling disappear after about 10 days to leave a dark-brown patch which remains for several months (*see* p. 264).

BULLOUS DRUG REACTIONS

Bullae at the site of pressure can occur in unconscious patients due to the following drugs:–

- barbiturates
- methadone
- nitrazepam
- imipramine
- meprobamate.

Bullous pemphigoid can on occasions be induced by:–

- clonidine
- furosemide (frusemide)
- diclofenac
- ibuprofen.

A **pemphigus type** of drug reaction is seen with:–

- captopril
- rifampicin
- penicillamine.

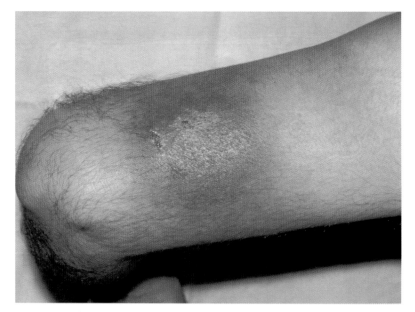

Fig. 7.15 Fixed drug eruption after taking Septrin.

TREATMENT FIXED DRUG ERUPTION

Stopping the drug will resolve the problem. You can confirm which drug is the cause as giving it again will produce the same reaction at the same site within 2 hours.

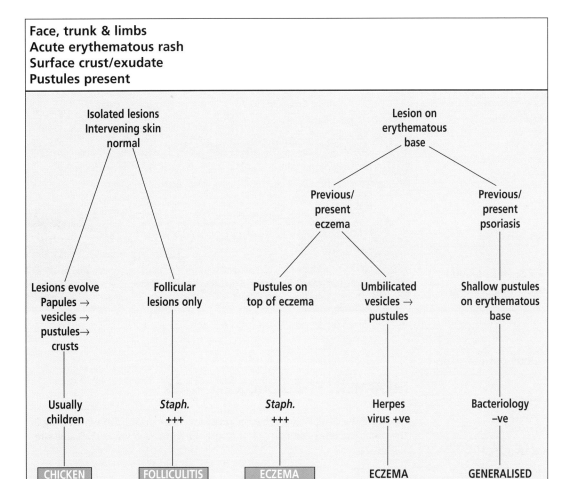

Face, trunk & limbs
Acute erythematous rash
Surface crust/exudate
Pustules present

Isolated lesions
Intervening skin
normal

Lesion on
erythematous
base

Previous/
present
eczema

Previous/
present
psoriasis

Lesions evolve
Papules →
vesicles →
pustules→
crusts

Follicular
lesions only

Pustules on
top of eczema

Umbilicated
vesicles →
pustules

Shallow pustules
on erythematous
base

Usually
children

Staph.
+++

Staph.
+++

Herpes
virus +ve

Bacteriology
−ve

CHICKEN POX	FOLLICULITIS	ECZEMA WITH FOLLICULITIS	ECZEMA HERPETICUM	GENERALISED PUSTULAR PSORIASIS

p. 161 — p. 162 — p. 162 — *see* p. 92 — *see* p. 168

CHICKENPOX (VARICELLA)

Chickenpox (*Herpes varicella zoster*) is a highly infectious illness spread by droplet infection from the upper respiratory tract. In urban communities most children under the age of 10 have been infected. The incubation period is usually 14–15 days. The prodromal illness is usually mild so that the rash is the first evidence of illness. The lesions start off as pink macules, which develop quickly into papules, tense vesicles, pustules and then crusts.

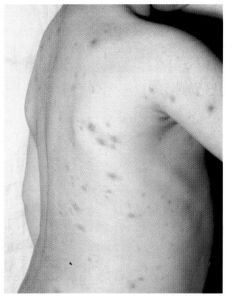

Fig. 7.16 Chickenpox on the trunk.

Crops of lesions occur over a few days so that there are always lesions at different stages of development present. The spots are very itchy and secondary infection may lead to pock-like scarring. Typically it occurs on the face and trunk rather than the limbs.

TREATMENT CHICKENPOX

In most instances chickenpox requires no treatment. In adults and immunocompromised patients treatment with famciclovir or valaciclovir will reduce the severity of attack (*see* p. 158 for doses).

FOLLICULITIS

Superficial infection of hair follicles is very common. A small bead of pus sits around a protruding hair and there may be slight erythema at the base. One or several follicles may be involved but there is no tenderness or involvement of the deep part of the follicle. It is usually due to *Staphylococcus aureus* which may be carried in the patient's nose or perineum. It can be caused by, or made worse by, the application of greasy ointments to the skin, tar preparations or plasters. The wearing of oily overalls may precipitate folliculitis of the thighs (**oil acne**).

TREATMENT FOLLICULITIS

Take swabs from a pustule and any possible carriage sites. Stop applying greasy ointments to the site. If this is the cause then nothing else is necessary. If folliculitis occurs in a patient with atopic eczema change the patient's steroid ointment to a cream for a few weeks.

Oral flucloxacillin or erythromycin 500mg four times a day for a week will clear most cases. Treat any infected carriage sites with topical mupiricin, fucidin or neomycin cream b.i.d. for 2 weeks.

Persistent folliculitis may require long-term suppressive treatment with low dose oral antibiotics (250mg twice a day for up to 6 months).

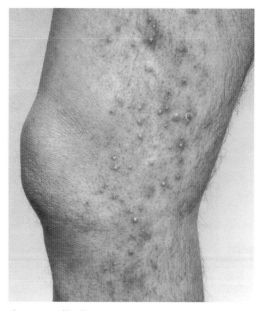

Fig. 7.17 Chickenpox on an adult's face.

Fig. 7.18 Folliculitis.

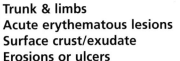

Trunk & limbs
Acute erythematous lesions
Surface crust/exudate
Erosions or ulcers

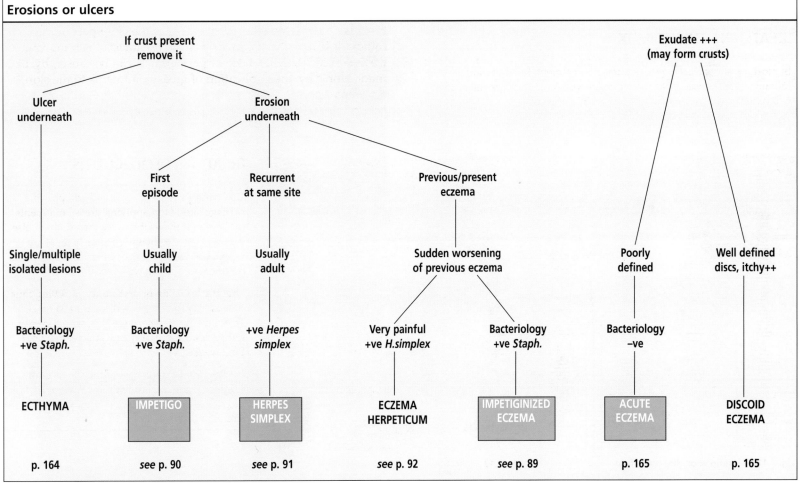

If crust present
remove it

Exudate +++
(may form crusts)

Ulcer
underneath

Erosion
underneath

First
episode

Recurrent
at same site

Previous/present
eczema

Single/multiple
isolated lesions

Usually
child

Usually
adult

Sudden worsening
of previous eczema

Poorly
defined

Well defined
discs, itchy++

Bacteriology
+ve *Staph.*

Bacteriology
+ve *Staph.*

+ve *Herpes
simplex*

Very painful
+ve *H.simplex*

Bacteriology
+ve *Staph.*

Bacteriology
–ve

ECTHYMA

IMPETIGO

HERPES
SIMPLEX

ECZEMA
HERPETICUM

IMPETIGINIZED
ECZEMA

ACUTE
ECZEMA

DISCOID
ECZEMA

p. 164

see p. 90

see p. 91

see p. 92

see p. 89

p. 165

p. 165

ECTHYMA

This is an infection of the full thickness of the epidermis and upper dermis (Fig. 7.19) by *Staphylococcus aureus* or *Streptococcus pyogenes* secondary to a break in the skin following an injury or insect bite. It presents as a round punched out ulcer with a thick crust on top. It is usually seen in children but may occur in adults, especially in hot humid climates. The lesions will heal with scarring.

TREATMENT ECTHYMA

Take swabs and give oral flucloxacillin or erythromycin by mouth, 125–500mg four times a day for 7–10 days depending on age. Do not treat with topical antibiotics, as the infection is deep and they will not work. The ulcer itself will take at least 4 weeks to heal, but antibiotics do not need to be continued for this long.

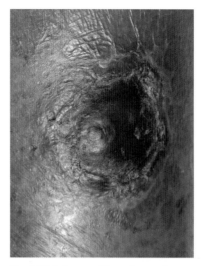

Fig. 7.20 Ecthyma with crust on surface.

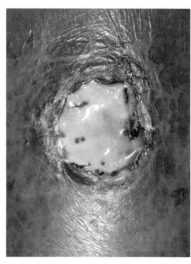

Fig. 7.21 Crust removed to reveal pus.

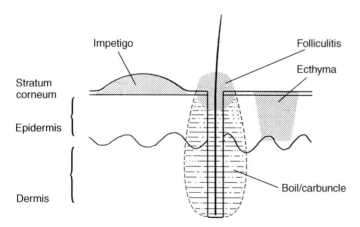

Fig. 7.19 Site of involvement of staphylococcal infection in the skin.

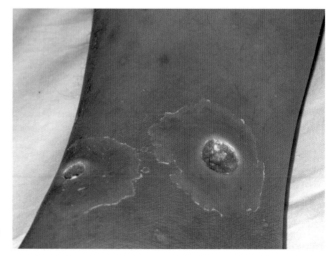

Fig. 7.22 Ecthyma on ankle secondary to insect bites.

ACUTE ECZEMA

Acute eczema clinically presents with tiny vesicles which burst to produce erosions, exudate and crusts. It may be due to an acute flare of chronic atopic eczema (*see* p. 206), or an allergic contact dermatitis. It may be difficult to distinguish from impetiginized eczema (*see* p. 89). A common mistake is to assume that weeping eczema is infected and treat it with antibiotics rather than topical steroids.

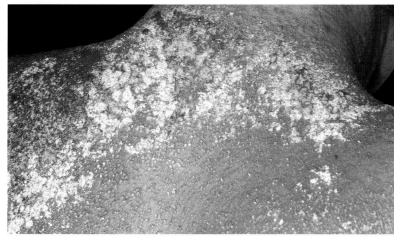

Fig. 7.23 Acute allergic contact dermatitis to an antihistamine cream.

DISCOID ECZEMA (WET TYPE)

Discoid eczema presents as well defined coin-shaped (nummular) plaques. The wet type is made up of coalescing erosions with exudate on the surface. The exudate dries to form crusts. There may be one or a number of lesions (*see also* p. 212).

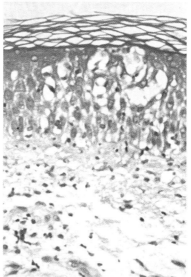

Fig. 7.24 Histology of acute eczema showing vesicles within the epidermis.

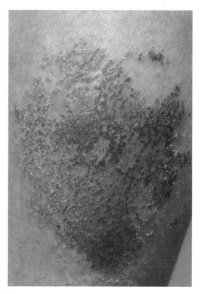

Fig. 7.25 Acute eczema with erosions and exudate.

TREATMENT ACUTE ECZEMA

It is no good trying to apply creams or ointments to an exuding rash because they are not able to penetrate the skin. First dry up the exudate with an astringent such as Burow's solution (aluminium acetate) or diluted potassium permanganate solution (1:10,000), *see* p. 26. The latter should be a light pink colour (*see* Fig. 2.01). Either put the solution in a bath or bowl and soak the affected area or soak a towel or flannel in the solution and apply it to the affected area for 10 minutes four times a day. After soaking, dry the skin with a towel and then apply a potent[UK]/group 2–3[USA] steroid ointment. If a contact allergy is suspected, refer the patient for patch testing once the rash has settled.

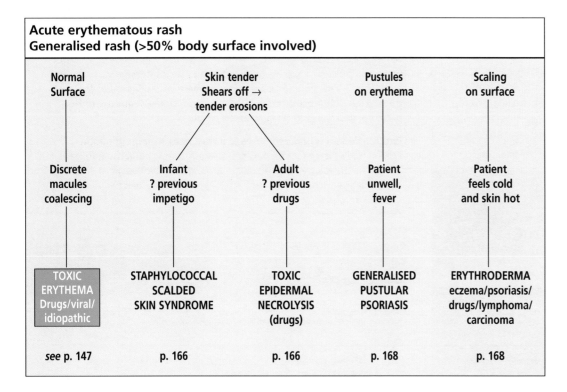

Acute erythematous rash
Generalised rash (>50% body surface involved)

Normal Surface	Skin tender Shears off → tender erosions		Pustules on erythema	Scaling on surface
Discrete macules coalescing	Infant ? previous impetigo	Adult ? previous drugs	Patient unwell, fever	Patient feels cold and skin hot
TOXIC ERYTHEMA Drugs/viral/ idiopathic	STAPHYLOCOCCAL SCALDED SKIN SYNDROME	TOXIC EPIDERMAL NECROLYSIS (drugs)	GENERALISED PUSTULAR PSORIASIS	ERYTHRODERMA eczema/psoriasis/ drugs/lymphoma/ carcinoma
see p. 147	p. 166	p. 166	p. 168	p. 168

STAPHYLOCOCCAL SCALDED SKIN SYNDROME

This is an infection due to phage type 71 *Staphylococcus aureus* which produces a toxin that causes a split in the upper part of the epidermis. It occurs almost entirely in infants and young children. The skin becomes red and very tender (like a scald) and then peels off. It often begins in the flexures but usually spreads to involve the whole body. The child will be screaming with pain. The source of infection is often an elder sibling with impetigo, infected eczema or scabies.

TREATMENT STAPHYLOCOCCAL SCALDED SKIN SYNDROME

Flucloxacillin elixir 62.5mg (children under age 2) or 125mg (age over 2 years) every 6 hours for 7 days. The pain will stop almost immediately. Other children in the family may require treatment for impetigo or infected eczema at the same time (*see* p. 90).

TOXIC EPIDERMAL NECROLYSIS

This is an uncommon but serious skin disease in which the whole of the epidermis dies and shears off. There is a mortality of around 30%, due to fluid loss or septicaemia.

It is most commonly due to drugs:–

- allopurinol
- barbiturates
- carbamazepine
- NSAIDS
- phenytoin
- sulphonamides
- thiacetazone

but can also occur in patients with a lymphoma and HIV infection. In some cases no cause can be found.

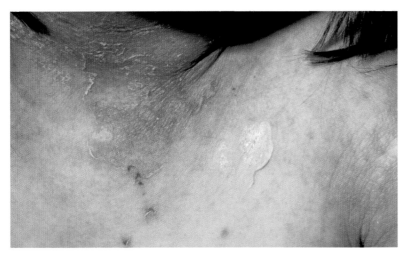

Fig. 7.26 Staphylococcal scalded skin syndrome in a young child.

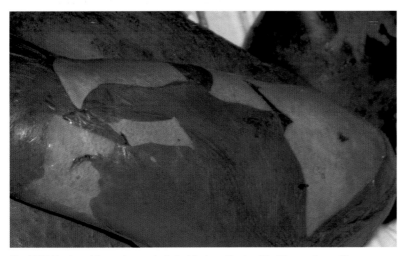

Fig. 7.27 Toxic epidermal necrolysis in black patient with skin peeling off.

TREATMENT TOXIC EPIDERMAL NECROLYSIS

Stop the suspected drug. The extensive skin loss will need to be treated just like a burn and admission to a burns unit or intensive care unit is advisable. Management includes replacement of fluid and electrolyte loss, prevention of infection and septicaemia, and careful handling of the patient's skin which tends to tear off easily.

Early treatment with large doses of intravenous immunoglobulin (2g/kg body weight given daily for 3–4 days) may switch the disease off and be life-saving. The immunoglobulins inhibit Fas-mediated epidermal cell death and allow the epidermis to recover. Systemic steroids do not help.

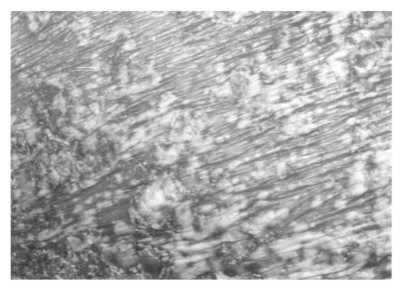

Fig. 7.28 Generalised pustular psoriasis – sheets of shallow pustules on an erythematous background.

GENERALISED PUSTULAR PSORIASIS

This acute, serious and unstable form of psoriasis is often precipitated by withdrawal of systemic or very potent topical steroids. Sheets of erythema studded with tiny sterile pustules come in waves associated with fever (*see* Fig. 7.28) and general malaise. This is the main reason why psoriasis should not be treated with either topical or systemic steroids.

ERYTHRODERMA

(EXFOLIATIVE DERMATITIS)

Erythroderma is the term used when >90% of the body surface is red and scaly. It can be due to:–

- Eczema
- Psoriasis
- A drug reaction, e.g. due to:–

  allopurinol   cimetidine
  barbiturates   gold
  captopril   isoniazid
  carbamazepine   nalidixic acid
  chlorpromazine   phenytoin
  chloroquine
  sulphonamides

- Sézary syndrome (mycosis fungoides)
- An underlying carcinoma.

TREATMENT GENERALISED PUSTULAR PSORIASIS (GPP)

This is a dermatological emergency and carries a significant mortality. The patient should be admitted to hospital for bed rest and sedation. Initially the skin will be treated with emollients (e.g. equal parts white soft paraffin & liquid Paraffin[UK]/petrolatum[USA]). Hypothermia should be prevented by nursing under a 'space blanket'. The associated fever is not due to infection, so there is no need for antibiotics. Both topical and systemic steroids are contraindicated. If the patient fails to improve on the above measures systemic treatment will be needed with methotrexate or ciclosporin.

TREATMENT ERYTHRODERMA

These patients should be managed in hospital both to find the cause and to prevent hypothermia, congestive cardiac failure or renal failure. Initially the skin should be treated with emollients such as white soft paraffin[UK]/petrolatum[USA]. Specific causes should be treated, e.g. psoriasis can be treated with methotrexate, or eczema with topical steroids. Stop any drugs and look for an underlying carcinoma or lymphoma.

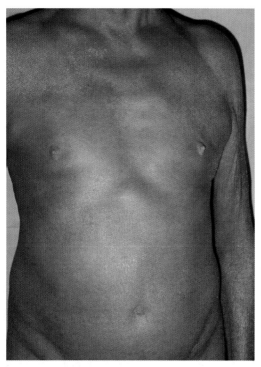

Fig. 7.29 Erythroderma due to carcinoma pancreas.

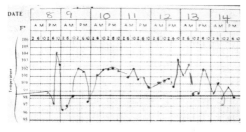

Fig. 7.30 Temperature chart of patient with GPP.

Chronic erythematous rash on the trunk

8

Normal surface

Scaly surface

Crust/exudate/excoriated surface

Trunk & limbs
Chronic erythematous rash
Surface normal/smooth
Multiple papules – no pustules (pustules present *see* p. 174)

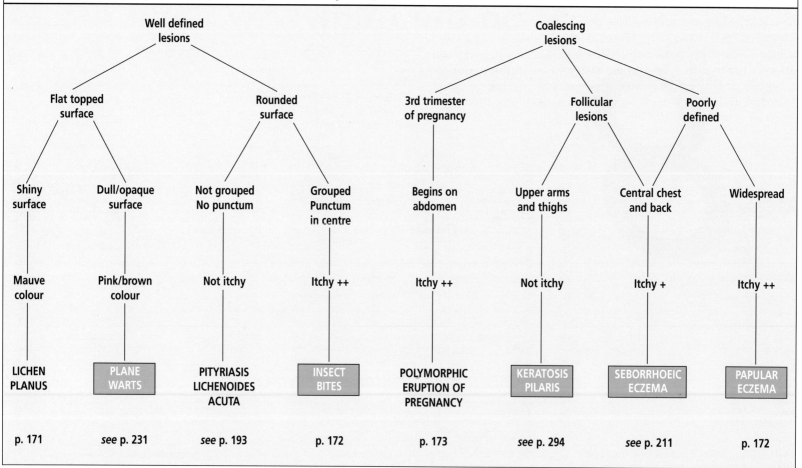

LICHEN PLANUS

The lesions in lichen planus are small mauve, flat-topped, shiny papules which sometimes have white streaky areas on the surface (Wickham's striae). The most characteristic place to look for the rash is on the flexor aspect of the wrist, but it is usually widespread on the trunk and limbs, and may occur at sites of trauma (Köebner phenomenon). Although it is very itchy, scratch marks are not usually seen. As the rash gets better the colour of the papules changes from mauve to brown (*see* Fig. 1.65, p. 14). The buccal mucosa may be involved with a white lace-like streaky pattern (*see* Fig. 6.12, p. 131).

The rash tends to last 9–18 months before disappearing. There may be some residual post-inflammatory hyperpigmentation for a time.

TREATMENT LICHEN PLANUS

Topical treatment will not make the rash go away any quicker, but the application of a potent[UK]/group 2–3[USA] topical steroid will control the itching.

Patients with extensive blistering (bullous) or severe erosive mucous membrane lichen planus may require treatment with systemic steroids and should be referred urgently to a dermatologist.

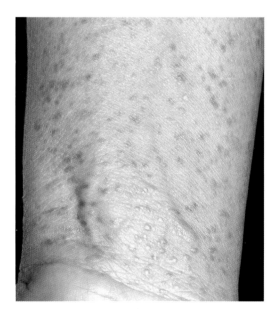

Fig. 8.01 Lichen planus. Flat topped shiny papules on flexor aspect of the wrist.

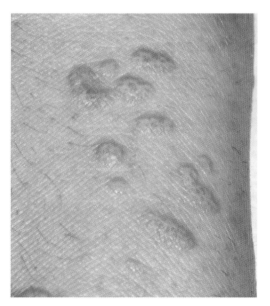

Fig. 8.02 Lichen planus. Wickham's striae.

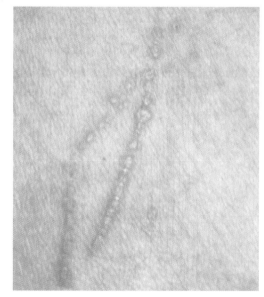

Fig. 8.03 Lichen planus. Köebner phenomenon.

INSECT BITES (Papular urticaria)

Insect bites present as itchy papules with a central punctum. If there are groups or rows of 3 or 4, think of flea bites. Single very large lesions on the face or hands are suggestive of bed bugs, particularly where new lesions are found each morning. Numerous other insects can also bite humans. Sometimes large blisters follow insect bites.

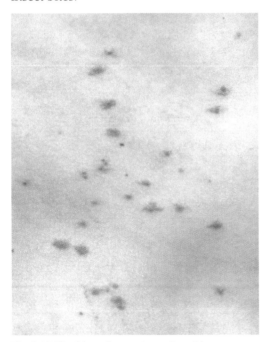

Fig. 8.04 Flea bites. Grouped papules with intervening skin normal.

Insect repellents

Mosquitoes can be discouraged from biting by using an insect repellent. DEET (NN-diethyl-m-toluamide) is the most effective insect repellent available at the moment, but it can cause irritation on the skin and should not be used around the eyes. It is available as a lotion, stick or spray. In children the insect repellent is applied to clothing near to the exposed skin, rather than on the skin itself so there will be no local irritation and no risk of the child getting it in his eyes.

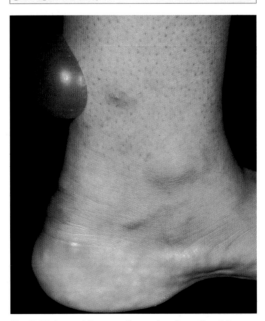

Fig. 8.05 Large blister on lower leg from flea bite. Note ordinary bite nearby.

TREATMENT INSECT BITES

Most patients will have acquired cat or dog fleas from their pets. Cats and dogs catch the fleas from other pets and bring them into the home, predominantly during the summer months, and occasionally during spells of warm weather at other times of the year. Successful treatment involves treating the animal and its sleeping place rather than the human. Regular spraying of the animal's fur, every 7–14 days throughout the summer months, with *Nuvantop* (111 trichloro-ethane, fenitrothion & bichlorvos) will keep them relatively flea-free (only available from veterinary surgeons). In addition the animal's bedding, and any of the armchairs or beds that the pet sleeps on, can also be sprayed.

For the patient, itching can be relieved by the application of 10% crotamiton cream (*Eurax*) or calamine lotion applied 2 or 3 times a day. If itching keeps the patient awake at night, use a sedating oral antihistamine at bed time.

PAPULAR ECZEMA

Eczema sometimes may present as papules which remain discrete rather than coalescing into poorly defined plaques.

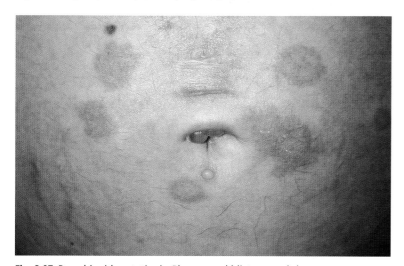

Fig. 8.06 Polymorphic eruption of pregnancy on abdomen.

Fig. 8.07 Pemphigoid gestationis. Plaques and blisters on abdomen.

POLYMORPHIC ERUPTION OF PREGNANCY

This is a common rash (about 1:150 pregnancies) that usually occurs in the 3rd trimester of pregnancy. It is a very itchy condition which starts on the abdomen. It is made up of urticated papules, plaques and sometimes vesicles. It clears up within 2–3 weeks of delivery and does not reoccur in subsequent pregnancies. It needs to be distinguished from the more serious pemphigoid gestationis (*see* Table below & p. 225).

TREATMENT POLYMORPHIC ERUPTION OF PREGNANCY

Apply a moderately potent[UK]/group 4–5[USA] topical steroid cream b.i.d. to relieve the itching. Occasionally an oral antihistamine will also be needed, such as chlorphenamine (*Piriton*) 4–8mg every 4 hours (maximum 24mg in 24 hours).

Polymorphic eruption	Pemphigoid gestationis
Common	Very rare
Urticated papules, vesicles, plaques	Tense vesicles & bullae
Cause unknown	Due to antibodies to basement membrane of skin
Very itchy	Very itchy
Usually primigravida	Reoccurs in each subsequent pregnancy
Occurs 3rd trimester	2nd and 3rd trimesters
Clears within 2–3 weeks after delivery	May take weeks–months to clear
Baby not affected	Baby may be born with same rash

Table 7.01 Comparison of polymorphic eruption of pregnancy and pemphigoid gestationis.

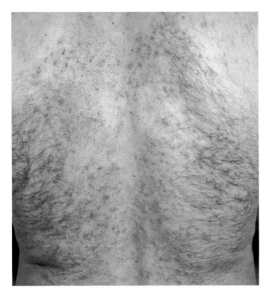

Fig. 8.08 Pityrosporum folliculitis on back.

Fig. 8.09 Close up of follicular papules.

SEBORRHOEIC DERMATITIS

On the trunk seborrhoeic dermatitis usually presents with poorly defined red scaly plaques on the centre of the chest and back (*see* p. 211). A less common pattern is extensive follicular papules and pustules (**pityrosporum folliculitis**). This rash tends to come and go. The diagnosis is made by the association with typical seborrhoeic dermatitis on the face (p. 118) and scalp (p. 74). For treatment *see* p. 212.

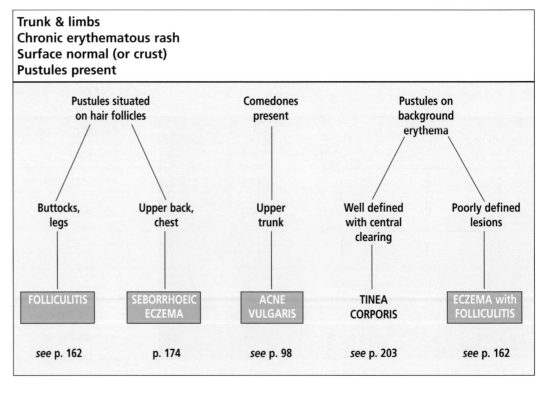

Trunk & limbs
Chronic erythematous rash
Surface normal (or crust)
Pustules present

Pustules situated on hair follicles		Comedones present	Pustules on background erythema	
Buttocks, legs	Upper back, chest	Upper trunk	Well defined with central clearing	Poorly defined lesions
FOLLICULITIS	SEBORRHOEIC ECZEMA	ACNE VULGARIS	TINEA CORPORIS	ECZEMA with FOLLICULITIS
see p. 162	p. 174	*see* p. 98	*see* p. 203	*see* p. 162

Trunk & limbs
Chronic erythematous rash/multiple lesions
Normal/smooth surface
Large patches & plaques (all lesions >2 cm)   **(For macules & small patches and plaques see p. 188)**

Lesions come and go	Ring shape/ annular (see also p. 176)				Round or irregular shape			Linear lesions (see also p. 179)	
Lesions expand over hours	Lesion expanding over few days	Lesions expand over weeks		Lesions fixed over site & time	Well defined fixed lesions		Poorly defined lesions	Stretch marks	Previous injury/ surgery
Peripheral red/white flare	Central clearing Fine scale inside ring	Central punctum ? previous tick bite	Accentuated border/ central clearing	Ring of papules	Red/ purple plaque	Lesion empties on compression		Teenager Pregnancy Obesity	
		+ve Lyme serology	Mycology +ve		Biopsy				
URTICARIA	ANNULAR ERYTHEMA	LYME DISEASE	TINEA INCOGNITO	GRANULOMA ANNULARE	SARCOID/ JESSNER'S/ LYMPHOMA	HAEM- ANGIOMA	ECZEMA	STRIAE	SCAR
see p. 150	p. 177	p. 176	p. 178	p. 177	pp. 180/111/182	see p. 278	p. 178	p. 179	see p. 180

CAUSES OF ANNULAR LESIONS

With normal surface Annular erythema (p. 177)
Erythema chronicum migrans (Lyme disease)
Erythema multiforme (p. 153)
Granuloma annulare (p. 177)
Jessner's lymphocytic infiltrate (p. 111)
Urticaria (p. 150)

With crust or scale Annular psoriasis (p. 196)
Discoid eczema (p. 212)
Porokeratosis (p. 290)
Pityriasis rosea (p. 191)
Tinea corporis (p. 203)

LYME DISEASE

A single lesion of gradually expanding erythema (**erythema chronicum migrans**) with or without a central punctum is likely to be Lyme disease. It is due to a tick bite which transmits a spirochaete (*Borrelia burgdorferi*) into the skin. Outbreaks of Lyme disease tend to occur in late May and early June when the ticks leave the ground vegetation to feed on their animal hosts (deer and sheep); they may wander onto humans as they walk through the countryside.

If treatment is delayed patients can go on to develop arthritis (initially intermittent swelling of large joints and later a chronic erosive arthritis), meningoencephalitis, facial nerve palsy and heart problems (conduction defects, myocarditis and pericarditis) weeks or months later. If suspected the diagnosis can be confirmed by finding antibodies to the spirochaete in the patient's serum. There should be a fourfold rise in antibody titre over 2–3 weeks. The antibody (ELISA) test can be done at your local hospital.

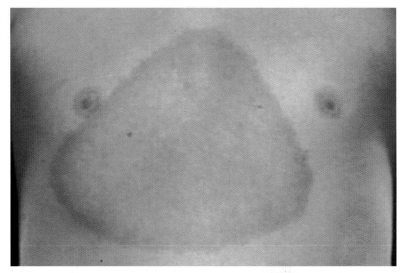

Fig. 8.10 Erythema chronicum migrans (Lyme disease).

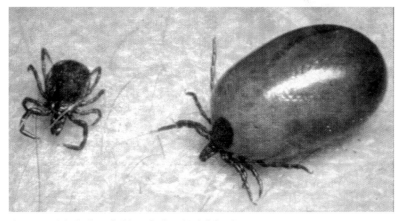

Fig. 8.11 Ticks before (left) and after (right) feeding.

TREATMENT LYME DISEASE

Oral oxytetracycline 250mg four times a day for 10–14 days is the treatment of choice. In children under the age of twelve give phenoxymethylpenicillin (Penicillin V), 50mg/kg body weight/day in divided doses instead. If children are allergic to penicillin, they can be given erythromycin 50mg/kg body weight/day in divided doses for 10–14 days.

ANNULAR ERYTHEMA

This describes areas of erythema which are annular or figurate in shape. Over a period of days the areas of erythema gradually expand or change. The lesions are often scaly just inside the spreading edge. In most instances no cause can be found, but very rarely some patients may have an underlying neoplasm (lymphoma or leukaemia). No treatment is available unless there is an underlying cause.

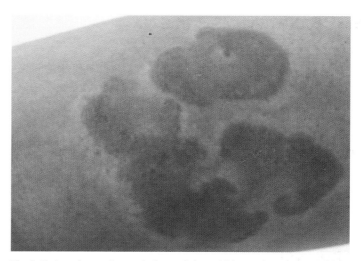

Fig. 8.12 Annular erythema: indurated ring which may have a central scale.

GRANULOMA ANNULARE

Granuloma annulare can present in one of two ways:–

1. Small pink papules which join together to form rings. There is never any scale on the surface so it should not be confused with tinea. It is usually seen on the dorsum of hand, elbows and knees, but can occur anywhere.

2. A flat pink or mauve patch often seen on the thighs, upper arms, trunk or dorsum of the foot (Fig. 8.14).

Both types may occur separately or be present together on different parts of the body.

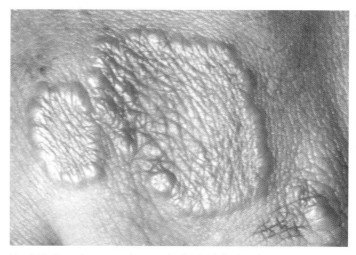

Fig. 8.13 Granuloma annulare on the back of the hand.

TREATMENT GRANULOMA ANNULARE

If it is asymptomatic, which it usually is, the patient can be reassured that it is harmless and will eventually go away on its own. It may take quite a long time – months or even years rather than weeks. If it is painful, injection of triamcinolone 5–10 mg/ml intralesionally will stop the pain and may make it go away.

TINEA INCOGNITO

Tinea incognito develops when tinea corporis (ringworm) is inadvertently treated with topical steroids. This alters the clinical appearance so that the lesions have no appreciable scale, and may be distributed symmetrically. Nevertheless scraping the edge will reveal fungus.

TREATMENT TINEA INCOGNITO

Stop applying any topical steroids. Terbinafine cream applied daily for 10 days or any imidazole cream for 14 days will be effective (*see also* p. 39).

ECZEMA

Any poorly defined itchy rash with macules and papules becoming confluent is likely to be eczema. The scaling in eczema may not be obvious but is usually there if carefully looked for. In addition rashes that vary over weeks rather than days and are itchy are likely to be eczema (*see* p. 204).

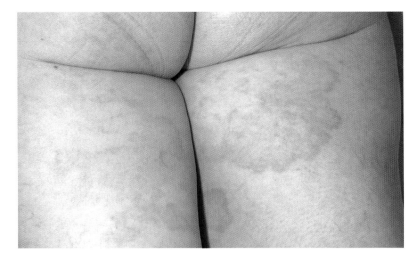

Fig. 8.14 Granuloma annulare: patch of erythema on the back of the thigh.

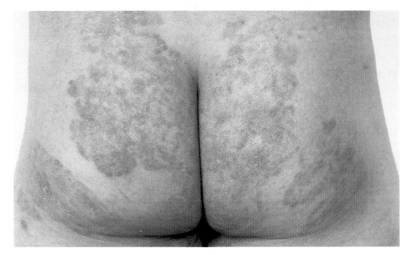

Fig. 8.15 Tinea incognito. Symmetrical non-scaly plaques (*see* Fig. 13.36, p. 379).

LINEAR LESIONS

Linear lesions occur in the following:–

With a normal surface
- Striae or stretch marks (see right)
- Surgical scars – normal, keloid or hypertrophic
  – sarcoid can occur in old scars
- Köebner phenomenon – when due to a scratch will be linear, e.g. in psoriasis, lichen planus, plane warts
- Along the line of blood vessels or lymphatics:–
  - thrombophlebitis – inflammation of superficial veins
  - lymphangitis – inflammation of lymphatics associated with cellulitis
  - sporotrichosis – deep fungal infection in which nodules occur along the course of a lymphatic vessel (*see* p. 364)
- Larva migrans – larvae leave a serpiginous track (p. 380)
- Linear morphoea (pp. 66, 248)
- Dermatomyositis – erythema over metacarpals and along fingers (p. 114).

With a surface scale or warty change
- Köebner phenomenon – psoriasis & plane warts
- Present from birth or early childhood down the length of a limb or around the side of the trunk:–
  - epidermal naevus (p. 283)
  - inflammatory linear verrucous epidermal naevus
  - lichen striatus.

With blistering, exudate or erosions
- Linear contact dermatitis:–
  - phytophotodermatitis due to sunlight and plant sap brushed onto the skin (p. 158)
  - allergic contact dermatitis due to plant sap (p. 159)
  - Berloque dermatitis due to sunlight and a psoralen (from cosmetics) in contact with skin (p. 159)
- Dermatomal – herpes zoster (p. 157)
- Dermatitis artefacta – self-inflicted (p. 227).

STRIAE

Linear red/purple plaques occur commonly on the thighs and lumbosacral regions in teenagers. With time they flatten off and become atrophic. Similar lesions occur on the abdomen and breasts in pregnancy, and in the flexures in patients on systemic steroids or those using potent topical steroids. No treatment will get rid of them.

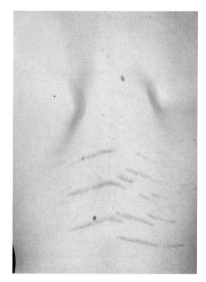

Fig. 8.16 Striae. Linear stretch marks on the back of a teenager.

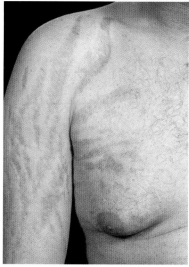

Fig. 8.17 Striae in patient with psoriasis who has used excessive topical steroids.

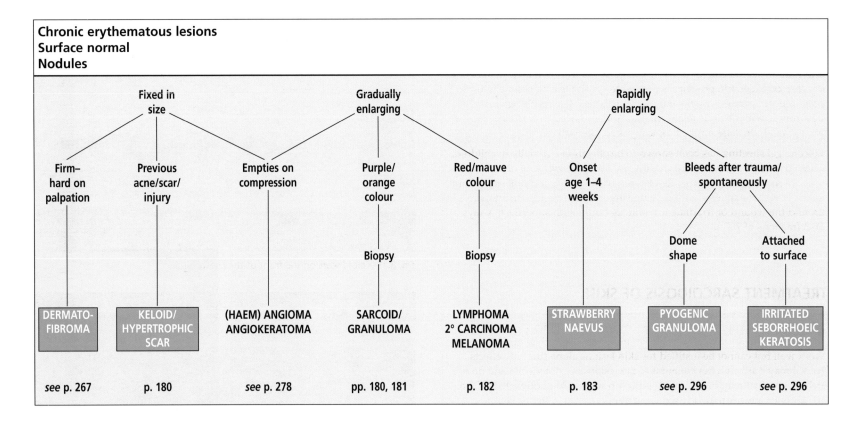

Chronic erythematous lesions
Surface normal
Nodules

Fixed in size	
Gradually enlarging	
Rapidly enlarging	

- Firm–hard on palpation → **DERMATO-FIBROMA** — *see p. 267*
- Previous acne/scar/injury → **KELOID/ HYPERTROPHIC SCAR** — *p. 180*
- Empties on compression → **(HAEM) ANGIOMA ANGIOKERATOMA** — *see p. 278*
- Purple/orange colour → Biopsy → **SARCOID/ GRANULOMA** — *pp. 180, 181*
- Red/mauve colour → Biopsy → **LYMPHOMA 2° CARCINOMA MELANOMA** — *p. 182*
- Onset age 1–4 weeks → **STRAWBERRY NAEVUS** — *p. 183*
- Bleeds after trauma/spontaneously
  - Dome shape → **PYOGENIC GRANULOMA** — *see p. 296*
  - Attached to surface → **IRRITATED SEBORRHOEIC KERATOSIS** — *see p. 296*

KELOID & HYPERTROPHIC SCARS

Hypertrophic scars are an overgrowth of scar tissue confined to the site of injury, while keloid scars grow out beyond the original site of injury. The commonest sites for keloid scarring are on the front of the chest, around the shoulders and on the ear lobes (*see also* p. 144).

SARCOID

Multiple mauve/purple papules or plaques on the trunk and limbs may be due to sarcoid especially if old scars are affected. The clinical appearance can be very varied including hypopigmented patches. X-ray the chest and do a skin biopsy to confirm the diagnosis.

TREATMENT KELOID SCARS

Injection of triamcinolone 10mg/ml directly into the scar will flatten it off and reduce the red colour. Use a 23 gauge needle rather than a smaller one because considerable pressure is needed to get the triamcinolone into the scar. Repeat every 4–6 weeks until the scar is flat. The resulting scar will be atrophic with obvious telangiectasia. You will need to warn the patient about this. *Haelantape* applied topically is an alternative.

Silicone gel sheeting has been shown to be effective, especially in children. The pulsed dye laser will improve the pruritis and erythema of scars but will not reduce the thickness. Re-excision of the scar is contraindicated but sometimes this may work if following surgery you inject triamcinolone around the wound or irradiate it within 24 hours with superficial X-rays (1–3 fractions of 7Gy).

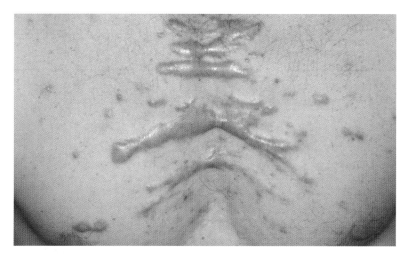

Fig. 8.18 Keloid scars on the front of the chest.

TREATMENT SARCOIDOSIS OF SKIN

Whether or not you treat the skin lesions will depend on whether there is sarcoid elsewhere. Topical steroids are not of any help. Sytemic steroids work well but cannot be justified for skin lesions alone (the side effects [p. 42] may outweigh the benefits). If the lesions are not visible and do not itch, the patient may be prepared to put up with it. Methotrexate 10–25mg (p. 43) once a week may be used as an alternative to systemic steroids.

GRANULOMATOUS INFILTRATES IN THE SKIN

A granuloma is strictly a histological term referring to a collection of monocytes, macrophages, epithelioid and giant cells in the dermis. It occurs in response to a persistent irritant such as a

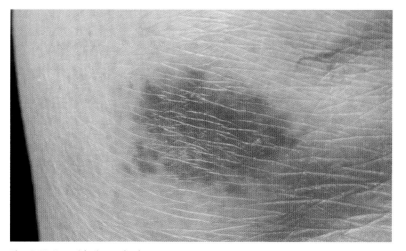

Fig. 8.19 Sarcoidosis on the knee.

foreign body (lipid, oil, glass fibre, talc, silica, metals) or infection (tuberculosis, leprosy, atypical mycobacterium, fungi). Quite often no obvious cause for a granuloma is found. Clinically granulomas are indurated nodules, orange to purple in colour with a normal surface. They tend to grow very slowly. Diagnosis is made by skin biopsy for histology and culture looking for atypical mycobacteria (incubate at <30°C), tuberculosis or fungi. A foreign body can be identified on histology by using polarised light. Treat any infection (atypical mycobacteria p. 364, tuberculosis p. 111, leprosy p. 250, fungus p. 39) and surgically excise any foreign bodies.

LYMPHOMA/CARCINOMA/SARCOMA/AMELANOTIC MELANOMA

A lymphomatous infiltrate usually presents as a rapidly growing red/purple indurated nodule with no surface changes. There may be one or several lesions. Diagnosis is confirmed by skin biopsy. A granuloma, metastatic carcinoma in the skin, a soft tissue sarcoma or an amelanotic malignant melanoma can all look the same. Diagnosis can only be made by skin biopsy. Treatment depends on the diagnosis.

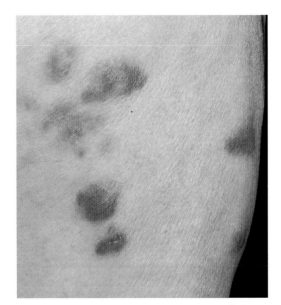

Fig. 8.20 Granulomas secondary to insulin injection in the thigh. A lymphoma would look the same.

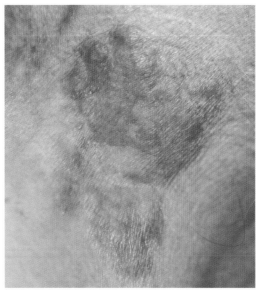

Fig. 8.21 Metastatic breast carcinoma on the neck.

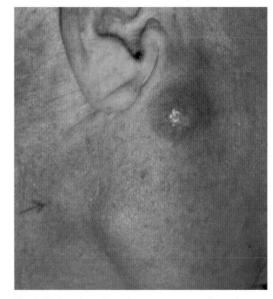

Fig. 8.22 Amelanotic melanoma – note enlarged lymph gland in neck (arrowed).

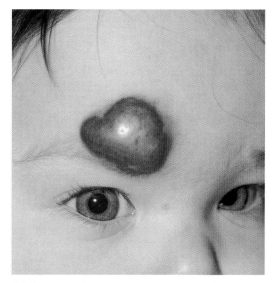

Fig. 8.23 Strawberry neavus at age 14 months.

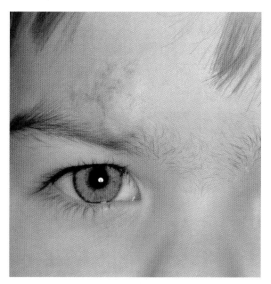

Fig. 8.24 Same patient at the age of 5 years.

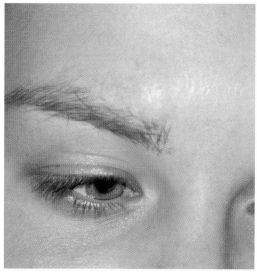

Fig. 8.25 Same patient at the age of 13 years.

STRAWBERRY NAEVUS

These red nodules are quite unmistakable. They are not present at birth but appear during the first 4 weeks of life. They grow quite quickly up to the age of 12–15 months, and then gradually and spontaneously involute. During this phase the colour becomes blue/purple, and as the nodule shrinks the overlying skin becomes slightly flaccid. Most lesions resolve completely by the age of 10 years but may leave some residual flaccidity of the skin. The main problem is a cosmetic one, but if traumatised, haemorrhage and ulceration can occur. Very rarely platelet comsumption can occur causing thrombocytopenia (**Kasabach–Merritt syndrome**).

TREATMENT STRAWBERRY NAEVUS

Most lesions will resolve spontaneously so they should be left alone to do so. Treatment is only needed when there are complications such as bleeding, thrombosis or interference with function (e.g. eyesight, eating, defaecation). The treatment options then include treatment with the pulse dye laser (a few treatments [2–4] will result in a reduction in size or growth), high dose oral steroids (prednisolone 40mg on alternate days) or surgical removal.

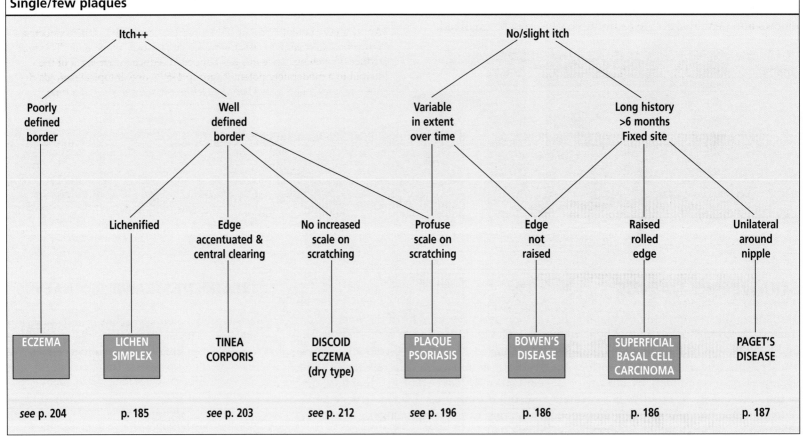

Trunk & limbs
Chronic erythematous rash
Scaly surface
Single/few plaques

Itch++

No/slight itch

Poorly
defined
border

Well
defined
border

Variable
in extent
over time

Long history
>6 months
Fixed site

Lichenified

Edge
accentuated &
central clearing

No increased
scale on
scratching

Profuse
scale on
scratching

Edge
not
raised

Raised
rolled
edge

Unilateral
around
nipple

ECZEMA

LICHEN
SIMPLEX

TINEA
CORPORIS

DISCOID
ECZEMA
(dry type)

PLAQUE
PSORIASIS

BOWEN'S
DISEASE

SUPERFICIAL
BASAL CELL
CARCINOMA

PAGET'S
DISEASE

see p. 204   p. 185   see p. 203   see p. 212   see p. 196   p. 186   p. 186   p. 187

LICHEN SIMPLEX

Lichen simplex is a well defined itchy plaque with increased skin markings on the surface (lichenification) due to persistent scratching. The commonest sites are the occiput, ankles, elbows and genitalia. Single or multiple sites may be involved.

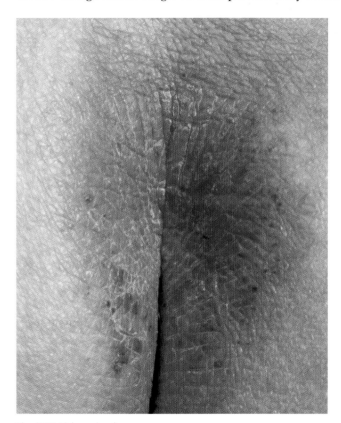

Fig. 8.26 Lichen simplex on sacrum.

TREATMENT LICHEN SIMPLEX

If the patient stops scratching it will get better, but this is often easier said than done. The patient may need to look at the circumstances in his life which are causing him to scratch and deal with or come to terms with them.

Apply a very potent[UK]/group 1[USA] topical steroid such as 0.05% clobetasol propionate (*Dermovate*[UK]/*Temovate*[USA]) b.i.d., or *Haelan* tape daily. This will reduce the itching. Once this has happened reduce the strength of the steroid to a moderately potent[UK]/group 4–5[USA] one. If topical steroids do not work, try an occlusive bandage left in place for a week at a time.

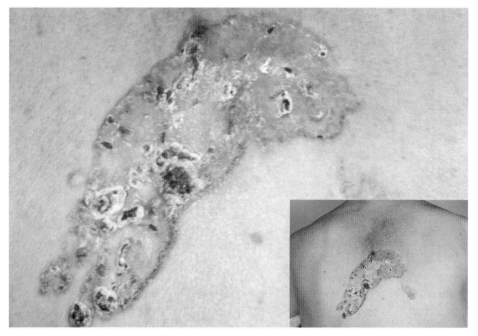

Fig. 8.27a & b (inset) Large superficial BCC which has been present for more than 10 years.

SUPERFICIAL BASAL CELL CARINOMA

On the trunk basal cell carcinomas often spread superficially and slowly over several years, presenting as a flat scaly plaque (Fig. 8.27). The edge of the lesion is just like a BCC elsewhere with a slightly raised, rolled edge; this can be seen more easily if the skin is put on the stretch (Fig. 1.81, p. 16). The centre of the lesion may be scaly and can be confused with Bowen's disease, or even eczema. A biopsy will distinguish between them.

TREATMENT SUPERFICIAL BASAL CELL CARCINOMA

If the lesion is small excision is the best option. Lesions bigger than 2cm or where excision is difficult can be treated with one of the following:–

1. Photodynamic therapy using methyl aminolaevulinate (*Metvix*) cream and a red light source (*see* p. 51).
2. Imiquimod 5% (*Aldara*) cream 3 times a week for up to 12 weeks.

Both produce an inflammatory reaction leading to resolution of the lesion (for imiquimod *see* p. 258).

BOWEN'S DISEASE

Bowen's disease is an intra-epidermal squamous cell carcinoma (*in-situ*). It presents as a fixed red scaly plaque which looks like psoriasis or eczema. It does not respond to treatment with topical steroids but gradually expands in size over many months. It can occur on any sun exposed site but characteristically occurs on the lower legs. Multiple lesions are common. Change to an invasive squamous cell carcinoma is uncommon and only occurs after many years.

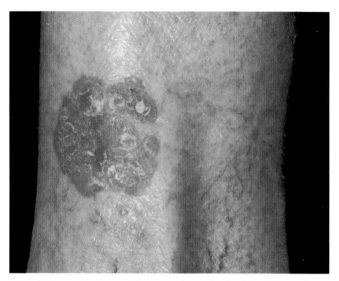

Fig. 8.28 Bowen's disease. Plaque on lower leg looking like psoriasis.

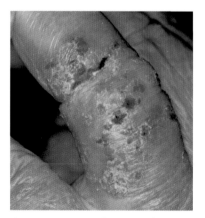

Fig. 8.29a Bowen's disease on finger.

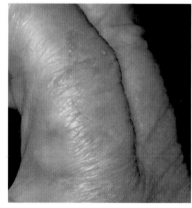

Fig. 8.29b After 4 weeks treatment with 5-fluorouracil cream.

TREATMENT BOWEN'S DISEASE

The options for treatment include:–

1. Cryotherapy
2. 5-fluorouracil (*Efudix*[UK]/*Effudex*[USA]) cream b.i.d. for 4 weeks (*see* p. 291)
3. Imiquimod (*Aldara*) cream 3 times a week for 12 weeks (*see also* p. 258)
4. Photodynamic therapy (*see* p. 51)
5. Curettage and cautery
6. Excision

Which you choose will depend on the size and site of the lesion, what facilities are available and the convenience of the patient. Care should be taken on the lower legs because all these options can lead to leg ulceration.

PAGET'S DISEASE OF THE NIPPLE

This is due to invasion of the skin around the nipple by malignant cells derived from an intraductal carcinoma. There is a unilateral red scaly plaque surrounding the nipple with or without crusting. It gradually increases in size and is often mistaken for eczema. The fact that is it unilateral and does not respond to topical steroids should alert you to the diagnosis which can be confirmed by a skin biopsy. Patients should be referred to a breast surgeon.

ECZEMA OF THE NIPPLE & AREOLA

Eczema of the areola and nipple is much more common than Paget's disease and may or may not be associated with atopic eczema. A red scaly itchy rash confined to the nipple and areola of one or both breasts is quite common in teenagers and young women particularly in Africans. Treatment is the same as for eczema elsewhere (*see* p. 208).

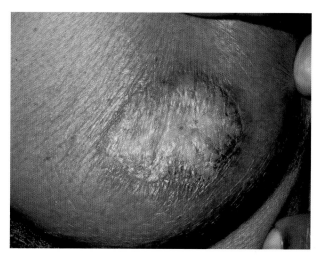

Fig. 8.30 Paget's disease of the nipple.

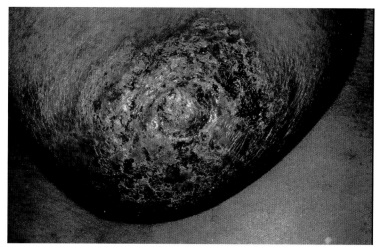

Fig. 8.31 Eczema of the nipple and areola in an African lady.

Trunk & limbs
Chronic erythematous rash
Scaly (or normal) surface
Multiple macules, papules, small patches & small plaques (all lesions <2cm)

SCRATCH LESIONS FIRMLY WITH NAIL, PALPATE WITH FINGER TIPS, NOTE COLOUR

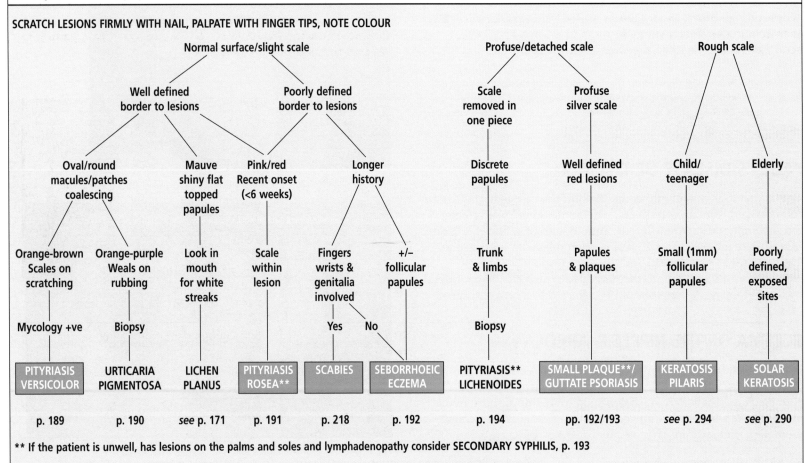

PITYRIASIS VERSICOLOR	URTICARIA PIGMENTOSA	LICHEN PLANUS	PITYRIASIS ROSEA**	SCABIES	SEBORRHOEIC ECZEMA	PITYRIASIS** LICHENOIDES	SMALL PLAQUE**/ GUTTATE PSORIASIS	KERATOSIS PILARIS	SOLAR KERATOSIS
p. 189	p. 190	*see* p. 171	p. 191	p. 218	p. 192	p. 194	pp. 192/193	*see* p. 294	*see* p. 290

** If the patient is unwell, has lesions on the palms and soles and lymphadenopathy consider SECONDARY SYPHILIS, p. 193

PITYRIASIS VERSICOLOR

The word pityriasis means 'bran-like' and here means a scaly rash; versicolor means different colours. Pityriasis versicolor is a scaly rash of different colours. In different individuals it may be white, orange-brown or dark brown. The lesions are small, less than 1cm in diameter, usually round and always scaly when scratched. Some may join together to form larger lesions or confluent plaques. It is a disease of young adults and occurs predominantly on the upper trunk. It is due to an infection with a yeast, *Pityrosporum orbiculare*, which we all have on our skin as a harmless commensal. Under certain conditions, the yeast produces hyphae and becomes pathogenic. It is then known as *Malassezia globosa*. The depigmentation is due to inhibition of tyrosinase by dicarboxylic acids produced by the *pityrosporum* yeast leading to suppression of melanin production.

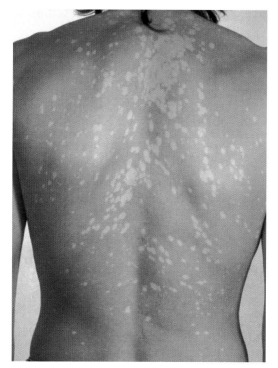

Fig. 8.32 Pityriasis versicolor, white variety.

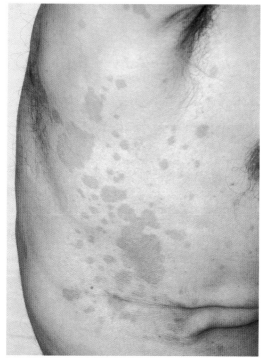

Fig. 8.33 Pityriasis versicolor, orange-brown colour.

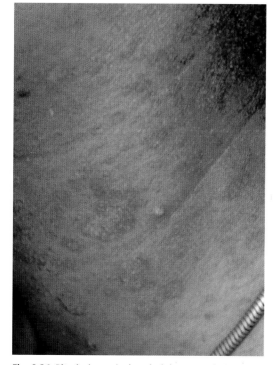

Fig. 8.34 Pityriasis versicolor, dark brown colour.

Most people with the rash have picked up the pathogenic form of the organism from someone else with it when on holiday in a warm climate; it is possible to transform your own commensal organisms if you are on steroids or other immunosuppressive therapy.

The orange-brown variety can be confused with pityriasis rosea but the diagnosis can be easily confirmed by scraping off the scales, mixing them with a mixture of equal parts of 20% potassium hydroxide solution and Parker blue-black ink. The organism takes up the blue colour of the ink and shows both spores and hyphae.

TREATMENT PITYRIASIS VERSICOLOR

If the rash is localised use an imidazole cream such as clotrimazole b.i.d. for 2 weeks. If it is extensive then a single dose of ketaconazole 400mg works well. An alternative is itraconazole 100 mg/day for 5 days. Griseofulvin and terbinafine do **not** work.

It is important to tell the patient that any hypopigmented areas will look the same after treatment. It usually takes 3 months for the pigment to return to normal. Patients with the pigmented variety will look normal immediately after treatment.

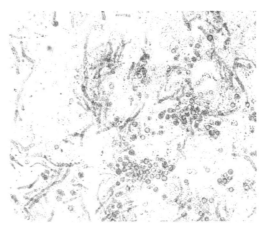

Fig. 8.35 Direct microscopy of scale in pityriasis versicolor ('spaghetti and meat balls').

URTICARIA PIGMENTOSA

This rare condition is due to increased mast cells in the skin. Orange-brown pigmented macules and small patches appear in children and young adults. The lesions may coalesce to form larger patches. The surface is not scaly but on rubbing a weal appears (Darier's sign) due to release of histamine from the mast cells. Most patients are asymptomatic but do not like the appearance of the rash; some patients may itch. Systemic symptoms of histamine release (flushing, headaches, dyspnoea, wheeze, diarrhoea or syncope) are extremely rare.

TREATMENT URTICARIA PIGMENTOSA

Avoid any mast cell degranulating agents (aspirin, alcohol, morphine, codeine). Antihistamines (both H_1 and H_2-antagonists) can be tried. If the patient is itching PUVA therapy is helpful and the tan it produces will mask the rash.

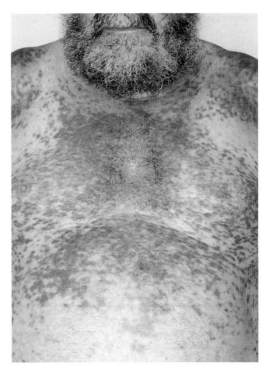

Fig. 8.36 Urticaria pigmentosa.

PITYRIASIS ROSEA

This condition is a viral infection due to the human herpes virus-7 (HHV-7). It occurs in otherwise fit and healthy children or young adults, and lasts about 6 weeks. First a single oval scaly plaque 2–3cm in diameter appears on the trunk or on a limb. This is the 'herald patch' which can sometimes be misdiagnosed as ringworm. A few days later, the rest of the rash appears. It consists of 2 different kinds of lesions; firstly petaloid lesions which are similar to the herald patch but smaller in size consisting of oval

Fig. 8.39 Pityriasis rosea. Scale within lesion and small follicular papules.

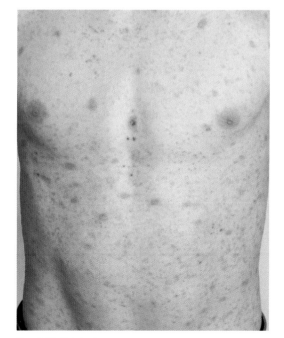

Fig. 8.37 Pityriasis rosea.

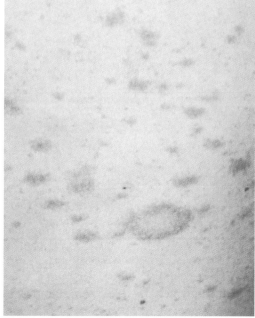

Fig. 8.38 Pityriasis rosea on the trunk of a young adult; herald patch and numerous petaloid lesions.

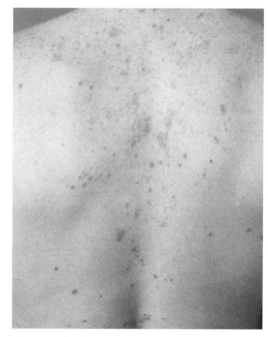

Fig. 8.40 Seborrhoeic eczema with scattered papules and small plaques on the back.

pink scaly papules or plaques where the scale is just inside the edge of the lesion, and secondly small pink follicular papules.

If the herald patch is on the trunk, the rest of the rash is confined to the vest and pants area, and the individual lesions follow Langer's lines giving a 'Christmas tree' pattern. If the herald patch is on a limb, the rash may be mainly on the limbs; if the herald patch is on the neck, most of the rash may be on the face and trunk.

TREATMENT PITYRIASIS ROSEA

It is usually asymptomatic and needs no treatment other than reassurance that it is harmless and will get better on its own in about 6 weeks. If it is particularly itchy you can use calamine lotion or 1% hydrocortisone cream b.i.d.

SEBORRHOEIC ECZEMA

There is a pattern of seborrhoeic eczema that is similar to pityriasis rosea. The clue to the diagnosis is that it has been present for more than 6 weeks and there is other evidence of seborrhoeic eczema such as scaling around the nasolabial folds (p. 118) and on the scalp (p. 74).

SMALL PLAQUE PSORIASIS

Psoriasis can be composed of multiple small plaques. This is not the same as guttate psoriasis where all the lesions are the same size. Here the plaques are of different sizes and do not get better spontaneously. *See* pp. 197 & 199 for treatment.

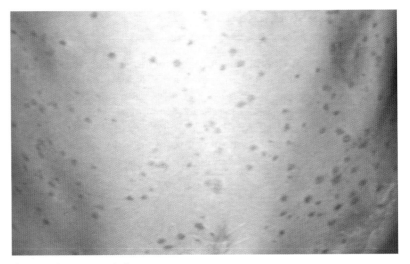

Fig. 8.41 Guttate psoriasis.

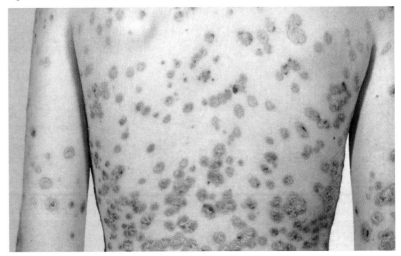

Fig. 8.42 Small plaque psoriasis.

GUTTATE PSORIASIS

This is an acute form of psoriasis that appears suddenly 10–14 days after a streptococcal sore throat. The individual lesions are typical of psoriasis, being bright red and well demarcated with silvery scaling, but all the lesions are uniformly small (0.5–1.0cm in diameter). The rash may be very widespread, appearing more or less overnight. It gets better spontaneously after 2–3 months. It may be the first manifestation of psoriasis or it can occur in someone who has had psoriasis for years. Since it is usually not itchy, it can be confused with pityriasis rosea and secondary syphilis. For treatment *see* p. 199.

SECONDARY SYPHILIS

Secondary syphilis occurs about 6 weeks after a primary infection with *Treponema pallidum*. The skin lesions are preceded by a flu-like illness and painless lymphadenopathy. The rash is very variable and may consist of macules, papules, pustules and plaques ranging in colour from pink to mauve, orange to brown. There are often lesions on the palms and soles, patchy alopecia and flat warty lesions on the genitalia and perianal skin (condylomata lata, *see* p. 313). The diagnosis can be confirmed by a +ve VDRL which distinguishes it from all the other non-itchy rashes on the skin.

TREATMENT SYPHILIS

Give a single dose of benzathine penicillin 2.4 megaunits intramuscularly or if allergic to penicillin use erythromycin 500mg 6 hourly for 21 days. Patients with syphilis should be seen in a department of genitourinary medicine so that other sexually transmitted diseases and HIV infection can also be screened for and any sexual contacts traced.

PITYRIASIS LICHENOIDES ACUTA

This rash is uncommon and presents with a polymorphic rash – pink papules, necrotic papules, some with ulceration and crusting on the surface (Fig. 8.45). Some lesions may be scaly like those found in the chronic form.

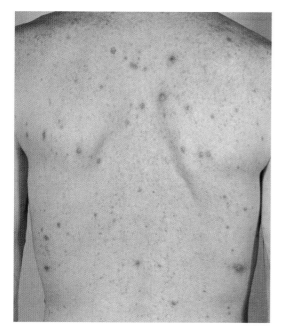

Fig. 8.43 Secondary syphilis. Rash on trunk.

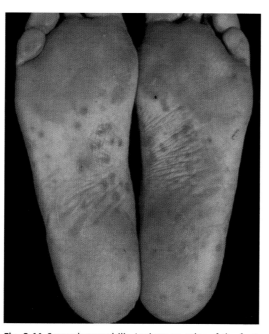

Fig. 8.44 Secondary syphilis. Lesions on soles of the feet.

PITYRIASIS LICHENOIDES CHRONICA

This rash is probably quite common but is rarely recognised by non-dermatologists. It consists of widepread small red-brown scaly papules, from which the scale can be 'picked off' in one piece (the 'mica scale'). It occurs mainly in children and young adults and lasts for several months. It often improves in the sun.

TREATMENT PITYRIASIS LICHENOIDES

This responds well to ultraviolet light. In the summer the patient can get out into the sunshine and expose the affected skin for half an hour each day. Alternatively UVB 3 times a week for 6–8 weeks clears it up. Rarely PUVA treatment needs to be given (p. 49). Tetracycline 500mg 4 times a day for 3 weeks may also be helpful in adults.

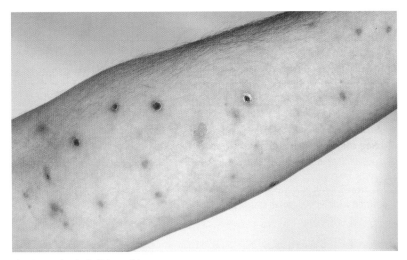

Fig. 8.45 Pityriasis lichenoides acuta.

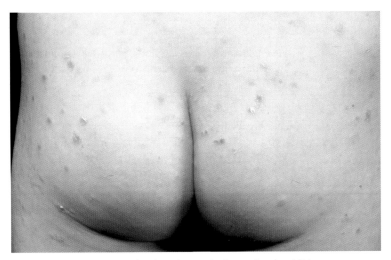

Fig. 8.46 Pityriasis lichenoides chronica on the buttocks of a child.

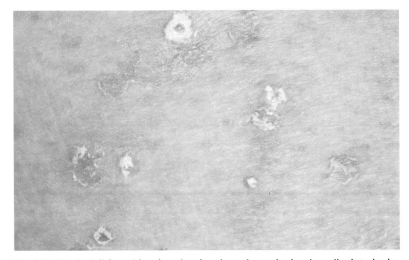

Fig. 8.47 Pityriasis lichenoides chronica showing mica scale that is easily detached.

Trunk & limbs
Chronic erythematous rash
Scaly surface
Large plaques (>2cm) present (lesions <2cm may be present as well)

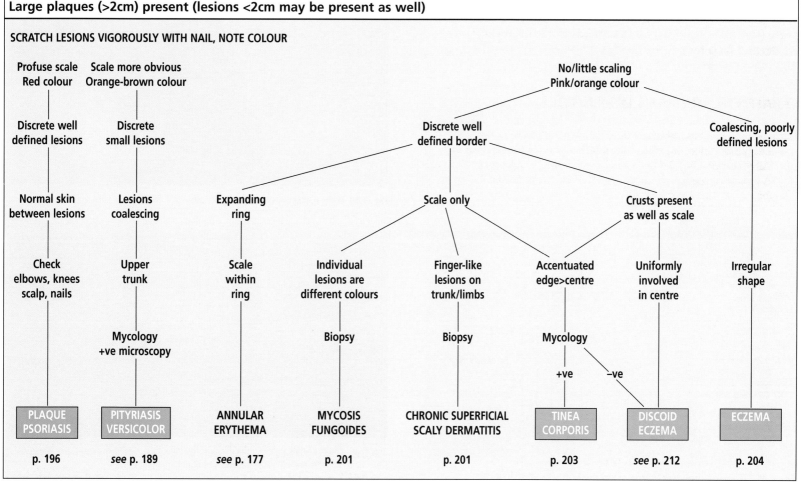

SCRATCH LESIONS VIGOROUSLY WITH NAIL, NOTE COLOUR

Profuse scale / Red colour → Discrete well defined lesions → Normal skin between lesions → Check elbows, knees scalp, nails → **PLAQUE PSORIASIS** — p. 196

Scale more obvious / Orange-brown colour → Discrete small lesions → Lesions coalescing → Upper trunk → Mycology +ve microscopy → **PITYRIASIS VERSICOLOR** — see p. 189

No/little scaling / Pink/orange colour

Expanding ring → Scale within ring → **ANNULAR ERYTHEMA** — see p. 177

Discrete well defined border

Scale only → Individual lesions are different colours → Biopsy → **MYCOSIS FUNGOIDES** — p. 201

Finger-like lesions on trunk/limbs → Biopsy → **CHRONIC SUPERFICIAL SCALY DERMATITIS** — p. 201

Accentuated edge>centre → Mycology → +ve → **TINEA CORPORIS** — p. 203

Crusts present as well as scale

Uniformly involved in centre → −ve → **DISCOID ECZEMA** — see p. 212

Coalescing, poorly defined lesions → Irregular shape → **ECZEMA** — p. 204

CHRONIC PLAQUE PSORIASIS

Psoriasis is a common disease which affects about 2% of the population worldwide. The inheritance of psoriasis is probably controlled by several genes, so that the occurrence within families is variable. It may be precipitated by hormonal changes, infection (e.g. streptococcal sore throat), trauma and emotional stress.

It can occur at any age but most often begins between the ages of 15 and 25 years. The clinical features can be explained by the pathology (Fig. 8.48). The lesions are bright red in colour, have clearly defined borders (edges) and a silvery scale. The scale becomes more obviously silvery when scratched (*see* Figs 1.45 & 1.46, p. 11), and the scale comes off easily and may make a mess on the floor.

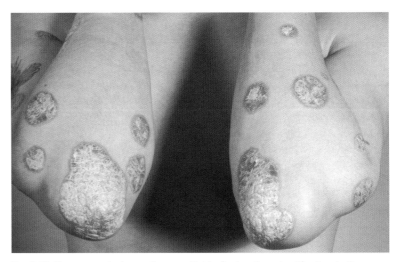

Fig. 8.49 Plaque psoriasis on elbows suitable for treatment with vitamin D₃ analogues or dithranol.

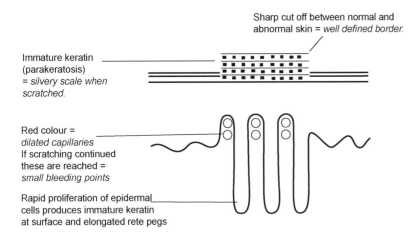

Fig. 8.48 Correlation of pathology of psoriasis with physical signs.

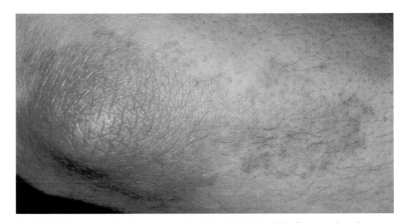

Fig. 8.50 Treatment of elbow psoriasis with calcitriol, which flattens the plaque and removes the scale, but often leaves residual erythema.

Characteristically the lesions are symmetrical, commonly affecting the elbows, knees, sacral area and lower legs, but any part of the skin can be involved including the scalp and nails. Most patients only have a few plaques but psoriasis can become very extensive. A small proportion of patients will have involvement of their joints as well (psoriatic arthropathy). The severity of the psoriatic arthropathy is often unrelated to the extent of the skin disease.

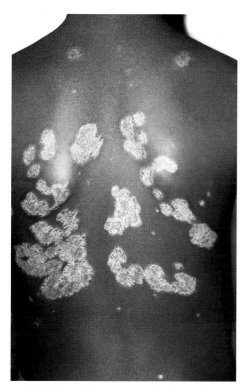

Fig. 8.51 Psoriasis in black skin. Note prominent silver scale but little erythema.

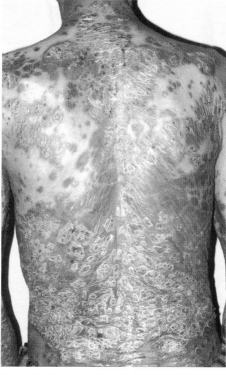

Fig. 8.52 Widespread psoriasis which requires ultraviolet light treatment or systemic therapy.

TREATMENT PLAQUE PSORIASIS

Treatment of psoriasis on the face, trunk and limbs depends on the **type**, **size** and **number** of lesions. The options for treatment are:–

FEW LARGE PLAQUES – topical treatment with:–
- Salicylic acid ointment or emollients
- Vitamin D_3 analogues
- Dithranol
- Tar
- Topical steroids
- Retinoids
- Lasers – excimer and pulsed dye lasers, *see* pp. 52–54

MULTIPLE SMALL PLAQUES, p. 199
- Emollients
- Tar
- UVB

EXTENSIVE LARGE PLAQUES, p. 200
- Out-patient or home narrow-band UVB
- In-patient or day treatment with tar (Goekerman's)
- In-patient or day treatment with dithranol (Ingram's)
- Systemic therapy (see below)

SYSTEMIC TREATMENT, p. 201
- PUVA, methotrexate, acitretin, ciclosporin, azathioprine, hydroxycarbamide (hydroxyurea)

TREATMENT PSORIASIS – FEW LARGE PLAQUES

1. SALICYLIC ACID & MOISTURISERS

Many patients are content to reduce the scaling of psoriasis with emollients or salicylic acid ointment (2–10%).

2. VITAMIN D₃ ANALOGUES

- Calcitriol (*Silkis*) ointment apply b.i.d.
- Calcipotriol[UK]/calcipotriene[USA] (*Dovonex*) cream or ointment apply b.i.d.
- Tacalcitol (*Curatoderm*) ointment apply once daily

These are the first-line treatment for most patients with psoriasis because they are not messy to use. The main problem is that they can irritate the skin of the face and flexures (calcitriol less so than the others). An improvement in the rash should begin to be seen in 2–4 weeks. Three-quarters of patients improve but complete clearance is likely in only 10%. In the remainder the plaques become flat and red, but do not completely clear (*see* Fig. 8.50).

They can be combined with a potent[UK]/group 2–3[USA] topical steroid (applied separately or as *Dovobet* = calcipotriol + betamethasone dipropionate). The combination is more effective than the vitamin D₃ analogue alone, but it should not be used for more than 4 weeks because of the long-term side effects of topical steroids.

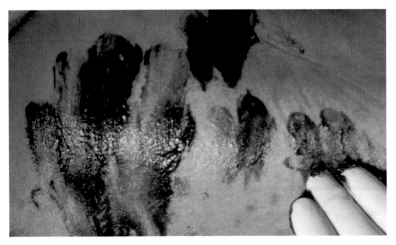

Fig. 8.53 Application of crude coal tar ointment.

3. DITHRANOL[UK]/ANTHRALIN[USA]

Dithranol[UK]/anthralin[USA] is a synthetic derivative of anthracene. It is a yellow powder which can be made up into a cream, ointment or paste. The major problems with dithranol are:–

- irritation and burning of normal skin
- brown discolouration of the skin and mauve/purple staining of the patient's clothes which will not wash out.

It needs to be applied carefully to the individual plaques without getting it on the surrounding normal skin and so is used mainly when there are a few large plaques of psoriasis. There are two ways of using dithranol:–

1. **Short contact therapy**. Start with the 0.1% cream (*Dithrocream*[UK]/ *Drithocreme*[USA]) and apply by rubbing it carefully on to the individual plaques. Leave on for 30 minutes and then wash off with soap and water. If no irritation occurs, the strength of dithranol cream can be increased every 2–3 days from 0.1% to 0.25%, to 0.5%, to 1.0% and finally to 2%. When the psoriatic plaques go brown (*see* Fig. 8.54) stop using the treatment. The brown colour fades after 7–10 days. Alternatively use *Micanol* 1% & 3% cream, *Antra-Derm*[USA] or *Psorin*[UK] ointment.

2. In **Lassar's paste** *see* p. 200.

4. COAL TAR

For very superficial or very numerous small plaques of psoriasis tar is easier to use than dithranol because it can be rubbed all over the skin without taking any special care (Fig. 8.53). For superficial plaques use a proprietary cream containing coal tar solution (*see* p. 30). For thicker plaques crude coal tar* can be used. This is very messy and is usually used in a day care unit or as an in-patient (*see* p. 200).

*Available from Martindale Pharmaceuticals; Tel: 0800 137627.

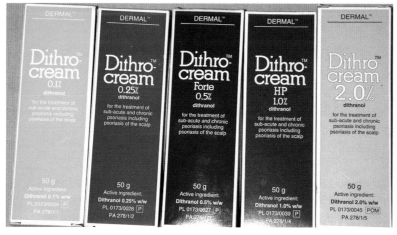

Fig. 8.54 Dithranol (Anthralin) staining.

Fig. 8.55 Strengths of Dithrocream^{UK}/Drithocreme^{USA}.

5. TOPICAL STEROIDS

Ideally topical steroids should be avoided completely in psoriasis because of the risk of causing a rebound of the psoriasis or even generalised pustular psoriasis on stopping. There are also all the dangers of long-term use which is inevitable in a chronic condition like psoriasis (*see* p. 28). They therefore should only be used on small areas of psoriasis, in the flexures (*see* p. 301) or on the scalp (*see* p. 74).

6. TOPICAL RETINOIDS

A topical retinoid, 0.05% & 0.1% tazarotene gel or cream (*Zorac*^{UK}/ *Tazorac*^{USA}) applied b.i.d. works by modifying abnormal epidermal differentiation. It can be effective but like all topical retinoids produces marked skin irritation. This can be reduced by applying it once daily.

TREATMENT PSORIASIS – GUTTATE & SMALL PLAQUE

For guttate psoriasis reassurance that it will clear in 2–3 months is all that is needed. If it is itchy use an emollient such as Aqueous cream^{UK}/ hydrophilic ointment^{USA} p.r.n.

Ultra-violet light therapy (*see* p. 48) or a tar cream are the most useful treatments when the patient has very numerous small plaques of psoriasis. Unfortunately refined coal tars (coal tar solution/liquor picis carbonis^{UK}/liquor carbonis detergens^{USA}) are not very effective. Crude coal tar works much better but is too messy for use at home, but can be used as part of day care treatment in a dermatology department.

TREATMENT PSORIASIS – EXTENSIVE LARGE PLAQUES

1. ULTRAVIOLET LIGHT THERAPY

Narrowband ultraviolet light therapy or PUVA are effective treatments for extensive larger plaque psoriasis, but the lifetime dose of treatment should be restricted (*see* p. 48).

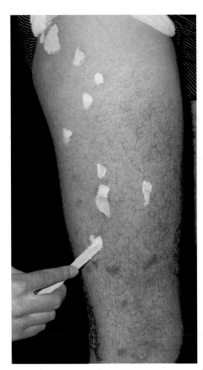

Fig. 8.56 Application of dithranol in Lassar's paste to plaques of psoriasis.

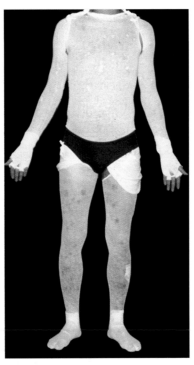

Fig. 8.57 Tubigauze suit covering the paste-treated skin to protect clothing.

2. DAY CARE OR IN-PATIENT TREATMENT

Ingram's or Goerckerman's regimen

1. Tar bath. The patient soaks in a bath containing 20–30ml of a tar emulsion (*Balnatar, Lavatar*[USA], *Polytar, Zetar*[USA]) for 10–15 minutes. While in the bath the scales can be rubbed off with a soft brush.

2. Ultraviolet light therapy. After getting out of the bath and patting dry the skin, the patient is exposed to a sub-erythema dose of UVB (*see* p. 48).

3a. INGRAM'S REGIMEN – Dithranol[UK]/anthralin[USA] in Lassar's paste is applied carefully to each psoriatic plaque (Fig. 8.56) and left on for 24 hours. Over a 3–4 week period the concentration of dithranol is gradually increased. Start with 0.1% dithranol and increase daily by increments of 0.1% up to 1% and then by increments of 1% up to 10%. Talcum powder is applied to the surface of the paste to stop it being smudged. The body is covered with *Tubigauze* or *Tubefast* to prevent staining of clothes and bedding (Fig. 8.57). The paste needs to be removed the next day with arachis oil.

Alternatively you can use:–

3b. GOERKERMAN'S REGIMEN – 2% crude coal tar in white soft paraffin or Lassar's paste is applied to the psoriasis and covered by a tubular dressing. The strength of tar is increased to 20% gradually over a 3–4 week period. 2% or 5% crude coal tar in Lassar's paste is a very effective treatment for psoriasis of the face.

4. The next morning (or later that day for day treatment) the paste is cleaned off with arachis oil or liquid paraffin[UK]/petrolatum[USA]. Tar ointment can be removed with ordinary soap and water.

5. Repeat the process daily until the psoriasis has cleared. It is usually possible to clear psoriasis in 3–4 weeks by these methods.

Do not use tar or dithranol in the flexures or in acutely erupting, erythrodermic or generalised pustular psoriasis.

TREATMENT PSORIASIS – SYSTEMIC THERAPY

Patients who fail to respond to in-patient or day unit treatment, frequently relapse or have very extensive disease require systemic treatment. The following are available:–

- PUVA (p. 49)
- Methotrexate (p. 43)
- Acitretin (p. 41)
- Ciclosporin (p. 44)
- Azathioprine (p. 45)
- Hydroxycarbamide (hydroxyurea, p. 45).

These all have serious side effects so should only be initiated by a dermatologist.

Newer drugs such as the anti-diabetic glitazones (e.g. pioglitazone 30mg daily), the fumaric acid esters (e.g. *Fumaderm*) which are available in Germany, and the biologicals such as alefacept (*Amevive*), efalizumab (*Rapitiva*), etanercept (*Enbrel*) and infliximab (*Remicade*), are available from dermatologists with a special interest in the treatment of psoriasis (*see* p. 45).

CHRONIC SUPERFICIAL SCALY DERMATITIS (Digitate dermatitis)

A pink scaly rash with oblong or finger-shaped patches/plaques around the trunk. The surface has a fine 'cigarette paper' wrinkling. It is usually asymptomatic. It differs from mycosis fungoides in that the lesions are all the same colour and a biopsy will show eczema and not a lymphoma.

TREATMENT SUPERFICIAL SCALY DERMATITIS

If it itches UVB phototherapy will stop the itching temporarily, but will not make the rash go away. It is given 2–3 times a week for 6–8 weeks. Topical steroids tend not to work.

Fig. 8.58 Chronic superficial dermatitis – note finger-shaped patches.

MYCOSIS FUNGOIDES

This uncommon disease is a T-cell lymphoma confined to the skin. It presents as itchy red scaly patches (Figs 8.59 & 8.60) that may mimic either eczema or psoriasis. The main differentiating feature is that individual lesions are of different colours, so that some patches are pink, others red or orangy-brown. The patches become more indurated to form plaques (Fig. 8.61). These stages of mycosis fungoides may persist for many years (>20 years).

Late in the course of the disease tumours develop (Fig. 8.62) from the plaques. The disease may then spread to other organs of the body and become more aggressive. The diagnosis is confirmed by skin biopsy and PCR to show that the abnormal cells are monoclonal.

TREATMENT MYCOSIS FUNGOIDES

All patients should be referred to a dermatologist for confirmation of the diagnosis. In the patches or plaque stage the options are:–

- A moderately potent[UK]/group 4–5[USA] topical steroid ointment or cream may be all that is needed for many years. This will alleviate the itching and keep the patient comfortable.
- PUVA (p. 49) given twice weekly for 8–10 weeks may make the rash go away for a period of months or years.

Once tumours have developed, radiotherapy or chemotherapy will be needed.

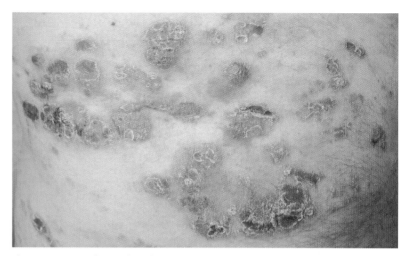

Fig. 8.61 Mycosis fungoides, plaque stage.

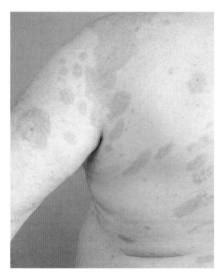

Fig. 8.59 Mycosis fungoides, patch stage.

Fig. 8.60 Close up of a patch.

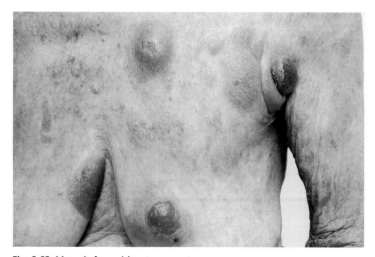

Fig. 8.62 Mycosis fungoides, tumour stage.

TINEA CORPORIS (Ringworm)

Ringworm of the body is due to dermatophyte fungi of the *Microsporum*, *Trichophyton* and *Epidermophyton* species. Dermatophytes live on keratin so the clinical picture is of one or more pink scaly papules or plaques, which gradually extend outwards healing from the centre, forming a ring. You should consider the diagnosis in any asymmetrical red scaly rash. If the lesion is viewed from a distance of about 6 feet, there is a definite border consisting of increased scaling or papules; outside this the skin is normal (*see also* Fig. 1.78, p. 16).

TREATMENT TINEA CORPORIS

Since the infection is in the keratin layer on the surface of the skin, topical treatment works better than systemic therapy. The options are:–

- Whitfield's ointment applied twice a day until the rash is clear and then for a further 2 weeks. This is the cheapest option.
- An imidazole cream applied twice a day for 2 weeks (*see also* p. 32).
- Terbinafine (*Lamisil*) cream applied daily for 7–10 days.

It is acceptable practice to treat a scaly rash which you think is due to a fungal infection with an anti-fungal cream **provided** you first take scrapings to be sent for mycology (*see* p. 19) where the fungal hyphae can be visualised by direct microscopy (*see* Fig. 10.03, p. 299) and cultured. The patient can be followed up after 4 weeks when the result of the mycology is known. If the mycology is –ve and the rash no better you should reconsider the diagnosis.

It is bad practice to treat scaly rashes with antifungal–steroid combinations to 'hedge your bets'. The steroid may make the fungal infection worse, and eczema will respond better to a moderately potent[UK]/group 4–5[USA] topical steroid alone.

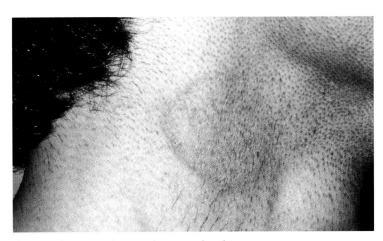

Fig. 8.63 Tinea corporis on neck; an annular plaque.

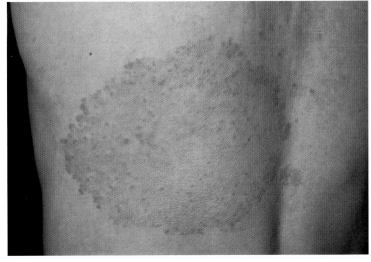

Fig. 8.64 Tinea corporis on back. Note well defined accentuated border.

Face, trunk & limbs
Chronic eczema

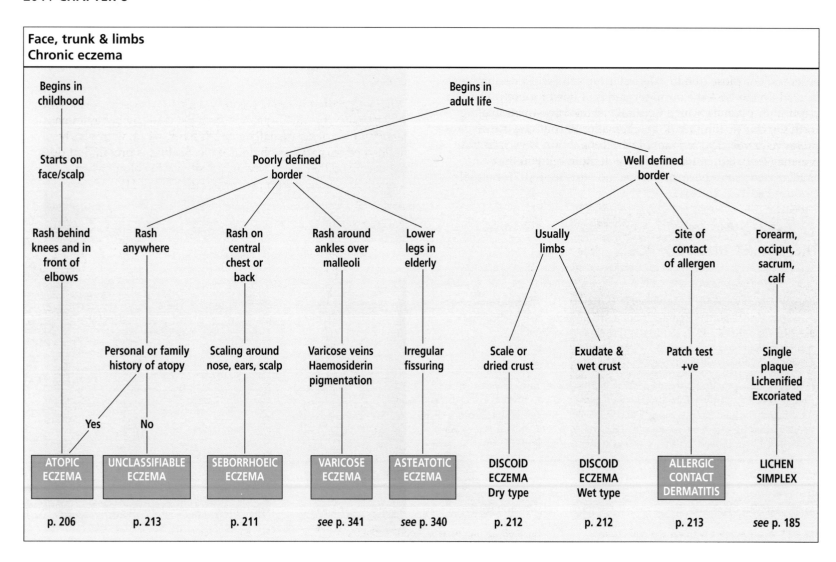

ATOPIC ECZEMA	UNCLASSIFIABLE ECZEMA	SEBORRHOEIC ECZEMA	VARICOSE ECZEMA	ASTEATOTIC ECZEMA	DISCOID ECZEMA Dry type	DISCOID ECZEMA Wet type	ALLERGIC CONTACT DERMATITIS	LICHEN SIMPLEX
p. 206	p. 213	p. 211	see p. 341	see p. 340	p. 212	p. 212	p. 213	see p. 185

CHRONIC ECZEMA/DERMATITIS

In this book the term eczema is used for the endogenous eczemas. For those due to external factors the word dermatitis is used. In the USA the term dermatitis is used for both. The word *eczema* comes from a Greek word meaning to bubble through, and the hall mark of eczema (or dermatitis) is the presence of vesicles. In practice vesicles are only seen in acute eczema (*see* p. 89), but the patient will often tell you that small blisters have been present in the past (*see* Fig. 7.24, p. 165),

and the remains of these are seen as small pinhead sized crusts.

What you normally see is a poorly defined pink scaly rash which is very itchy. It is distinguished from psoriasis by being much less vivid in colour (usually a nondescript pink), with poorly defined edges and less obvious scale. Scaling is present but does not become either more obvious or silvery in colour when scratched (compare with psoriasis, Fig. 1.46, p. 11).

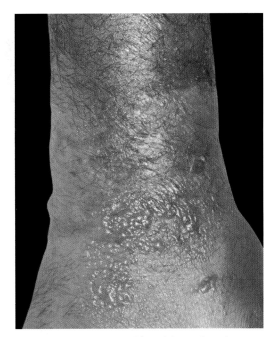

Fig. 8.65 Acute eczema with vesicles and erosions.

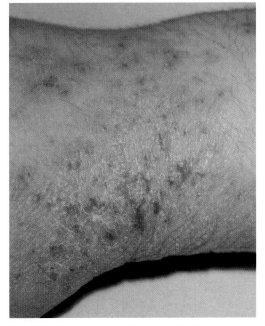

Fig. 8.66 Chronic eczema. Poorly defined pink plaques with surface scale and crust.

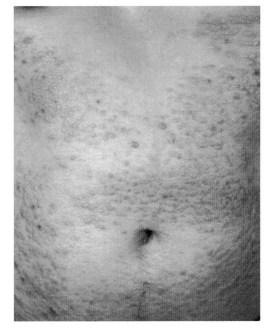

Fig. 8.67 Lichenified eczema.

ATOPIC ECZEMA

Atopy means an inherited predisposition to eczema, asthma or hay fever, and atopic individuals may have one or all of these manifestations. The eczema usually begins between the ages of 3 and 12 months, the asthma at age 3–4 years and the hay fever in the teens.

In infancy the eczema often begins on the scalp and face, and may or may not spread to involve the rest of the body. When children get older it may localise in the flexures, particularly the popliteal and antecubital fossae. It is very itchy so excoriations and lichenification may be seen, and if children rub rather than

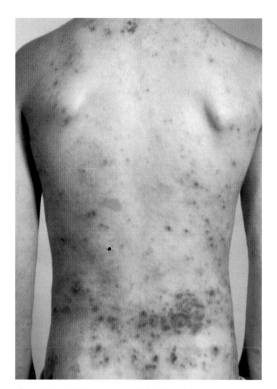

Fig. 8.68 Atopic eczema. Widespread excoriated lesions on the trunk.

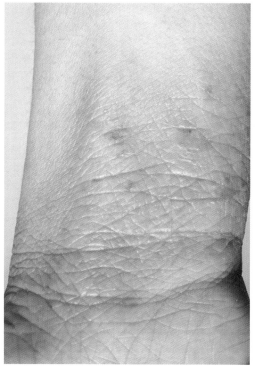

Fig. 8.69 Atopic eczema. Lichenification at wrist due to continual scratching.

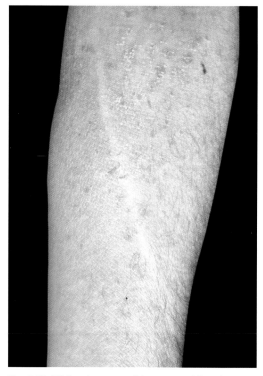

Fig. 8.70 White dermographism – scratching the eczematous skin produces a white line.

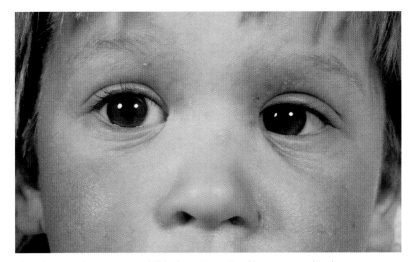

Fig. 8.71 Atopic eczema on child's face. Note the skin crease under the eyes.

scratch, the nails may become very shiny. 50% of such children will also have ichthyosis (dry scaly skin) with increased skin markings on the palms and soles. In 90% of children the eczema will clear spontaneously by puberty, but in a small minority it will persist into adult life. A few of these will have very extensive and troublesome eczema.

In adults a diagnosis of atopic eczema can be made if there is a history of infantile eczema, or if they also have or have had asthma, hay fever, ichthyosis, increased skin markings on the palms and soles or white dermographism (stroke gently with your finger nail through an area of eczema: after 30 seconds a white line appears, *see* Fig. 8.70). A positive history of atopic eczema or asthma in the immediate family (parents, siblings, children) is further evidence of atopy.

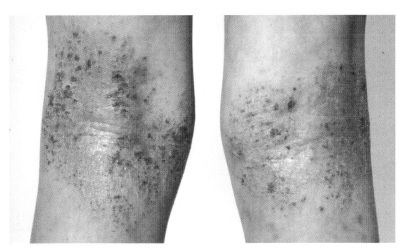

Fig. 8.72 Atopic eczema localised to the popliteal fossae.

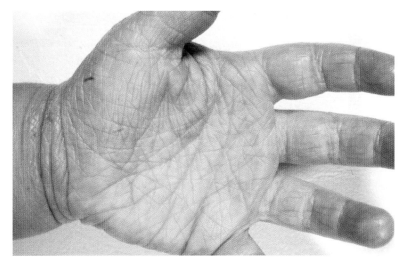

Fig. 8.73 Increased palmar markings in patient with ichthyosis vulgaris.

TREATMENT ATOPIC ECZEMA

Consider the following when planning treatment of atopic eczema:–

1. If the skin is dry – use emollients.
2. For the eczema itself – treat with topical steroids or topical immune-modulators.
3. If the patient is awake at night – use a sedative antihistamine.
4. If the eczema is weeping – dry it up with potassium permanganate or aluminium acetate soaks (p. 26).
5. If there is infection – use a systemic antibiotic.
6. Other considerations – diet, clothing, life-style, stress.
7. Wet wraps are useful in controlling acute flare ups or in preventing excessive scratching in young children.

1. EMOLLIENTS (MOISTURISERS)

Emollients are an important part of treatment if the patient has a dry skin as well as eczema. Soaking in a lukewarm bath for 10–15 minutes every day is helpful provided 10–20mls of one of the dispersable bath oils has been added (e.g. *Alpha Keri*[USA], *Aveeno*, *Balneum*[UK], *Dermol 500*[UK], *Diprobath*[UK], *Lubriderm*[USA], *Oilatum*). Aqueous cream[UK]/hydrophilic ointment[USA], or *Epaderm* may be used instead of soap for washing. If the patient wants something that looks like soap they can use *Aveeno*, *Oilatum* or *Sebamed* bars.

Topical emollients can be applied to the skin after getting out of the bath while the skin is still warm and moist. They can also be applied frequently during the day. Numerous emollients are available ranging from the very greasy white soft paraffin[UK]/petrolatum[USA] to *Boots' E45*[UK] cream, *Dermol 500*[UK], *Diprobase*[UK], *Doublebase*[UK], *Eucerin*[USA], *Keri lotion*[USA] (water-in-oil creams), to aqueous cream[UK] and *Ponds*[USA] cream (non greasy oil-in-water creams).

2a. TOPICAL STEROIDS

Topical steroid ointments are still the mainstay of treatment for atopic eczema. Use the *weakest one that works*. Patients or parents are often afraid of using topical steroids because of the widespread publicity about side effects. In most cases this fear is unjustified, but *see* p. 28 for the side effects of topical steroids.

You will need to explain that there are different strengths of steroids (*see* p. 27) and that the low potent[UK]/group 6–7[USA] topical steroids, such as 1% hydrocortisone, will not harm the skin (even if used over a long period of time). Start with 1% hydrocortisone ointment applied twice a day. Do not use anything stronger than this on the face however bad the eczema is.

On the trunk and limbs, if 1% hydrocortisone ointment is not working, either add 10% urea to the hydrocortisone (*Alphaderm* cream, *Calmurid HC* cream), or use a moderately potent[UK]/group 4–5[USA] topical steroid ointment instead. In some instances short courses of potent[UK]/group 2–3[USA] steroids may in fact result in a lower cumulative dose than chronic use of a weaker steroid.

Prolonged use of topical steroids can lead to tachyphylaxis (it becomes progressively less effective). One way round this is to rest the skin for 2 days each week, i.e. use a topical steroid for 5 days followed by a moisturiser only for 2 days.

Ointments work much better than creams since the grease forms an occlusive barrier preventing evaporation of water and delivering the steroid more effectively to the skin. They are best applied immediately after a bath. It is important to give the patient enough ointment so that it can be used regularly. To cover the whole body surface, infants will need approximately 10gm a day (70gm/week), a 7 year old 20gm a day (140gm/week) and adults 30gm a day (210gm/week).

2b. TOPICAL IMMUNE-MODULATORS

These drugs work by blocking the molecular mechanisms of inflammation in the skin (*see* p. 29). Two drugs are available – tacrolimus 0.1% & 0.03% (*Protopic*) ointment and pimecrolimus 1% (*Elidel*) cream. Both can cause a burning/stinging sensation when first used which stops after about 20 minutes and disappears altogether after a few days. Because they are relatively new and expensive drugs, they are not recommended as the first-line treatment for atopic eczema. They are very useful in the following situations:–

- Patients who have not responded to topical steroids or who are using too much steroid or too strong a steroid.
- Patients who have been on topical steroids for years and have developed steroid side effects (*see* p. 28).
- Patients with poor compliance with topical steroids because they are afraid of the side effects.
- Patients in whom you would otherwise be considering systemic treatment.

3. ANTIHISTAMINES

Sedative antihistamines are useful if the child is not sleeping at night and keeping the family awake. They will not stop the itching, but if given in adequate dosage the child will sleep through the night. Start with 5ml of promethazine (*Phenergan* 5mg/5ml) or alimemazine (trimeprazine, *Vallergan* 7.5mg/5ml) elixir an hour before bedtime. Double the dose each night till the child sleeps till morning. *Vallergan forte* is available as 30mg/5ml. Children surprisingly can tolerate much higher doses than adults. Neither are addictive and are quite safe.

In adults start with 10mg of promethazine or alimemazine and double the dose as necessary till the patient sleeps through the night.

Non-sedative antihistamines (p. 40) generally are ineffective in treating eczema and should not be used.

4. ASTRINGENTS

Astringents (*see* p. 26) dry up exudate by coagulating protein. Soak the affected areas in one of these solutions by applying moistened gauze swabs or by immersion in a bath or hand basin.

5. TREATMENT OF SECONDARY INFECTION

If the eczema becomes suddenly worse, infection with *Staphylococcus aureus* may be the cause. There will be associated pustules or yellow crusting. This is best treated with a systemic antibiotic such as flucloxacillin 125–250mg q.i.d. (or erythromycin if the patient is allergic to penicillin). Do not use topical antibiotics as these are often ineffective and are likely to cause an allergic contact dermatitis. Likewise do not use topical steroid–antibiotic mixtures.

If the pustules are umbilicated consider eczema herpeticum (*see* p. 92).

6. OTHER CONSIDERATIONS

Special diets and involved methods of removing house dust mite from the house are not usually helpful. Allergy testing (prick, RAST) are useful in patients with hay fever and asthma but do not identify the allergens that may make atopic eczema worse. If any particular foodstuff or material makes eczema suddenly worse (usually within 30 minutes), it would be prudent to avoid this in the future.

Cotton clothing worn next to the skin is comfortable, while wool is irritating. Cotton gloves or even a cotton suit using tubifast bandages (Fig. 8.74) will help prevent skin damage from scratching.

Patient and parent support can be provided by specialised dermatological nurses, the local dermatology department or the National Eczema Society.

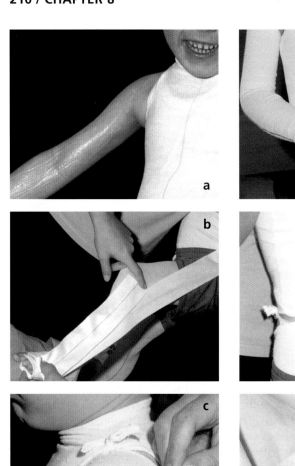

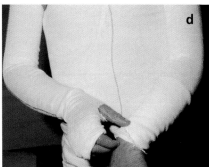

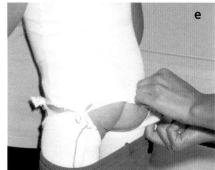

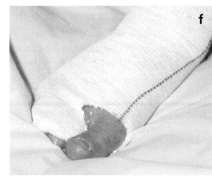

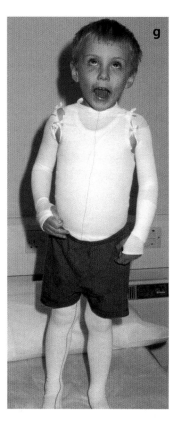

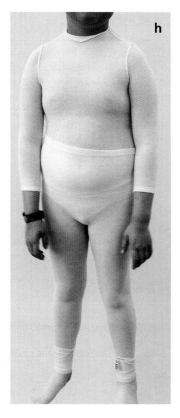

Fig. 8.74a Apply moisturiser thickly to skin.

Fig. 8.74b Measure out 1½ × length of arm & leg.

Fig. 8.74c Tie around shoulders.

Fig. 8.74d Cut hole for thumb and double back the layer of bandage.

Fig. 8.74e Tie around hips.

Fig. 8.74f Cut hole for big toe.

Fig. 8.74g Complete suit with pants over.

Fig. 8.74h Suit with arm/vest and pants/legs sewn together.

7. WET WRAPS

This is a bandaging technique which is useful for treating flares of atopic eczema. It improves the moisturisation of the skin, reduces the need for topical steroids and prevents scratching.

First the affected areas are treated with a topical steroid ointment, and then the whole body surface is covered with a suitable emollient (Fig. 8.74a). The limbs and trunk are wrapped in *Tubifast/Comfeel/Actifast* tubular bandages. Sizes are available for trunk, arms and legs suitable for adults and children (Fig. 8.75). Cut holes in the sides of the trunk bandage for the arms (Fig. 8.74a). Measure one and a half lengths for each arm and leg (Fig. 8.74b). The bandages next to the skin of the trunk and limbs are soaked in warm water and then put on. The arms and legs are tied onto the trunk bandage with small ties made by cutting 2cm strips from left over bandages (Fig. 8.74c & e). A second layer of dry bandage is put over the wet layer to prevent rapid drying. Holes are cut for the thumb and big toe to prevent the bandages slipping upwards (Fig. 8.74d & f).

In babies and infants a double layer is used for arms and legs. Half is moistened and twisted at the finger tips or toes and the dry portion is pulled back on itself and tied at the shoulders or hips. In this way the hands are covered and the child is unable to scratch directly with their finger nails. The face can be wrapped using the trunk (yellow line) bandage with holes cut for eyes, nose and mouth.

Instead of tubular bandages, moistened cotton pyjamas can be used.

Although an effective treatment, children do not like it and may need to be persuaded to wear them. However once they realise the benefit, compliance is usually better. This may be improved by using the recently available *Tubifast suits* with vest/arms and pants/legs already sewn together (Fig. 8.74h). They are more acceptable for children to wear and easier for mothers to put on.

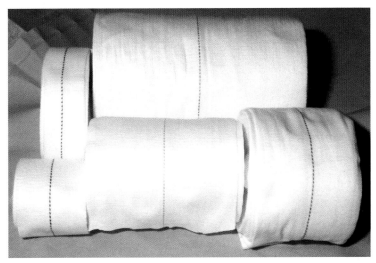

Fig. 8.75 Tubifast bandages:
Grey & yellow for trunk   Green for arms & legs (under age 5)
Blue for legs (over age 5)   Red for baby's arms

SEBORRHOEIC ECZEMA

Seborrhoeic eczema (dermatitis) is due to an overgrowth of pityrosporum yeasts in the skin. The diagnosis is made on the distribution of the rash. The scalp is always involved with scaling and/or redness. The eyebrows, eyelashes, external ears and naso-labial folds are often also involved (*see* p. 118). Pink or orangy-brown poorly defined scaly plaques are present on the centre of the chest or back (Fig. 8.76), and occasionally in the flexures. Alternatively a follicular rash is seen, sometimes with tiny pustules, affecting the back, shoulders and chest (pityrosporum folliculitis, *see* p. 174).

TREATMENT SEBORRHOEIC ECZEMA

Use an imidazole cream, e.g. ketoconazole (*Nizoral*), 1% hydrocortisone cream or a mixture of a topical imidazole plus hydrocortisone (*Daktacort, Canestan HC*). If this is ineffective you can give the imidazole orally (ketoconazole 200mg or itraconazole 100mg daily) for 2 weeks. There is a tendency for seborrhoeic eczema to come and go. Use the treatment when it is there and leave it off once it has cleared. Treat the scalp with ketoconazole shampoo (*see* p. 74).

DISCOID (Nummular) ECZEMA

This differs from other forms of eczema in that it presents as well demarcated round, oval or annular red scaly plaques. It can be wet or dry. The wet type consists of plaques made up of numerous vesicles which break to produce exudate and crust on the surface. The dry type is similar but has a scale as well as crust on the surface. In young adults the commonest site is the dorsum of hands and fingers. In older individuals it is more usual on the

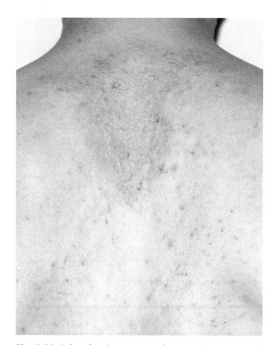

Fig. 8.76 Seborrhoeic eczema. Plaque in the centre of the upper back.

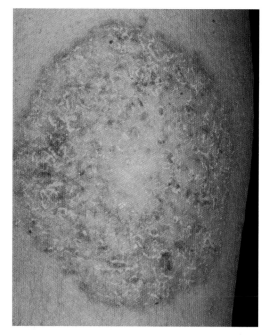

Fig. 8.77 Discoid eczema. Dry scaly plaque on the lower leg.

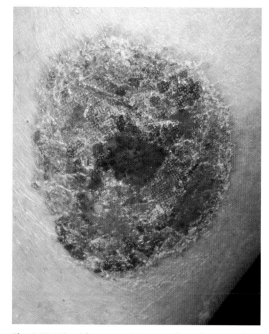

Fig. 8.78 Discoid eczema. Wet exuding plaque with surface crust on the calf.

lower legs. Some patients with atopic eczema, allergic contact dermatitis or unclassifiable eczema also have discoid plaques of eczema. Non-dermatologists often misdiagnose discoid eczema as tinea.

TREATMENT DISCOID ECZEMA

Use a potent[UK]/group 2–3[USA] topical steroid ointment applied b.i.d. The response is variable – sometimes discoid eczema can be quite resistant to treatment or relapse quickly on stopping topical steroids. If that is the case tar often works better. Try 2% crude coal tar in white soft paraffin[UK]/petrolatum[USA] but this is messy for the patient to use.

ALLERGIC CONTACT DERMATITIS

A well defined plaque of eczema may be due to contact with an allergen such as nickel in buckles or jean studs, colophony in elastoplast or chrome in leather straps. Creams containing parabens, antibiotics, antihistamines or even a topical steroid may also cause an allergic contact dermatitis.

UNCLASSIFIABLE ECZEMA

Any symmetrical eczema (diagnosis made by morphology of the lesions – ill-defined papules and plaques which tend to be variable in site and extent over time) on the trunk and limbs which does not fit one of the recognisable patterns (i.e. atopic, seborrhoeic, discoid, varicose, hand & foot) is called unclassifiable eczema. This is really quite common (for treatment, *see* atopic eczema, p. 208).

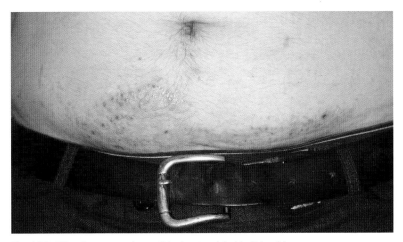

Fig. 8.79 Allergic contact dermatitis due to nickel belt buckle.

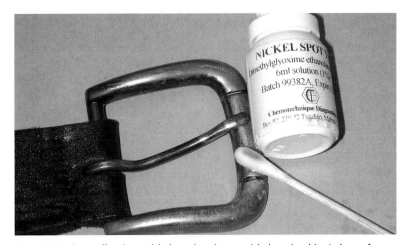

Fig. 8.80 Patients allergic to nickel can be given a nickel testing kit. A drop of dimethylglyoxime and ammonia on a cotton wool bud rubbed onto the buckle stains pink.

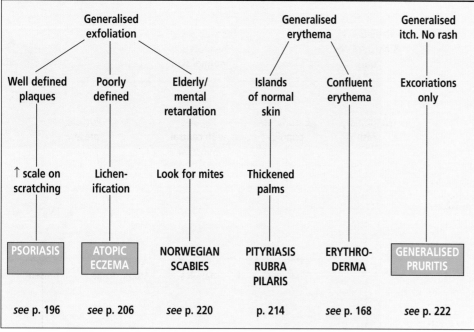

Trunk & limbs
Chronic erythematous rash
Normal or scaly surface
Generalised rash/itching (>50% body surface)

Generalised exfoliation			Generalised erythema		Generalised itch. No rash
Well defined plaques	Poorly defined	Elderly/ mental retardation	Islands of normal skin	Confluent erythema	Excoriations only
↑ scale on scratching	Lichen-ification	Look for mites	Thickened palms		
PSORIASIS	ATOPIC ECZEMA	NORWEGIAN SCABIES	PITYRIASIS RUBRA PILARIS	ERYTHRO-DERMA	GENERALISED PRURITIS
see p. 196	see p. 206	see p. 220	p. 214	see p. 168	see p. 222

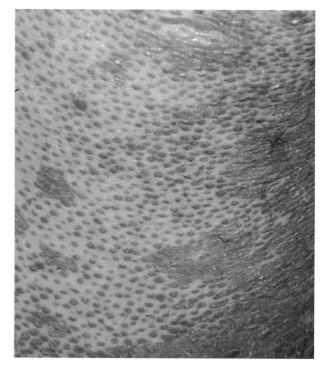

Fig. 8.81 Pityriasis rubra pilaris. Follicular macules and papules coalescing into generalised erythema.

PITYRIASIS RUBRA PILARIS

A rare condition of unknown cause. Red macules appear around follicles and gradually coalesce to areas of widespread erythema. Characteristically there are islands of spared normal skin. The palms and soles become hyperkeratotic and orange in colour and the nails thicken and discolour distally.

TREATMENT PITYRIASIS RUBRA PILARIS

The majority of cases resolve spontaneously in 1–3 years. Treatment with a systemic retinoid such as acitretin 0.75mg/kg or isotretinin 1mg/kg will hasten this (*see* p. 41). Topical steroids are not effective but emollients are useful.

Trunk & limbs
Chronic erythematous rash
Surface crust/excoriation
Widespread papules/plaques/small erosions – no blisters present

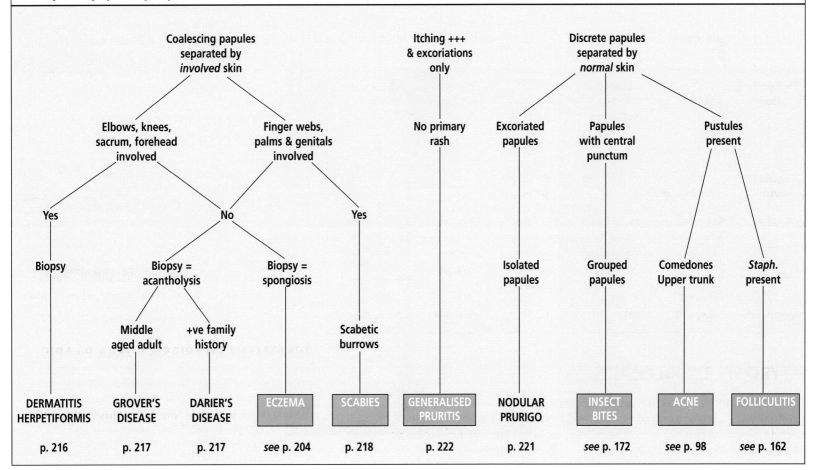

DERMATITIS HERPETIFORMIS

This is a disease of young adults and presents with severe itching particularly at night. Grouped vesicles in the distribution of psoriasis (elbows, knees, sacrum, scalp) are quickly scratched away to leave pink excoriated papules and plaques. It is unusual to see blisters and the rash can be confused with eczema. It is an important, if uncommon, disease because it is associated with a gluten enteropathy.

The diagnosis can be confirmed by finding:–

- anti-gliadin and anti-endomysial antibodies in the blood
- a sub-epidermal blister containing polymorphs on skin biopsy
- deposits of IgA in the upper dermis on immunofluorescence of normal skin.

TREATMENT DERMATITIS HERPETIFORMIS

Initial treatment with dapsone, 50–150mg daily is required. This will stop the itching within a few hours and is usually dramatic. Check a full blood count before starting dapsone because it causes haemolysis of red blood cells. This normally occurs within a few days of starting treatment, so the blood count should be repeated after one week. Most patients will show some haemolysis and methaemoglobinaemia. The side effects can be minimised by giving cimetidine 400mg t.d.s. with the dapsone.

A gluten-free diet will eradicate the IgA from the dermal papillae in 9–12 months and the itching will then stop. Although not pleasant, patients should be encouraged to stick to a gluten-free diet so that the dapsone may be stopped and to prevent the long-term risk of small bowel lymphoma from developing (the risk same as for Coeliac disease).

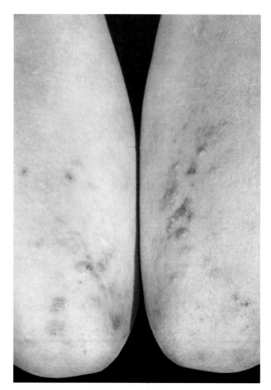

Fig. 8.82 Dermatitis herpetiformis: grouped vesicles.

Fig. 8.83 Dermatitis herpetiformis: more usual picture with excoriated papules on elbows.

GROVER'S DISEASE (Acantholytic dermatosis)

This is a very itchy rash which occurs on the trunk (usually middle-aged men). It is made up of itchy papules with an eroded surface. Individual papules are discrete and usually 2–3mm in size. The rash lasts from 2 weeks to many months and tends to remit and relapse. Diagnosis is established by skin biopsy which shows acantholysis (loss of cohesion) of the epidermal cells. Treatment is unsatisfactory.

DARIER'S DISEASE

This rare condition is inherited as an autosomal dominant trait. The rash consists of follicular papules that coalesce into plaques affecting the trunk, upper arms, face and flexures. The surface is covered with a yellow-brown greasy crust. A skin biopsy is diagnostic. Other changes are longitudinal ridging of the nails (Fig. 14.06, p. 390), pits on the palms and soles, and plane wart-like papules on the dorsum of hands and feet.

TREATMENT DARIER'S DISEASE

For localised areas use 0.025% retinoic acid cream or a topical steroid–antibiotic mix twice a day. For extensive disease use acitretin 0.5–1mg/kg/day which will need to be prescribed by a dermatologist.

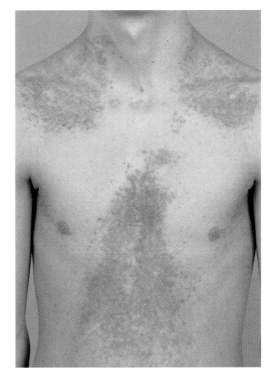

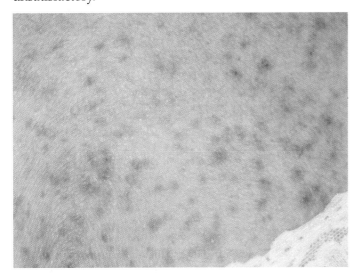

Fig. 8.84 Grover's disease. Individual papules remain discrete.

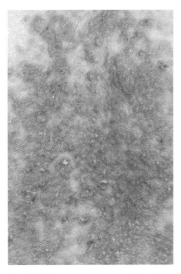

Fig. 8.85 Darier's disease. Follicular papules coalescing to form plaques.

Fig. 8.86 Darier's disease on the trunk.

SCABIES

Scabies is an infestation with the human scabies mite *Sarcoptes scabei*. It is transmitted by prolonged skin to skin contact with someone who has it (usually by lying next to someone in bed all night or by holding hands). A fertilized female has to be transferred for infestation to take place. She will then find a place to lay her eggs (a burrow); 4–6 weeks later a secondary hypersensitivity rash occurs. This is characterised by intense itching particularly at night. The rash is made up of excoriated papules scattered over the trunk and limbs but sparing the face (except in infants). The diagnosis is confirmed by finding one or more burrows (often there are fewer than 10 in total to be found). These are linear S-shaped papules, 3–5mm in length usually along the sides of the fingers or on the front of the wrists. Less commonly they can be found along the sides of the feet, around the nipples, on the buttocks or on the genitalia. There is almost always a rash on the hands, and in males papules on the penis and scrotum. Other members of the family or sexual partners may also be itching.

A similar rash without any burrows can be due to **animal scabies** where mites are found on the pet (usually a dog) and the diagnosis is confirmed by brushing the animal's fur on to a sheet and sending the brushings to the local microbiology laboratory to identify the mites.

TREATMENT HUMAN SCABIES

It is essential to treat not only the patient but anyone else who has been in close contact, even if they are asymptomatic. In practice this means all individuals living in the same house and any sexual partner(s). If there are children in the family, grandparents, aunts and uncles, baby-sitters, neighbours and anyone else who has been holding the children will also need treating.

The idea of treatment is to kill all stages of the life cycle of the scabies mite (eggs, larvae, nymphs and adults) at the same time. 5% permethrin cream (*Lyclear*[UK]/*Elimite*[USA]) or 0.5% malathion lotion (*Derbac-M*) can be used. The cream or lotion is applied to the whole body surface except the face and scalp (including the skin between the fingers and toes, the genitalia and the soles of the feet). Treatment is applied at night before the patient goes to bed and left on for 24 hours. The whole family and other contacts should be treated at the same time. Twenty-four hours later the patient can have a bath and wash the scabicide off. He should then change his underwear, pyjamas and the sheets on his bed. The clothes should be washed and ironed to kill any wandering acari, although in practice it is very unlikely that any will be left alive at this stage. There is no need to go to elaborate means to fumigate the house or bedding. 15g of permethrin cream or 30ml of malathion lotion will be needed for a single application (for an adult), so you can work out how much to prescribe for the whole family. Any residual itching can be treated with calamine lotion or crotamiton (*Eurax*) cream twice a day.

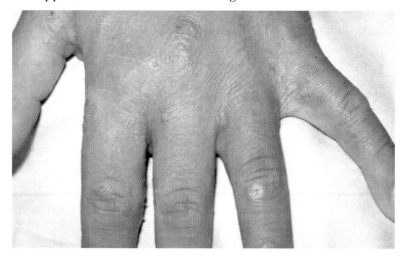

Fig. 8.87 Scabies. Rash involving the finger webs.

Treatment failure in scabies is due to:–

- The scabicide not being applied over the whole body.
- The contacts not being treated.
- The wrong diagnosis.

Treatment animal scabies

Wash the dog in 1% lindane lotion or monosulphuram soap (*Tetmosol*). Carpets and soft furnishings should be vacuumed and the floor washed with lindane emulsion. Treat the patient with crotamiton (*Eurax*) cream b.i.d. until the itching stops.

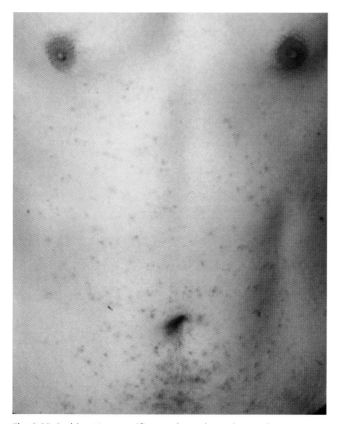

Fig. 8.88 Scabies. Non-specific papular rash on the trunk.

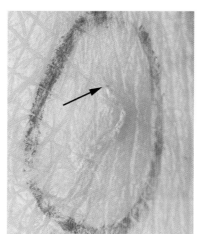

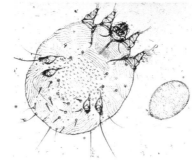

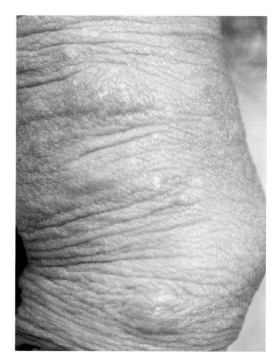

Fig. 8.89 (above centre) Close up of scabies burrow (arrow shows site of mite).

Fig. 8.90 (below centre) Scabies mite and egg (×350).

Fig. 8.91 (above right) Scabies. Typical papules on shaft of penis.

NORWEGIAN SCABIES (Crusted scabies)

This is an infestation with the human scabies mite in an individual with lowered immunity, mental retardation or sensory loss. The host response is abnormal leading to the presence of thousands of mites all over the skin. These are shed into the environment eventually infecting other people. Thick hyperkeratotic scale occurs on palms, soles, flexures and under the nails. Eventually a wide-spread scaly rash occurs all over the body which is often mis-diagnosed as eczema. The diagnosis usually comes to light when those in contact with the patient develop an itchy rash (which is diagnosed as ordinary scabies). To confirm the diagnosis remove some of the thick scale from the patient and/or collect up scales and other debris from the bed, and examine under the microscope. Numerous eggs, larvae, nymphs and adult mites will be seen.

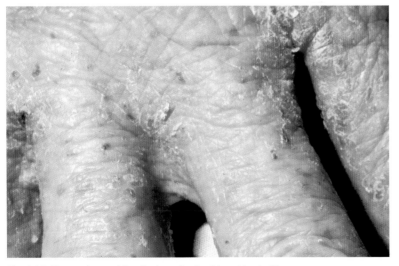

Fig. 8.92 Norwegian scabies. Rash on back of hand looks like eczema.

TREATMENT NORWEGIAN SCABIES

Treatment in an old people's home

1. Identify the patient with Norwegian scabies.
2. Identify a single room where he/she can be isolated and empty that room of all furniture and soft furnishings apart from a bed. Clean the room thoroughly and wash the floor and walls with 1% lindane emulsion. Make up the bed with freshly washed and ironed bedding.
3. Treat the patient with permethrin (*Lyclear*) cream as a single application all over (including the face and scalp).
4. After treatment put the patient into the cleaned single room.
5. The home should be closed to new residents and visitors until stages 7–9 have been carried out.
6. Explain to the staff (whether or not they have had direct physical contact with the patient) what is happening. Explain that the patient has Norwegian scabies and that whether or not they are itching, they will almost certainly have caught it and will need treatment. Explain that the variety they have caught is ordinary scabies and not the very infectious kind that the patient has. Explain that they are only infectious to very close contacts, i.e. immediate family or those with whom they share a bed.
7. Explain what is happening to the other residents and tell them that they will not be able to go out or have visitors until they have been treated. Treat them once with permethrin cream over the whole of the skin except the face and scalp. Leave it on the skin for 24 hours.
8. To remove any mites from the environment wash and iron all bedding, curtains and other soft furnishings in the patient's bedroom and any public rooms that he has used. Wash or spray the floors, walls and other hard surfaces in all the rooms where he has been with 1% lindane emulsion.
9. All staff and their husbands, wives, boyfriends, girlfriends and children must be treated with permethrin cream as directed on p. 218.
10. Once 7–9 above have been done the home can be reopened to visitors.

Treatment Norwegian scabies in a children's home.

If the infestation has arisen in a children's home rather than an old people's home, the procedure is basically the same. But, since children from a single home may attend a variety of schools and be in different classes, help from the local medical officer of health will be needed to ensure that all the relevant individuals are identified and treated. As well as the children and staff in the children's home, the children, teachers and school helpers in all the classes which have children from the home in them will need treatment as will their families.

NODULAR PRURIGO

Nodular prurigo is a rash which is caused by the patient scratching and picking his skin. Numerous discrete intensely itchy pink, mauve or brown papules or nodules occur. They are excoriated and heal to leave white scars which sometimes have very obvious follicular openings within them. It can sometimes be associated with eczema.

TREATMENT NODULAR PRURIGO

In order to get this better the patient somehow has got to stop scratching and picking the skin. A potent^{UK}/group 2–3^{USA} topical steroid ointment applied twice a day may help control the itching. Flurandrenolone (*Haelan*) tape may be applied to individual lesions and left on for several days at a time. Sometimes a sedative antihistamine at night may be needed. If it is confined to the arms and legs, they can be wrapped up in an occlusive paste bandage (*Ichthopaste* or *Zipzoc*) covered with Tubifast for a week at a time. Unfortunately when the bandages are taken off the patient will often begin to scratch again. Severe cases may need hospitalisation to break the itch-scratch cycle. Thalidomide can be used in intractable cases.

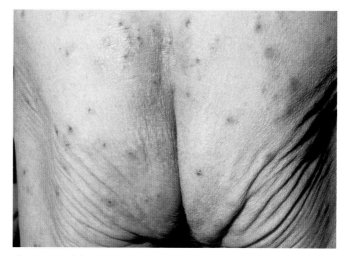

Fig. 8.93 Nodular prurigo lesions on the buttocks of an elderly man.

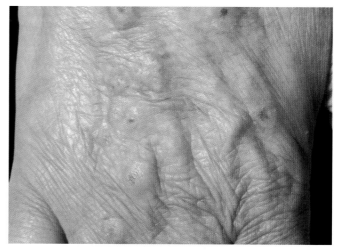

Fig. 8.94 Nodular prurigo on the dorsum of the hand.

GENERALISED PRURITIS

If someone is itching all over but no rash is seen other than excoriations consider:–

- Anaemia, especially iron deficiency – check **serum iron** and **ferritin** levels.
- Polycythemia rubra vera (itching especially in a hot bath) – check **FBC**.
- Uraemia (also seen in 80% patients on maintenance haemodialysis) – check **urea & creatinine**.
- Obstructive jaundice (may occur in patients with primary biliary cirrhosis before jaundice occurs) – check **liver function tests** and **auto-immune profile**.
- Thyroid disease – both hypo and hyperthyroid – check T_4 & **TSH**.
- Lymphoma – especially in young adult – check for **enlarged lymph nodes clinically** and on **chest X-ray**.
- Carcinoma, especially in old age – **good history, full physical examination, chest X-ray, occult bloods**, and if indicated, **abdominal ultrasound** and **CAT scan**.
- HIV/AIDS – check **HIV ELISA** test.
- Drying out of the skin especially in the elderly.
- Body lice – look for lice and nits in the seams of underwear.
- Psychological – look for evidence of depression, anxiety or emotional upset.

TREATMENT PRURITIS

Any specific cause found (*see* above) needs treating. In the elderly prescribe emollients. If no cause is found treatment will need to be symptomatic. Start with 10% crotamiton (*Eurax*) cream twice a day. If it does not help use a moderately potent^{UK}/group 4–7^{USA} steroid ointment or cream. If the topical steroids do not adequately control the itching and it is interfering with sleep, a sedative anti-histamine such as alimemazine (*Vallergan*, 10–20mg) or promethazine (*Phenergan*, 25–50mg) taken about an hour before going to bed may help. The patient will, of course, need to be careful about driving the next day. Other measures worth trying include doxepin cream or 0.5% menthol in aqueous/hydrophilic cream. In patients with uraemia or HIV infection, UVB therapy 2–3× a week may be helpful (*see* p. 48).

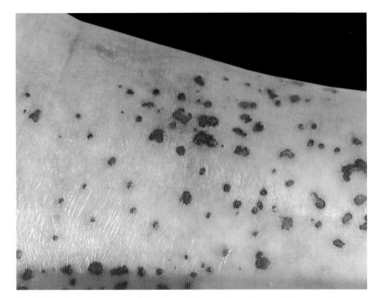

Fig. 8.95 Generalised pruritis: excoriations only with no obvious rash.

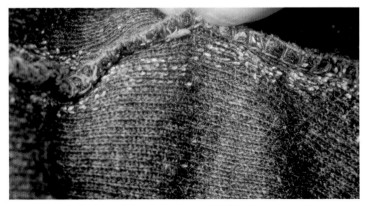

Fig. 8.96 Body louse and nits along the seam of a sweater.

Trunk & limbs
Chronic erythematous rash
Surface crust or exudate
Widespread vesicles/bullae/large erosions

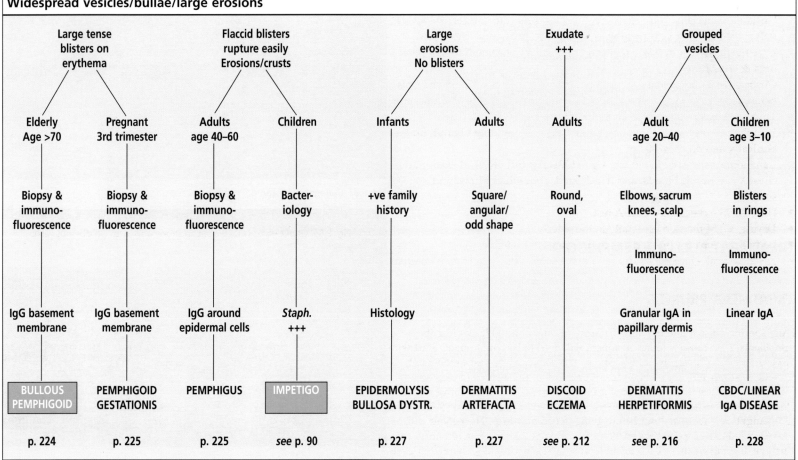

BULLOUS PEMPHIGOID

Bullous pemphigoid is an autoimmune disease which usually begins with a non-specific itchy rash that does not look quite right for either eczema or urticaria. Weeks or months later blisters occur. Here the separation of the skin is at the dermo-epidermal junction (with localisation of IgG antibodies here). Antibodies to basement membrane are also found in the blood. The roof of the blister is made up of the full thickness of the epidermis, so blisters may become large, haemorrhagic and remain intact for several days. It is often localised to one part of the body for a while, but like pemphigus will eventually become widespread. It is the commonest cause of blisters in the elderly.

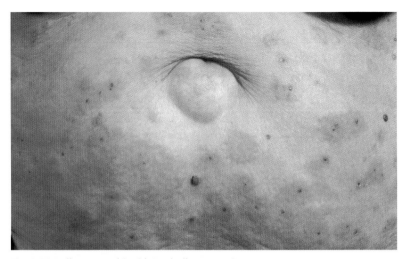

Fig. 8.97 Bullous pemphigoid. Pre-bullous eruption.

TREATMENT BULLOUS PEMPHIGOID

Localised areas can be treated with a potent^{UK}/group 2–3^{USA} topical steroid ointment or cream applied b.i.d. Widespread blistering requires treatment with systemic steroids (e.g. prednisolone 30–40mg/day) until the blistering stops. The dose can be reduced by 5mg weekly down to 15mg and then by 2.5mg weekly. If blistering starts up again the dose is put up and steroid-sparing agents such as azathioprine 50mg t.d.s. may need to be added. Long-term maintenance with around 5mg of prednisolone is usually necessary.

Topical steroids are given for **pemphigoid gestationis** (*see* p. 225) especially if near term. If it occurs earlier and itching is intolerable systemic steroids (prednisolone 30mg/day) may be needed.

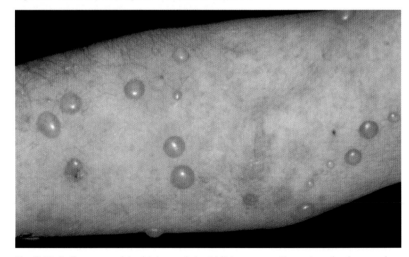

Fig. 8.98 Bullous pemphigoid. Large intact blisters on erythematous background.

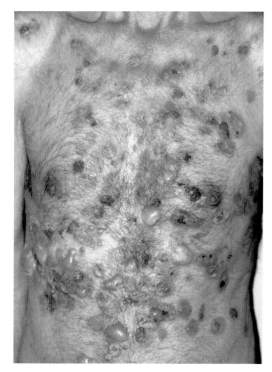

Fig. 8.99 Bullous pemphigoid. Large intact blisters, some haemorrhagic.

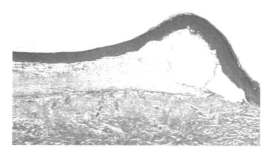

Fig. 8.100 Histology of bullous pemphigoid. Blister occurs at the dermo-epidermal junction.

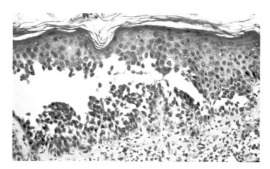

Fig. 8.101 Histology of pemphigus vulgaris. Individual epidermal cells have separated from each other causing a blister within the epidermis.

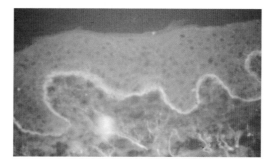

Fig. 8.102 Immunofluorescence of pemphigoid. IgG antibodies localised to epidermal basement membrane.

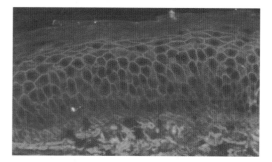

Fig. 8.103 Immunofluorescence of pemphigus vulgaris. IgG antibodies localised around epidermal cells.

PEMPHIGOID (HERPES) GESTATIONIS

This is a very rare condition occurring in pregnancy. It is a very itchy rash looking like either widespread erythema multiforme or bullous pemphigoid. It needs to be differentiated from the much more common polymorphic eruption of pregnancy (p. 173).

PEMPHIGUS VULGARIS

This is an autoimmune disease in which circulating IgG antibodies target desmosomal proteins (Desmoglein 3 +/– Desmoglein 1). The epidermal cells come apart from one another (acantholysis) resulting in an intra-epidermal blister. These are always very superficial so are unable to stay intact for very long. You therefore see mainly erosions and crusts. The blisters are never haemorrhagic. The skin shears easily if rubbed producing an erosion (Nikolsky sign). It most commonly begins with erosions in the mouth and it may be weeks or months before the tell-tale blisters appear on the skin. It may spread very rapidly and be life-threatening. Diagnosis is confirmed by histology (Fig. 8.101), immunofluorescence (Fig. 8.103), and high titres of serum antibodies.

PEMPHIGUS FOLIACEUS

Here the split is just below the granular layer so the blisters are very superficial. Clinically widespread crusted erosions on the face, scalp and upper trunk are seen. It is often misdiagnosed as seborrhoeic eczema as no blisters are seen. It is less common than pemphigus vulgaris in Europe and the USA, but commoner in Africa and South America. Here the antigen is Desmoglein 1. The diagnosis can be confirmed by skin biopsy and immuno-fluorescence. Treat as for bullous pemphigoid, *see* p. 224.

TREATMENT PEMPHIGUS VULGARIS

Immediate referral to hospital is recommended. Sometimes it is necessary to treat the patient in a burns unit if large areas of skin are eroded. Treatment is started with prednisolone 120mg daily until the blisters stop. The dose is then gradually reduced to a maintenance dose of 5–10mg a day.

What often happens is that the blisters dry up initially, but once the dose is down to 50mg a day, new blisters appear. Steroid-sparing agents such as azathioprine, ciclosporin or methotrexate may well be needed as well. Complications caused by high-dose steroids or secondary infection can result in considerable mortality.

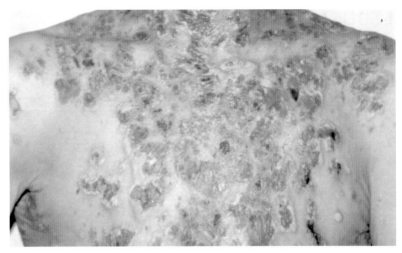

Fig. 8.104 Pemphigus vulgaris. Flaccid blisters, erosions and crusts.

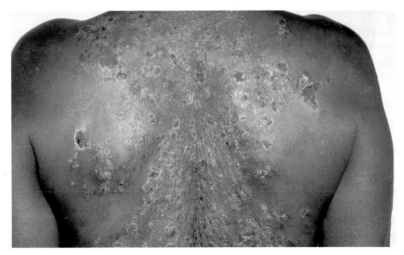

Fig. 8.105 Pemphigus foliaceus. Scaling and crusts on upper back.

EPIDERMOLYSIS BULLOSA (DYSTROPHIC)

This is a group of inherited diseases where blisters and erosions appear in response to trauma. Dystrophic EB is due to a split below the epidermal basement membrane. Many patients do not survive the first two years of life, while others are disabled by the skin shearing off easily. Secondary scarring, milia formation, infection and binding together of fingers and toes can occur. Patients will need referral to a dermatology department for confirmation of diagnosis by skin biopsy and electron microscopy.

TREATMENT EPIDERMOLYSIS BULLOSA

Treatment is a wound care problem. Exudate should be dried up with potassium permanganate or Burow's solution (*see* p. 26). Raw areas need to be dressed with a non-stick dressing (*see* p. 38). The skin should be moisturised with emollients and protected from injury by hydrocolloid dressings. Shoes and clothing should not be allowed to rub. Pain and secondary infection need treatment and genetic counselling and parent support will be necessary.

DERMATITIS ARTEFACTA

These lesions are self-induced. The clue is that instead of being round or oval like most naturally occurring rashes they have straight sides – square, rectangular or triangular (Fig. 1.84, p. 17). They occur anywhere that the patient can reach and damage the skin with finger nails, scissors, nail files, phenol, acids, household cleaners etc. The open wounds exude serum then form crusts.

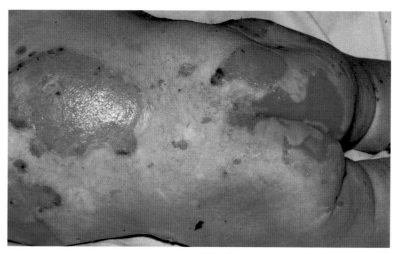

Fig. 8.106 Recessive dystrophic epidermolysis bullosa in a newborn infant.

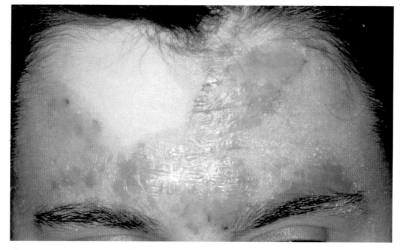

Fig. 8.107 Dermatitis artefacta. Straight rather than rounded outline to rash.

TREATMENT DERMATITIS ARTEFACTA

This is very difficult to treat because the patient (often female) is not willing to admit to producing the lesion(s) or to the idea that treatment involves facing up to the problem or conflict in her life which is causing her to damage her own skin. If the lesions are occluded so that the patient cannot get at them, they will usually heal very quickly.

These patients need psychiatric help. Unfortunately psychiatrists are not always interested in helping them. Direct confrontation usually leads to the patient seeking help elsewhere.

CHRONIC BULLOUS DISEASE OF CHILDHOOD (CBDC) (Linear IgA disease)

A rare disease of young children (usually begins age 3–5) with grouped blisters around the genitalia, umbilicus and on the face. It is not itchy and gets better spontaneously after 3–4 years. Histology shows a subepidermal blister and on direct immunofluorescence a linear band of IgA is seen along the basement membrane of the epidermis. Linear IgA disease is the adult version of CBDC. Usually the blisters occur in rings.

TREATMENT CHRONIC BULLOUS DISEASE OF CHILDHOOD/LINEAR IgA DISEASE

Oral dapsone 25–100mg/day is given until it remits spontaneously. Check the FBC regularly for haemolysis. Add cimetidine 400mg t.d.s. if haemolysis or methaemoglobinaemia occurs.

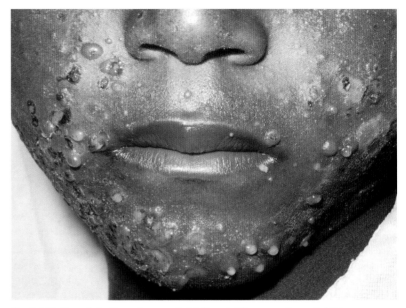

Fig. 8.108 Chronic bullous disease of childhood. Blisters on face of child.

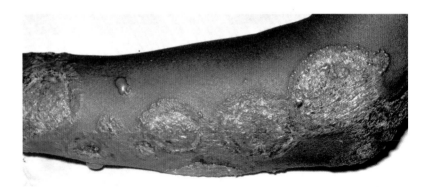

Fig. 8.109 Linear IgA disease. Blister in rings on arm.

Non-erythematous lesions

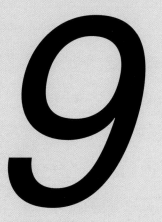

Normal surface

Warty surface

Scaly/keratotic surface

Crust/ulcerated surface

Non-erythematous lesions
Normal surface
Skin colour/pink/yellow
Papules

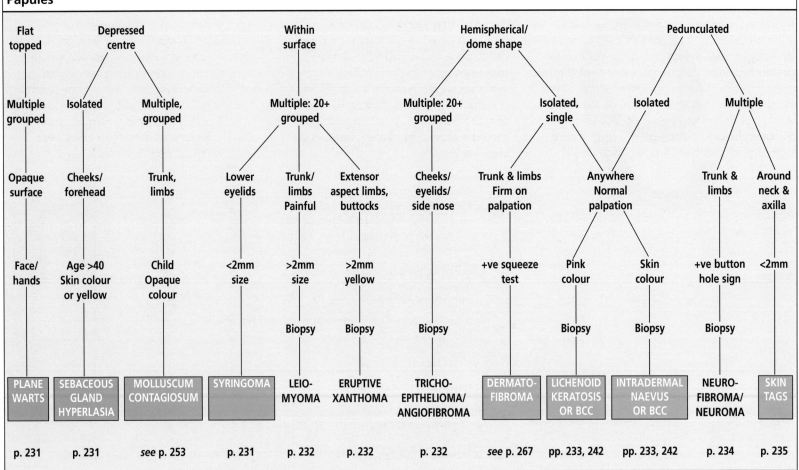

PLANE WARTS

These are small flat-topped papules but unlike the papules of lichen planus are not shiny on the surface. They are not rough to the touch like common warts. They are skin coloured, pink or brown, and may be found in straight lines at sites of trauma (Köebner phenomenon). They occur mainly in children on the face and dorsum of the hands. They eventually resolve spontaneously. Treatment tends not to be very effective. You can try 5% salicylic acid ointment or a light freeze with liquid nitrogen (few seconds only).

SEBACEOUS GLAND HYPERPLASIA

This is a common benign lesion due to enlargement of sebaceous glands around a single hair follicle on the face. It is a small (2–5mm diameter) skin coloured–yellow papule with telangiectasia running over the surface and a central punctum (the opening of the hair follicle). It is sometimes confused with a small basal cell carcinoma since both occur on the face of middle aged or elderly individuals. They can be removed by cautery under local anaesthetic.

SYRINGOMA

These small (1–5mm) round dome-shaped translucent papules on the lower eyelids are very common and completely harmless. They are benign tumours of sweat glands which are inherited as an autosomal dominant trait. They appear after puberty. Cautery with a fine loop will ablate them. Rarely multiple lesions may be seen elsewhere on the face and trunk.

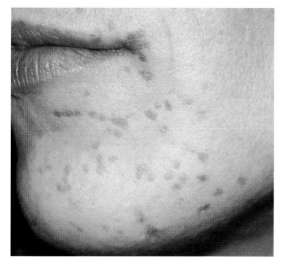

Fig. 9.01 Plane warts. Flat topped papules with opaque surface.

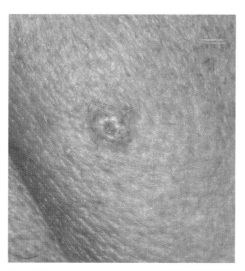

Fig. 9.02 Sebaceous gland hyperplasia.

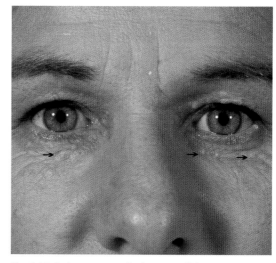

Fig. 9.03 Syringomas on the lower eyelids.

LEIOMYOMA

This is a benign smooth muscle tumour of the erector pili muscle. Multiple pink, red or brown papules are grouped together on the trunk or on a limb in young adults. They can be painful in the cold or when knocked. Diagnosis is confirmed by skin biopsy. They can be removed by surgical excision but if the lesions are extensive then excision may not always be practical.

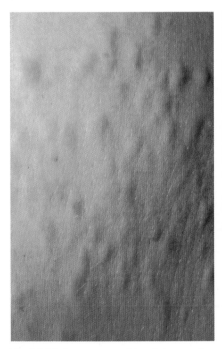 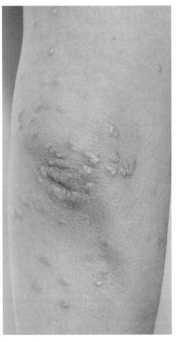

Fig. 9.04 Leiomyoma on side of chest wall.

Fig. 9.05 Eruptive xanthomas on the elbow.

ANGIOFIBROMAS (Adenoma sebaceum)

These are multiple very firm, discrete, translucent papules with a telangiectatic surface affecting the nasolabial folds and spreading out on to the cheeks and chin. They appear in early childhood (age 3–4) and are a sign of tuberous sclerosis (epiloa). **Tuberous sclerosis** is an autosomal dominant disorder affecting many organs. Other skin lesions are oval or ash-leaf shaped white patches which are present from birth, the Shagreen patch (a connective tissue naevus) and periungual and subungual fibromas which appear after puberty. Other features of the syndrome include mental retardation, epilepsy and occasionally tumours affecting the heart and kidneys.

TRICHOEPITHELIOMA

Single or multiple translucent papules around the eyes or on the naso-labial folds appear after puberty. They look similar to angiofibromas but can be distinguished on biopsy. They are benign hair follicle tumours (also known as **epithelioma adenoides cysticum**), which are inherited as an autosomal dominant trait.

ERUPTIVE XANTHOMA

Eruptive xanthomas are yellow papules containing lipid deposits secondary to hypertriglyceridaemia. They commonly occur on the buttocks and extensor surface of limbs. Most of these patients are diabetic so check the blood sugar as well as lipid levels. The lesions will clear once the underlying diabetes and hyperlipidaemia are treated.

TREATMENT ANGIOFIBROMAS/ TRICHOEPITHELIOMAS

A few lesions can be removed by shave and cautery under local anaesthetic. Widespread lesions present a problem. Extensive debridement can be tried using a carbon dioxide laser, shave or curettage and cautery under general anaesthetic. Unfortunately there is a tendency for the lesions to recur.

LICHENOID KERATOSIS

This is a variety of a solar lentigo which is a pink papule with a smooth surface. On histology a lichenoid infiltrate is present. It can be confused clinically with an early basal cell carcinoma.

INTRADERMAL NAEVUS

This is a skin coloured melanocytic naevus. All the naevus cells are in the dermis so pigment is no longer seen on the surface (*see* p. 269). It is a small, round, dome-shaped or papillomatous papule. Occasionally telangiectasia can be seen on the surface, but the lack of growth, long history and symmetrical dome shape distinguish it from a basal cell carcinoma. They are sometimes pedunculated (*see* Fig. 3.42, p. 80), and can be difficult to distinguish from neurofibromas or skin tags.

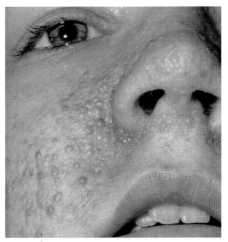
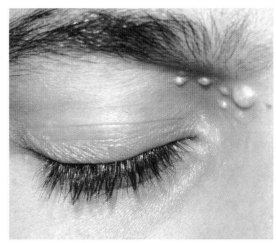

Fig. 9.06 Angiofibromas in tuberose sclerosis.   **Fig. 9.07** Trichoepitheliomas.

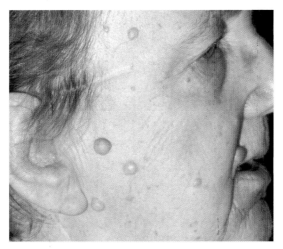
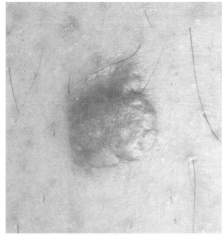

Fig. 9.08 Numerous intradermal naevi on the cheek.   **Fig. 9.09** Lichenoid keratosis on the leg.

TREATMENT INTRADERMAL NAEVUS

Reassure that they are harmless. If they are very unsightly, small lesions can be sliced off flush with the surface, and the bleeding stopped using 20% aluminium chloride hexahydrate antiperspirant (*Anhydrol*, *Drichlor*UK/*Drysol*USA), cautery or a hyfrecator. This gives a better result than excision. Always send the lesion for histology.

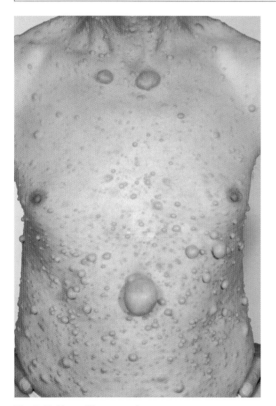

Fig. 9.10 Neurofibromatosis.

NEUROFIBROMAS (VON RECKLINGHAUSEN'S DISEASE)

Multiple skin coloured, pink or red papules and nodules appear anywhere on the skin after puberty. If you press on the surface, the lesions are found to be soft with a hole at the base (like a button hole). They vary in size from 1–2mm to several cm in diameter. Some are sessile, some pedunculated. The patient will also have multiple (>5) café-au-lait patches (*see* p. 260) and axillary freckling. Lisch nodules (pigmented iris hamartomas) are seen on slit-lamp examination and help confirm the diagnosis. Various endocrine and neurological abnormalities can also be present. This condition is inherited as an autosomal dominant trait, the gene being on chromosome 17.

TREATMENT NEUROFIBROMAS

Single lesions can be removed by excision or shave and cautery. It is impossible to remove all the lesions in von Recklinghausen's disease, but any particularly unsightly ones can be excised.

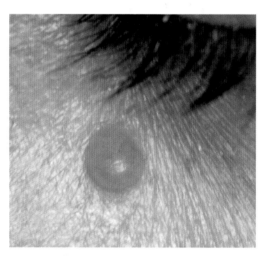

Fig. 9.11 Pallisading encapsulated neuroma.

PALLISADING ENCAPSULATED NEUROMA (PEN)

These are solitary small skin coloured papules which look like intradermal naevi. Diagnosis is usually made on histology after removal. These lesions have nothing to do with neurofibromatosis.

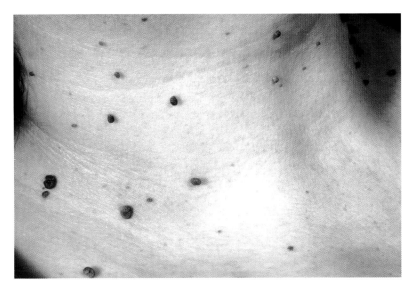

Fig. 9.12 Skin tags on the neck.

SKIN TAGS

These are small pedunculated, skin-coloured or brown papules around the neck, in the axillae or sometimes on the inner thighs.

TREATMENT SKIN TAGS

If the patient wants them removed, snip the tag off with a pair of sharp scissors without any local anaesthetic. Bleeding is stopped with aluminium chloride, a silver nitrate stick or cautery. Alternatively if they are very small, ablate with the hyfrecator.

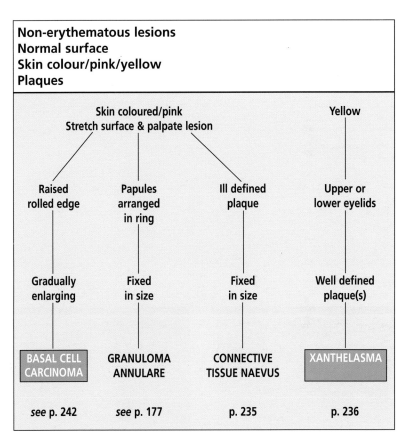

Non-erythematous lesions
Normal surface
Skin colour/pink/yellow
Plaques

Skin coloured/pink — Stretch surface & palpate lesion

Yellow

Raised rolled edge	Papules arranged in ring	Ill defined plaque	Upper or lower eyelids
Gradually enlarging	Fixed in size	Fixed in size	Well defined plaque(s)
BASAL CELL CARCINOMA	**GRANULOMA ANNULARE**	**CONNECTIVE TISSUE NAEVUS**	**XANTHELASMA**
see p. 242	*see* p. 177	p. 235	p. 236

CONNECTIVE TISSUE NAEVUS

A birth mark consisting of a skin coloured/yellowish plaque with a cobblestone surface (Fig. 9.13). It may be present alone or as part of tuberous sclerosis (*see* p. 232).

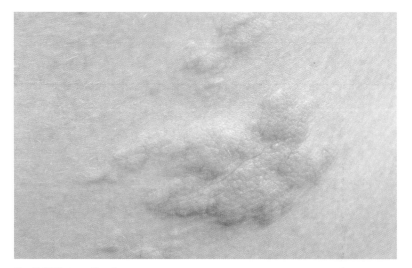

Fig. 9.13 Connective tissue naevus.

XANTHELASMA

These are yellow flat plaques usually found on the medial aspect of the eyelids. They are not necessarily associated with hyperlipidaemia.

TREATMENT XANTHELASMA

Dip a cotton wool bud in a saturated solution of trichloracetic acid (TCA) and lightly paint the surface of the xanthelasma making sure that it does not get onto normal skin. After a few seconds the surface goes white. Immediately smother the surface with surgical spirit – this quickly neutralises the acid. Any excess acid can also be washed away with copious amounts of water. The stinging caused by the acid should stop after just a few seconds. A week later the treated area scabs over and the skin will heal normally after about 6 weeks. Recurrences or residual areas can be retreated in the same way.

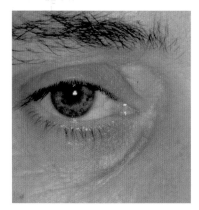

Fig. 9.14a Xanthelasma before treatment. Yellow plaques on inner eyelids.

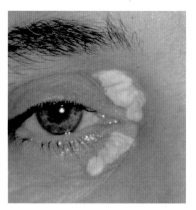

Fig. 9.14b Treatment of xanthelasma. Immediately after application of TCA.

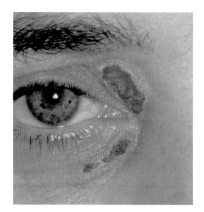

Fig. 9.14c Crusts have formed 7 days later.

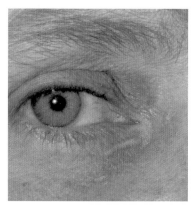

Fig. 9.14d Two months later there is just a faint erythema.

Non-erythematous lesions
Normal surface
Skin coloured/light pink
Large papules (>0.5cm) & nodules

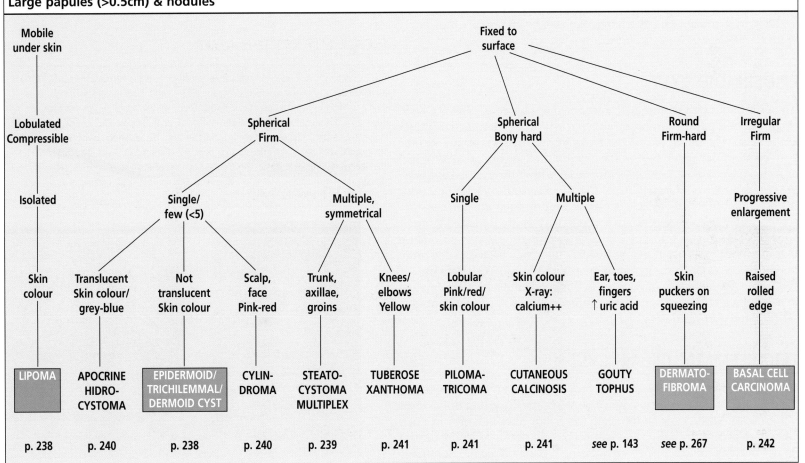

LIPOMA

This is a benign tumour of fat cells presenting as soft or firm sub-cutaneous nodules (you can move the skin over it), round or irregular in shape. They may be single or multiple and vary in size from ½–10cm in diameter. The overlying skin is normal. Usually they are of no significance.

EPIDERMOID CYST

An epidermoid cyst (commonly misnamed a sebaceous cyst) is a well circumscribed papule or nodule situated within the dermis (i.e. attached to the skin). The lining of the cyst looks like normal epidermis and it is derived from the upper part of the external root sheath of a hair follicle or from a sweat duct. The cheesy material within the cyst is keratin produced by the epidermal lining. Usually a central punctum marking the opening of the hair follicle is visible, and through this the cyst contents may become secondarily infected. They are inherited as an autosomal dominant trait but appear after puberty (usually 15–30 years). If epidermoid cysts occur before puberty they may be associated with polyposis coli (Gardner's syndrome) or with the basal cell naevus syndrome. Similar cysts may occur in patients with acne after damage to hair follicles, or after penetrating injuries where bits of epidermis are implanted in the dermis.

TRICHILEMMAL (PILAR) CYST

These are derived from the external root sheath of a hair follicle between the opening of the sebaceous duct and the bulge (insertion of the erector pili muscle). Most occur on the scalp (see p. 80), although they can occur anywhere except the palms and soles. They do not have a punctum so do not become infected. They are inherited as an autosomal dominant trait.

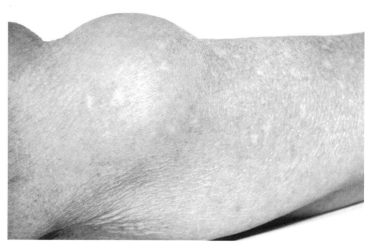

Fig. 9.15 Lipoma on arm.

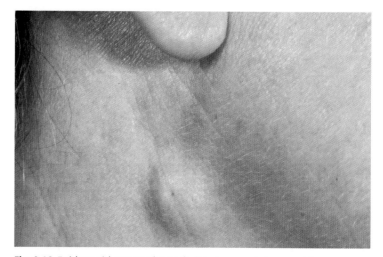

Fig. 9.16 Epidermoid cyst on the neck showing an obvious punctum.

DERMOID CYST

Dermoid cysts look like epidermoid cysts but they are present from birth or early childhood. They are due to the inclusion of epidermis and its appendages in the dermis at the time of embryonic skin closure. Most occur on the head and neck, either in the midline or at the lateral end of the eyebrow. They have an obvious punctum which may have hairs protruding from it.

STEATOCYSTOMA MULTIPLEX

Multiple, symmetrical, small skin-coloured, white or yellowish papules or nodules occur on the skin of young adults. In females they are mainly in the axillae and between the breasts. In males they are mostly on the trunk in a ◊-shaped area between the xiphisternum and umbilicus (Fig. 9.18) or on the back. They are inherited as an autosomal dominant trait.

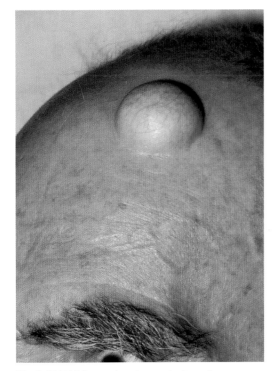

Fig. 9.17 Trichilemmal cyst on scalp (*see also* Fig. 3.41, p. 80).

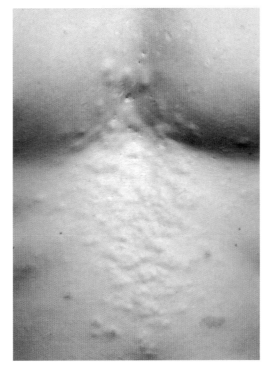

Fig. 9.18 Steatocystoma multiplex.

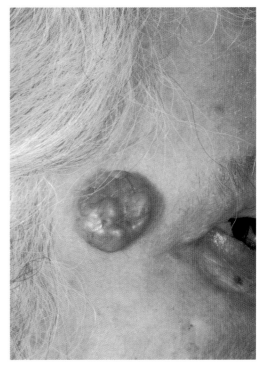

Fig. 9.19 Cylindroma.

CYLINDROMA

Single or multiple, spherical or lobulated, red, smooth nodules occur on the scalp or face (Fig. 9.19). They can grow to quite a large size. Sometimes they occur in association with multiple trichoepitheliomas (*see* p. 232). Alone or in combination they are inherited as an autosomal dominant trait. They are uncommon.

APOCRINE HIDROCYSTOMA

This is a solitary smooth, dome-shaped, cystic nodule which may be skin coloured or blue-grey in colour. It is found most commonly around the eyelids. It is probably not uncommon and is usually misdiagnosed as a basal cell carcinoma.

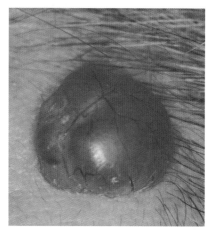

Fig. 9.20 Hidrocystoma. Translucent nodule filled with fluid.

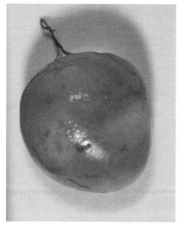

Fig. 9.21 Cyst removed and transilluminated.

TREATMENT LIPOMAS, CYSTS AND APPENDAGE TUMOURS

These can all be excised under local anaesthetic if they are large or a nuisance. **Lipomas** are removed by making an incision through the skin and shelling out an encapsulated tumour of fatty tissue.

Appendage tumours (hidradenomas, cylindromas, pilomatricomas) can be excised together with the overlying skin.

When removing **cysts** first excise an ellipse of skin over the cyst so that the upper surface of the cyst is visible (you will now be in the right plane to dissect out the cyst). The amount of skin you need to remove depends on how big the cyst is and how much redundant skin has been pushed up. The cyst is then dissected out using a pair of blunt curved scissors. If the resultant hole is large, close off the dead space with deep dissolving sutures before inserting ordinary interrupted sutures into the skin.

Epidermoid cysts are the most difficult to remove since they are often stuck down to the surrounding connective tissue, particularly if they have ever been inflamed. **Trichilemmal** cysts shell out very easily once you are in the right plane, since they have a connective tissue sheath around them. If huge numbers of **steatocystoma multiplex** cysts are present, they can be incised with a no. 15 scalpel blade, the contents squeezed out and the cyst lining removed by pulling out with a pair of artery forceps. You have to pull quite hard to remove them. This will normally need to be done under a general anaesthetic.

Do not remove cysts while they are actively inflamed. It is important to remove all of the cyst wall during the procedure; if any of it is left behind, the cyst will recur.

PILOMATRICOMA

A pilomatricoma is a benign tumour of the hair follicle most commonly occurring in children. It presents as a nodule resembling a cyst but is often pink-red in colour. It can be excised under local anaesthesia.

TUBEROSE XANTHOMA

These are firm lobulated tumours appearing at sites of pressure, usually the extensor surface of the knees or elbows in patients with hypercholesterolaemia. The lesions will regress slowly once the hyperlipidaemia has been treated.

CUTANEOUS CALCINOSIS

Deposition of calcium within the dermis can occur in:–

Localised lesions

- Various cysts (trichilemmal & pilomatricoma)
- Pinneal (ear) calcification
- Venous disease on the lower legs
- Cutaneous calculus (*see* p. 253)
- Scrotal calcinosis (*see* p. 323)

Generalised disease

- Chronic renal failure
- Dermatomyositis
- Hyperparathyroidism
- Sarcoidosis
- Systemic lupus erythematosus
- Systemic sclerosus (CREST syndrome)

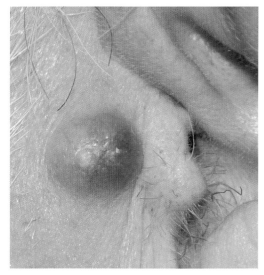

Fig. 9.22 Pilomatricoma in front of the ear.

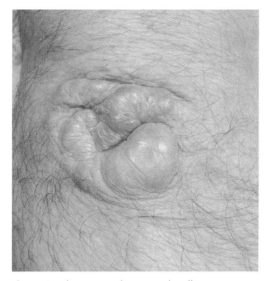

Fig. 9.23 Tuberose xanthoma on the elbow.

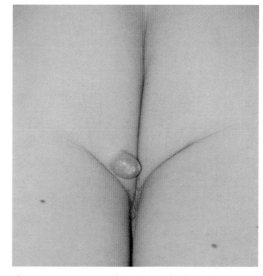

Fig. 9.24 Cutaneous calcinosis on the buttock.

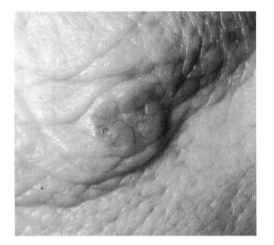

Fig. 9.25 Early BCC.

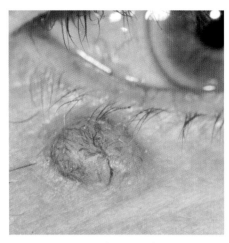

Fig. 9.26 Cystic BCC showing telangiectasia.

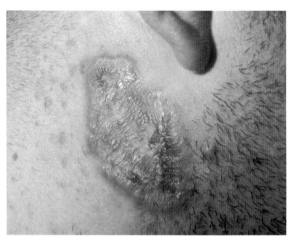

Fig. 9.27 Large BCC on the neck with a rolled edge and some crusting on the surface.

BASAL CELL CARCINOMA (BCC, Rodent ulcer)

This is the commonest malignant tumour of the skin. It usually occurs in middle-aged or elderly fair-skinned individuals who have worked out of doors all their lives, or who have spent a lot of time gardening, fishing, sailing etc. Although due to sun damage, they do not occur at the sites of maximum sun exposure, i.e. rarely on the bald scalp, lower lip or dorsum of the hands. Most occur on the face, some on the trunk and limbs.

A basal cell carcinoma starts as a small translucent (pearly) papule with obvious telangiectasia over the surface. It gradually increases in size, and the centre may then ulcerate and crust. Growth is very slow – some may reach a diameter of 1cm only after 5 years. If there is any doubt over the diagnosis, stretch the skin and you will see the raised rolled edge like a piece of string around the edge (*see* Fig. 1.81, p. 16).

TREATMENT BASAL CELL CARCINOMA

1. **Local excision** with a 2mm margin is the treatment of choice. If the lesion is completely excised recurrence is unlikely (<5%).

2. **Mohs micrographic surgery**. Removal of the lesion and assessment of the peripheral and deep margins by frozen section results in recurrence rates of less than 1%. Since this process is time consuming and requires the assistance of a pathology technician, Mohs surgery should be restricted to:–

   - Central facial lesions in those under the age of 45
   - Recurrent lesions (especially after radiotherapy) on the face
   - Lesions with indistinct margins
   - Morphoeic BCCs

(continued on p. 244)

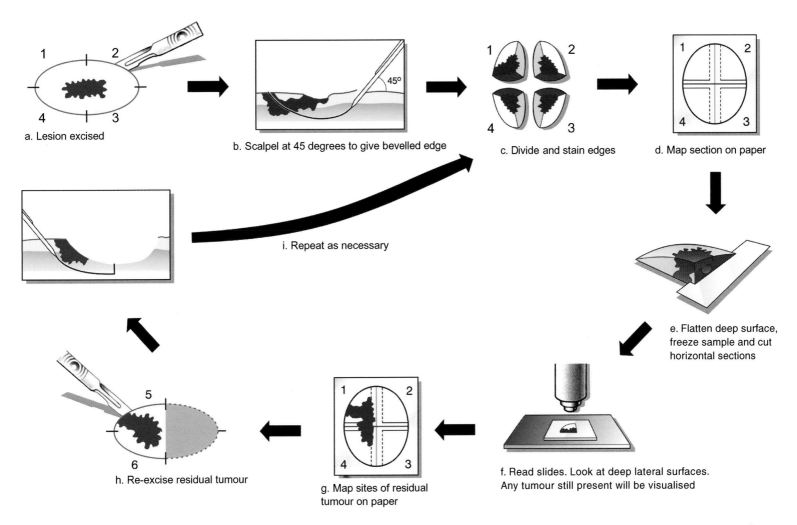

a. Lesion excised

b. Scalpel at 45 degrees to give bevelled edge

c. Divide and stain edges

d. Map section on paper

e. Flatten deep surface, freeze sample and cut horizontal sections

f. Read slides. Look at deep lateral surfaces. Any tumour still present will be visualised

g. Map sites of residual tumour on paper

h. Re-excise residual tumour

i. Repeat as necessary

Fig. 9.28 How Mohs surgery is carried out (adapted with permission from Rook A *et al.* [eds] *Textbook of Dermatology* 78:30, Seventh Edition, Blackwell Science, Oxford).

3. **Curettage and cautery** has a higher recurrence rate than excision but is useful in elderly patients with multiple tumours or when there are multiple lesions on the trunk. The lesion is curetted out and the margin cauterised for 1mm around. This is repeated three times to give a 3mm margin. The subsequent wound will heal by secondary intention over a period of 2–4 weeks. This should be cleaned daily with damp cotton wool and a topical antibiotic ointment applied.

4. **Radiotherapy** is only indicated when surgery is inappropriate, e.g. large lesions in the elderly. 10 daily fractions of 3.75Gy are given. If the patient is very frail, the time between fractions can be increased, so that 10 fractions are given over 10 weeks. This will cause virtually no local reaction and will be much more pleasant for the patient.

5. **Photodynamic therapy** is useful if the patient has numerous tumours. A photosensitiser is applied and this is irradiated with a red light source (*see* p. 51).

6. **Topical imiquimod** (*Aldara*) cream works for superficial BCCs on the trunk and limbs. The cream is applied to lesions 3× week for 12 weeks (*see* pp. 29 & 258).

7. **Cryotherapy** is not recommended since the recurrence rate is unacceptably high.

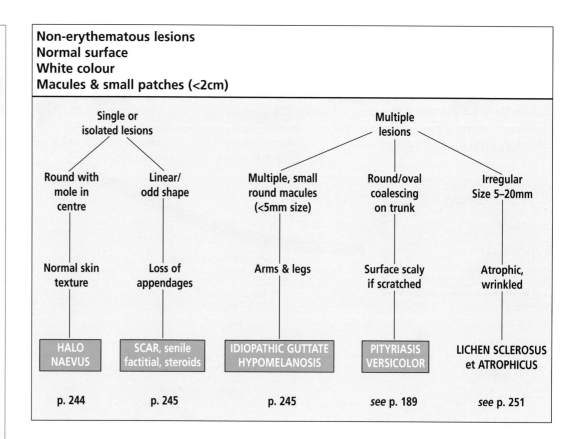

Non-erythematous lesions
Normal surface
White colour
Macules & small patches (<2cm)

Single or isolated lesions → Round with mole in centre → Normal skin texture → **HALO NAEVUS** — p. 244

Single or isolated lesions → Linear/ odd shape → Loss of appendages → **SCAR, senile factitial, steroids** — p. 245

Multiple lesions → Multiple, small round macules (<5mm size) → Arms & legs → **IDIOPATHIC GUTTATE HYPOMELANOSIS** — p. 245

Multiple lesions → Round/oval coalescing on trunk → Surface scaly if scratched → **PITYRIASIS VERSICOLOR** — *see* p. 189

Multiple lesions → Irregular Size 5–20mm → Atrophic, wrinkled → **LICHEN SCLEROSUS et ATROPHICUS** — *see* p. 251

HALO NAEVUS

An immunological reaction against the melanocytes in a mole produces a halo of depigmentation around it. Eventually the mole disappears. This reaction is common in children, quite benign and does not indicate that the mole has undergone malignant change.

IDIOPATHIC GUTTATE HYPOMELANOSIS

Numerous symmetrical small (1–5mm) white macules on the arms or legs are extremely common, especially in individuals with black or pigmented skin. Individual lesions have well defined borders and normal skin markings within them. Reassurance that they are harmless is all that is required.

SCARRING

Scars may be flat or raised: usually the patient will remember the cause. Scars due to an injury or operation are usually linear (*see* Fig. 1.37, p. 10); those with triangular or rectangular shapes may be due to self-inflicted damage; those that are crescent-shaped or star-shaped may be due to tearing of the skin after minor trauma in elderly patients or those taking oral corticosteroids or using potent topical steroids.

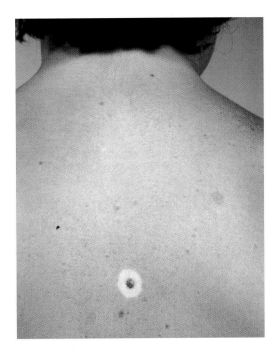

Fig. 9.29 Halo naevus.

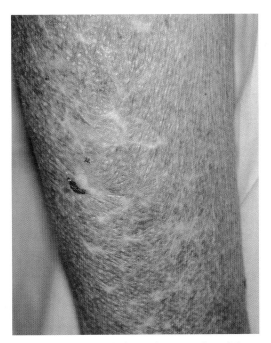

Fig. 9.30 Scarring on forearm due to tearing of the skin after minor trauma in a patient taking systemic steroids.

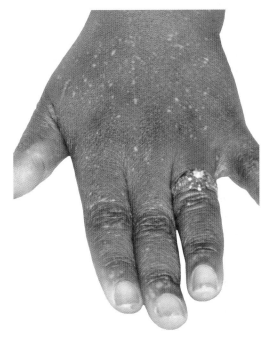

Fig. 9.31 Idiopathic guttate hypomelanosis.

Non-erythematous lesions
Normal surface
White colour
Large patches & plaques (>2cm size)

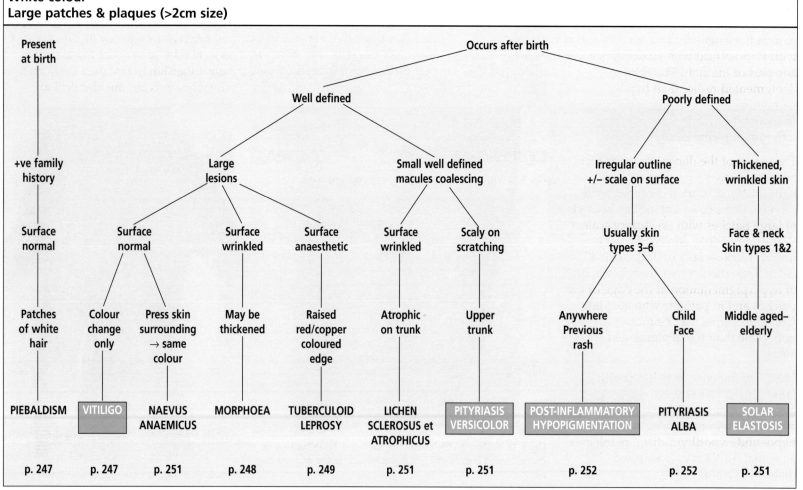

VITILIGO

Vitiligo is thought to be an autoimmune disease in which the melanocytes disappear from the epidermis. The patient presents
with symmetrical white patches on any part of the skin. The skin is depigmented rather than hypo-pigmented which distinguishes it from all other white skin lesions (other than piebaldism).

The extent of the depigmentation can be more easily seen using a Wood's light (p. 18). It is often confused with pityriasis versicolor but vitiligo consists of large patches with no surface scale. Vitiligo on visible skin can be very unsightly, especially in dark-skinned individuals. Sometimes there is a band of hyperpigmentation at the edge of the patches and in patients who are very fair skinned this may be more noticeable than the depigmented areas.

In 30% of patients there is a positive family history of vitiligo, and it may also be associated with the organ-specific auto-immune diseases such as hypo- and hyperthyroidism, pernicious anaemia, Addison's disease and diabetes mellitus.

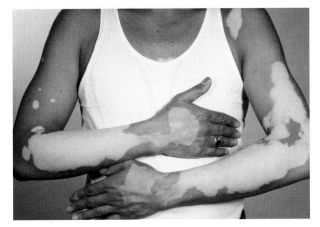

Fig. 9.32 Vitiligo: symmetrical areas of depigmentation.

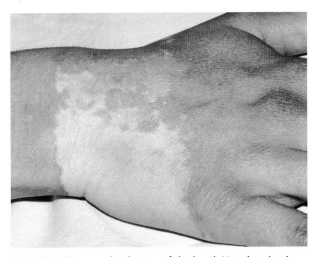

Fig. 9.33 Vitiligo on the dorsum of the hand. Note burning in depigmented areas and hyperpigmentation at the edge of the patches.

PIEBALDISM

This is an inherited condition (autosomal dominant) where white patches are present at birth and remain unchanged throughout life. It may be associated with a white forelock of hair if the skin in that area is affected. The white patches are identical to those of vitiligo.

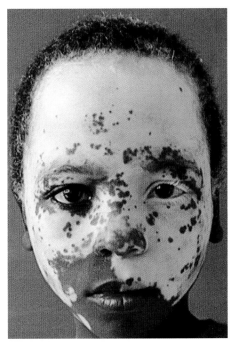

Fig. 9.34 Vitiligo on the face of an African girl.

TREATMENT VITILIGO

1. If it is spreading very rapidly you need to switch it off. This is best done with systemic steroids. In adults give three doses of 40mg triamcinolone IM at monthly intervals. In children give prednisolone 5–10mg/day for 2–3 weeks.

2. If the disease is stable you can try the following to promote repigmentation:–

   - Apply a potent[UK]/group 1–2[USA] topical steroid cream to the white areas in the morning followed by half an hour of sun exposure a day (or UVB at your local hospital in the winter).
   - PUVA therapy for up to 6 months (*see* p. 49).
   - Sunlight alone may help but it is best to use a high factor sunblock in very hot weather to prevent burning of the non-pigmented skin.

   When the vitiligo repigments it does so initially from the hair follicles so you will see small brown macules in the white patches.

3. Improve the cosmetic appearance by using cosmetic camouflage. This is especially useful on the face and hands. An alternative is to use dihydroxyacetone to colour the white areas. This can be purchased over the counter as an artificial suntan lotion.

4. Localised areas on the face in patients with pigmented skin may be repigmented using the excimer laser at 318nm.

5. In very extensive vitiligo depigmentation of the remaining normal skin can be attempted by using the monobenzyl ether of hydroquinone b.i.d. for several weeks.

In white skinned individuals the best advice is probably to keep out of the sun and to apply a high factor sunblock all over to prevent the normal skin from tanning and the depigmented skin from burning.

MORPHOEA

This is a localised thickening of the dermis due to excess collagen with loss of appendages (sweat glands and hair follicles). It occurs at any age (peak incidence from 20–40) and is more common in females. The lesions are firm oval plaques with a shiny smooth surface. The edge is often purple or brown while the centre is white or yellow. It feels thickened compared to the surrounding skin. Rarely it may be linear going down an arm or leg, or on the forehead (*see* p. 66).

In rare instances, morphoea can be extensive, and when involving large areas of the chest wall breathing may be impeded. It is not related to systemic sclerosis, which is a widespread multi-system disease. There is a rare and mutilating form of linear morphoea in children in which the underlying muscle and bone are involved as well as the skin, causing problems with growth and permanent deformity.

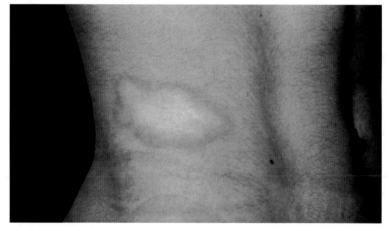

Fig. 9.35 Morphoea (*see also* Fig. 9.70, p. 265).

TREATMENT MORPHOEA

Both the plaque form and the linear form of morphoea will resolve spontaneously in time although it may take months or sometimes several years. Potent [UK]/group 1–2[USA] topical steroids or topical vitamin D_3 analogues under occlusion for 3 months may be useful in the inflammatory stage. High dose systemic steroids or ciclosporin may by necessary to halt the mutilating linear form of the disease.

LEPROSY

Leprosy is a chronic bacterial infection due to *Mycobacterium leprae*. It is spread by droplet infection and has a long incubation period (anything from 2 months to 40 years). It principally affects peripheral nerves and the skin. The clinical features

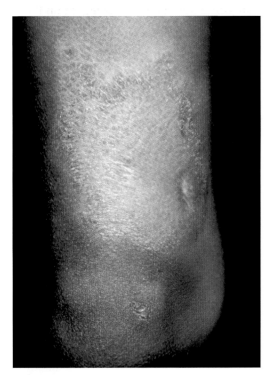

Fig. 9.36 Tuberculoid leprosy. Single anaesthetic hypo-pigmented plaque on arm with raised border.

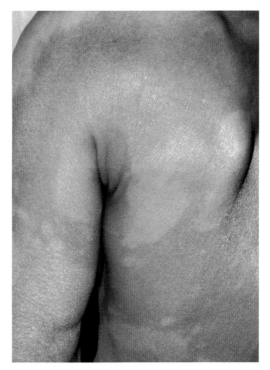

Fig. 9.37 Borderline leprosy. Multiple asymmetrical hypopigmented patches.

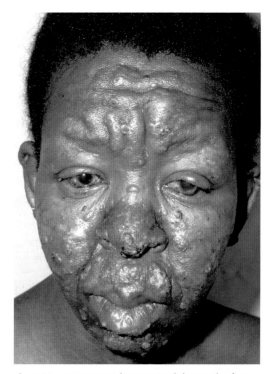

Fig. 9.38 Lepromatous leprosy. Nodules on the face.

are very variable depending on the patient's cell-mediated immunity to the leprosy bacillus.

In **tuberculoid (TT) leprosy** (where patients have good cell-mediated immunity) few/no bacteria are found in the skin (pauci-bacillary leprosy). There are 1–5 hypopigmented anaesthetic patches with a raised red-copper coloured border. Often this is associated with a single enlarged cutaneous nerve nearby. At the other end of the spectrum, in **lepromatous (LL) leprosy**, the patient has no cell-mediated immunity and consequently there are numerous organisms in the skin (multi-bacillary leprosy). Clinically there are multiple papules, nodules and plaques which are not anaesthetic, and a 'glove and stocking' peripheral neuropathy due to widespread nerve damage. In between are various forms of **borderline leprosy** (BT-borderline tuberculoid, BB-mid borderline, BL-borderline lepromatous) with clinical features gradually changing from tuberculoid to lepromatous.

The diagnosis is made by recognising the typical clinical features, doing slit skin smears looking for organisms or by doing a skin biopsy.

TREATMENT LEPROSY

Patients suspected of leprosy should be referred to a leprologist since management requires careful monitoring of the skin and nerve lesions and regular supervision. All patients must have multidrug therapy.

	TT & BT	BB, BL & LL
	Pauci-bacillary	*Multi-bacillary*
Duration of Rx	6 months	24 months
Rifampicin	600mg monthly	600mg monthly
Dapsone	100mg daily	100mg daily
Clofazimine		50mg daily & 300mg monthly

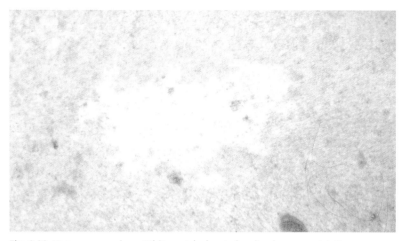

Fig. 9.39 Naevus anaemicus. White patch due to localised vasoconstriction.

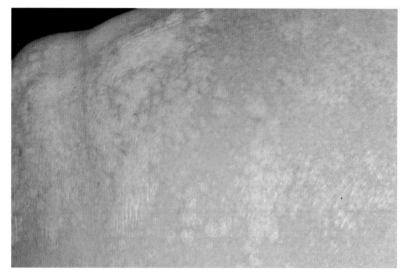

Fig. 9.40 Lichen sclerosus et atrophicus on the upper back.

NAEVUS ANAEMICUS

There is no structural abnormality in the skin; it is a pharmacological naevus with the blood vessels over-reacting to adrenaline[UK]/epinephrine[USA] and noradrenaline[UK]/norepinephrine[USA]. Pressure through the edge of the lesion will make the naevus disappear as the surrounding blood vessels are compressed.

LICHEN SCLEROSUS ET ATROPHICUS (LSA)

This condition usually presents with genital itching and is seen as white atrophic plaques in the perineum (*see* p. 327). Rarely the trunk and limbs may also be involved. Small flat white atrophic macules and papules with a shiny wrinkled surface occur, most commonly on the upper trunk. Fortunately they are usually asymptomatic. Trunk lesions tend to be unresponsive to treatment.

PITYRIASIS VERSICOLOR

White oval macules coalesce to form large hypopigmented patches on the upper trunk and proximal limbs in young adults with tanned or pigmented skin. The surface is always slightly scaly when scratched (*see* p. 189).

SOLAR ELASTOSIS

This is a yellowish discolouration of the skin with more obvious skin creases and follicular openings on the face and neck due to chronic sun damage. Both open and closed comedones can be found within solar elastosis (Favre–Racouchot syndrome, *see* Fig. 1.38, p. 10).

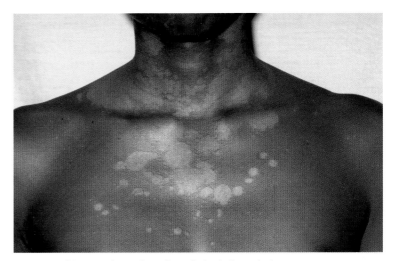

Fig. 9.41 White macules and patches of pityriasis versicolor.

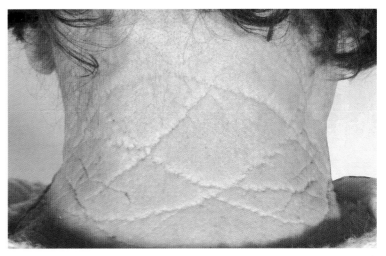

Fig. 9.42 Solar elastosis on the back of the neck.

POST-INFLAMMATORY HYPOPIGMENTATION

Partial loss of pigment may follow any inflammatory skin condition affecting the epidermis, e.g. eczema or psoriasis, just as some individuals develop hyperpigmentation in response to the same stimulus. It is distinguished from pityriasis versicolor in being more ill-defined and irregular in outline, and producing little or no scale on scratching the surface, and from vitiligo by being hypopigmented rather than depigmented.

PITYRIASIS ALBA

Multiple poorly defined hypopigmented, slightly scaly patches can occur on the face of children. In Caucasians they may only be visible in the summer when the normal skin tans. In dark-skinned individuals it is relatively common. It is considered to be a form of post-inflammatory hypopigmentation following mild eczema.

TREATMENT POST-INFLAMMATORY HYPOPIGMENTATION

Treat the underlying disease if it is still active, but reassure the patient that the pigmentation will return to normal in due course.

Fig. 9.43 Post-inflammatory hypopigmentation. Poorly defined white macules.

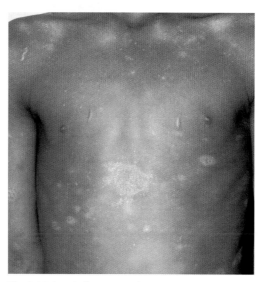

Fig. 9.44 Post-inflammatory hypopigmentation following atopic eczema in black skin.

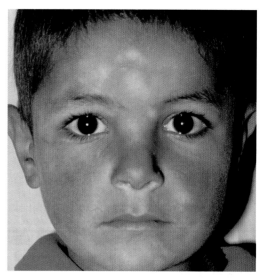

Fig. 9.45 Pityriasis alba. Poorly defined white patches on the face of a child.

Non-erythematous lesions
Normal surface
White colour
Papules

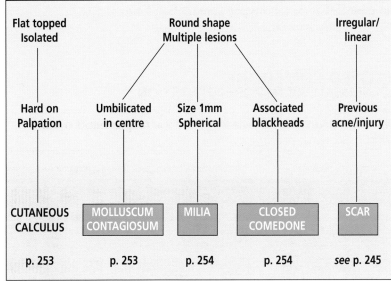

Flat topped Isolated		Round shape Multiple lesions			Irregular/ linear
Hard on Palpation	Umbilicated in centre	Size 1mm Spherical	Associated blackheads		Previous acne/injury
CUTANEOUS CALCULUS	MOLLUSCUM CONTAGIOSUM	MILIA	CLOSED COMEDONE		SCAR
p. 253	p. 253	p. 254	p. 254		*see* p. 245

MOLLUSCUM CONTAGIOSUM

This is a pox virus infection of the skin usually affecting children. Small 1–5mm white or pink umbilicated papules (Fig. 9.47) are found anywhere on the skin and there may be few or many. They can become inflamed and red in colour. They last 6–24 months and then disappear spontaneously. Isolated lesions in adults can be confused with a basal cell carcinoma.

CUTANEOUS CALCULUS

A single white, round, flat topped papule on the face of a child which feels firm to hard on palpation. It is harmless and is due to calcium deposited in the upper dermis.

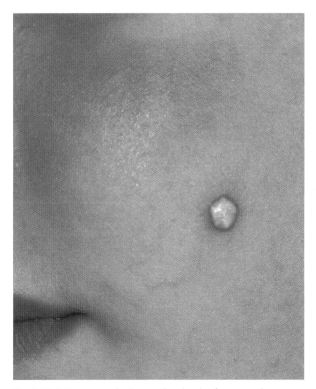

Fig. 9.46 Cutaneous calculus on the cheek of a young boy.

TREATMENT MOLLUSCUM CONTAGIOSUM

Trauma to individual lesions results in their resolution. They can be pricked by a sharpened orange stick dipped in phenol. Children do not take kindly to this but if you first apply EMLA anaesthetic cream to all the lesions under occlusion for 2 hours, they can be curetted off without discomfort. Do not cauterise as this is painful.

TREATMENT MILIA

Open the skin over each cyst with a sharp needle. Press on either side and it will pop out.

MILIA

These are very small superficial epidermoid cysts. They are small (1–2mm diameter only) white spherical papules protruding above the surface on the cheeks and eyelids. They can occur spontaneously or follow any acute sub-epidermal blister, e.g. after burns or other blistering diseases.

CLOSED COMEDONE

A closed comedone (whitehead) is a single blocked pilosebaceous follicle in which the follicular opening is not visible (*see* acne, p. 98).

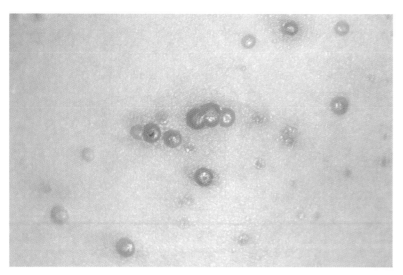

Fig. 9.47 Molluscum contagiosum.

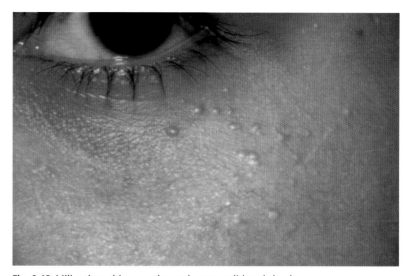

Fig. 9.48 Milia: tiny white papules on lower eyelid and cheek.

Non-erythematous lesions
Normal surface
Brown colour
Macules and small patches (<3cm size)

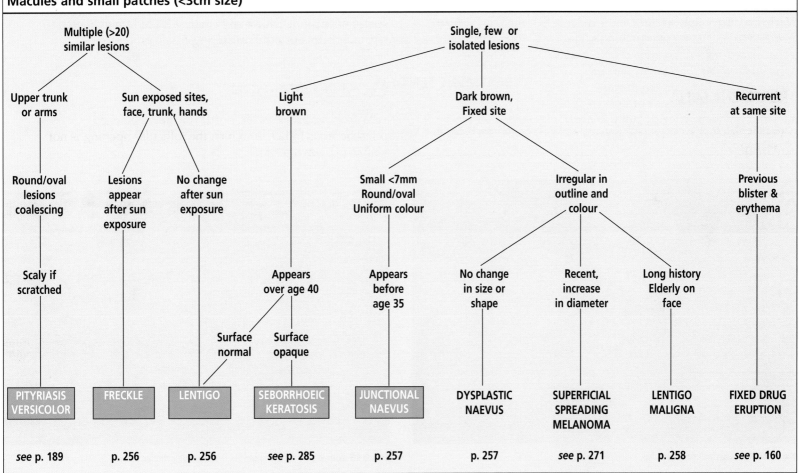

PITYRIASIS VERSICOLOR	FRECKLE	LENTIGO	SEBORRHOEIC KERATOSIS	JUNCTIONAL NAEVUS	DYSPLASTIC NAEVUS	SUPERFICIAL SPREADING MELANOMA	LENTIGO MALIGNA	FIXED DRUG ERUPTION
see p. 189	p. 256	p. 256	*see* p. 285	p. 257	p. 257	*see* p. 271	p. 258	*see* p. 160

FRECKLES (Ephelides)

These well demarcated, small (1–5mm in diameter) orangy-brown macules occur on sun exposed sites (face, dorsum hands and forearms). They appear after sun exposure in summer and disappear in winter. They occur in red-haired, blue-eyed individuals who burn rather than tan in the sun. Histologically they contain normal numbers of melanocytes but increased melanin pigment. They do not usually present a diagnostic problem or need any treatment.

LENTIGO

Lentigines are larger and darker than freckles and may have irregular edges. They occur mainly on the sun exposed skin of middle aged and elderly people and are present all the year round. They are caused by chronic sun exposure and if seen on the trunk in younger people (age <40) are evidence of too much sun exposure as a child. They are due to increased numbers of melanocytes in the basal cell layer of the epidermis.

TREATMENT LENTIGO

Skin lightening creams do not work. Reassure the patient that they are part of the normal ageing process. Individual lesions can be frozen with liquid nitrogen or treated with the Nd-YAG laser at 532nm.

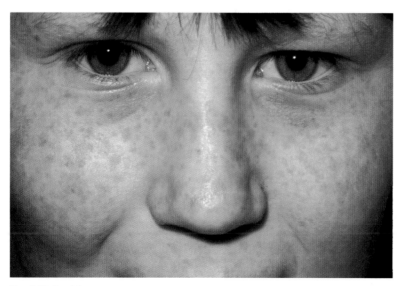

Fig. 9.49 Freckles.

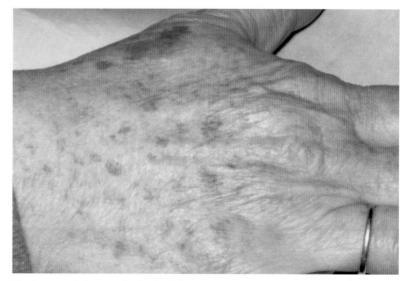

Fig. 9.50 Lentigines on the back of the hand.

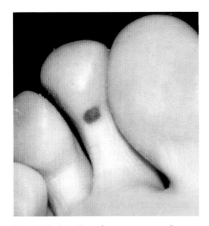

Fig. 9.51 Junctional naevus: round, symmetrical and evenly pigmented.

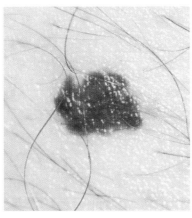

Fig. 9.52 Dysplastic naevus. Note the irregular shape.

JUNCTIONAL NAEVUS

A flat dark brown mole which is round or oval in shape is a junctional naevus. Most are smaller than 7mm in diameter. They can occur anywhere on the skin including the palms, soles and nail matrix (*see* p. 392). They appear at any age but usually before the age of 35. Histologically, groups of melanocytes are found in contact with the basal layer hence the term junctional naevus (*see* Fig. 9.78a, p. 269).

DYSPLASTIC (ATYPICAL) NAEVUS

A flat or slightly raised mole, often >7mm in diameter, which looks like a junctional naevus but has an irregular edge and different shades of brown within it.

The atypical mole (dysplastic naevus) syndrome

There are a small number of families where some members have large numbers of moles (often >100), most of which are dysplastic and a family history of malignant melanoma. Such individuals have an increased risk of developing multiple malignant melanomas.

TREATMENT JUNCTIONAL AND DYSPLASTIC NAEVI

Junctional naevi do not need to be removed unless there is doubt over the diagnosis, and indeed if lesions on the trunk are excised in young adults, the subsequent scarring can be unsightly. If the lesion has changed or developed any irregularity in colour, shape or border it should be excised and sent for histology to exclude a malignant melanoma. In patients with multiple dysplastic naevi, professional medical photographs taken of the whole body and given to the patient will help them identify any new or changing naevi.

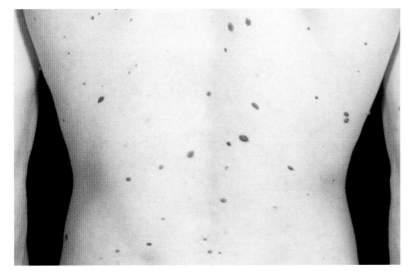

Fig. 9.53 Atypical mole syndrome. Numerous large and irregular naevi on the trunk.

LENTIGO MALIGNA

This looks very similar to an ordinary lentigo, but is larger (usually >20mm), has irregular margins and variation in pigment. It occurs only on sun damaged skin, most commonly on the cheeks of the elderly. It may be difficult to distinguish from a benign lentigo, but slow extension over several years is characteristic. The diagnosis should be confirmed by a skin biopsy which shows a malignant melanoma confined to the epidermis (melanoma-in-situ, *see* p. 270). These can sometimes progress to become an invasive malignant melanoma.

TREATMENT LENTIGO MALIGNA

Excision is the treatment of choice, although for very large lesions on the face this may be impractical. Mohs surgery (*see* p. 242) can be used to control margins. Topical 5% imiquimod (*Aldara*) cream applied 3× a week for 12 weeks is an alternative. This causes marked inflammation (*see* Fig. 9.57a) and the patient should be warned about this. Recurrence can occur so follow up is advisable.

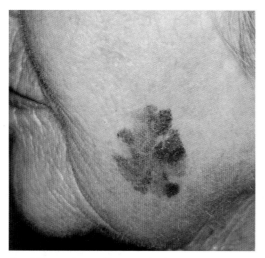

Fig. 9.54 Lentigo maligna on cheek.

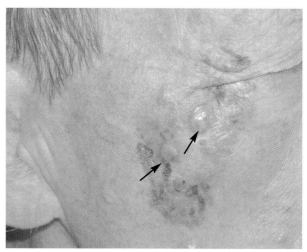

Fig. 9.55 Nodular melanoma arising in a lentigo maligna.

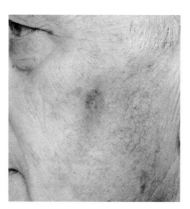

Fig. 9.56 Lentigo maligna on the cheek.

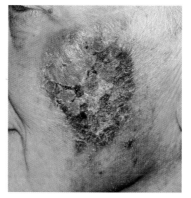

Fig. 9.57a Treatment with imiquimod produces an intense inflammatory reaction.

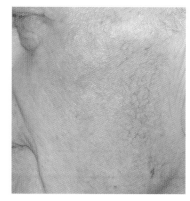

Fig. 9.57b Four weeks after completion of imiquimod treatment.

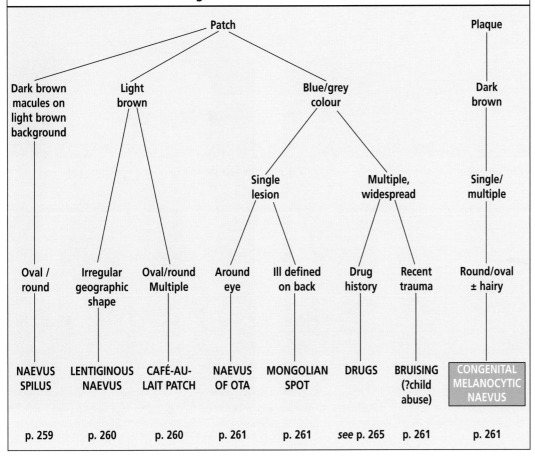

Non-erythematous lesions
Normal surface
Brown/blue/grey colour
Large patches & plaques (>3cm size)
Present from birth or before age 10

Patch — Plaque

Dark brown macules on light brown background — Light brown — Blue/grey colour — Dark brown

Single lesion — Multiple, widespread — Single/multiple

Oval / round — Irregular geographic shape — Oval/round Multiple — Around eye — Ill defined on back — Drug history — Recent trauma — Round/oval ± hairy

NAEVUS SPILUS — LENTIGINOUS NAEVUS — CAFÉ-AU-LAIT PATCH — NAEVUS OF OTA — MONGOLIAN SPOT — DRUGS — BRUISING (?child abuse) — CONGENITAL MELANOCYTIC NAEVUS

p. 259 — p. 260 — p. 260 — p. 261 — p. 261 — *see* p. 265 — p. 261 — p. 261

NAEVUS SPILUS

This is a birthmark where dark speckled macules or papules occur in a larger pale brown pigmented patch.

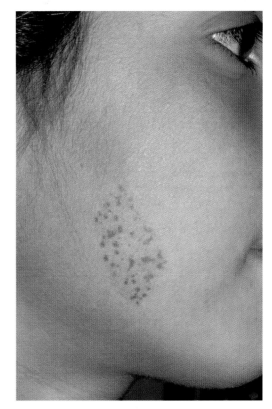

Fig. 9.58 Naevus spilus.

LENTIGINOUS NAEVUS

This is a flat pigmented birthmark, light or medium brown in colour and oval or geographic in outline. There is no surface abnormality.

CAFÉ-AU-LAIT PATCH

These are light brown patches, round or oval in shape, and often large (2–10cm diameter). They are present at birth or appear in early childhood. If more than six are found, or the patient also has freckles in the axillae and multiple neurofibromas in the skin or peripheral nerves the diagnosis of neurofibromatosis (von Recklinghausen's disease) can be made (*see* p. 234).

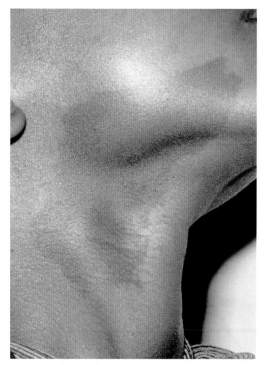

Fig. 9.59 Lentiginous naevus.

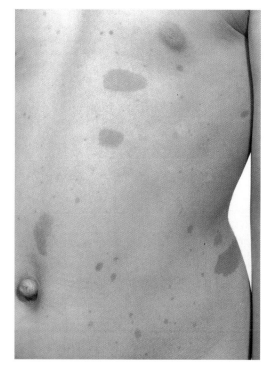

Fig. 9.60 Multiple café-au-lait patches.

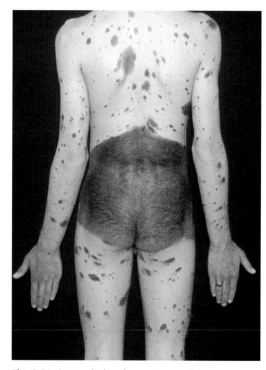

Fig. 9.61 Congenital melanocytic naevi. Large 'bathing trunk' naevus and multiple smaller naevi.

NAEVUS OF OTA

This is grey-blue patch of pigmentation around the eye and on the sclera on one side only. It is a type of blue naevus with the melanocytes situated deep within the dermis. It is common amongst the Japanese and is present from birth or early childhood. It remains present throughout life. A similar lesion on the shoulder is called a **naevus of Ito**.

MONGOLIAN SPOT

A large blue-grey patch on the back of an oriental baby is extremely common. It disappears spontaneously in the first year of life.

BRUISING (Child abuse)

Bruising can leave a blue-grey discolouration. In children the possibility of abuse always needs to be considered.

CONGENITAL MELANOCYTIC NAEVUS

Congenital melanocytic naevi are moles that are present at birth. They are normally >2cm in diameter. At birth they may be red, rather than brown, but within a few months are obviously pigmented. They may be flat or raised, hairy or warty. They may sometimes be very large covering up to ½ the body surface. For the very large naevi there is a 9% lifetime risk, greatest before puberty, of developing one or more malignant melanomas within the naevus.

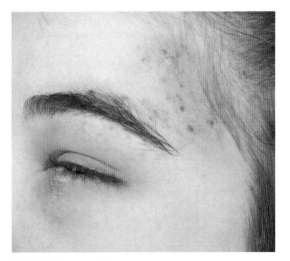

Fig. 9.62 Mongolian spot on buttocks and lower back.

Fig. 9.63 Naevus of Ota.

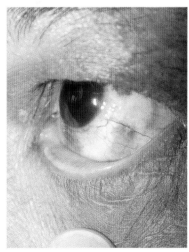

Fig. 9.64 Naevus of Ota on the sclera.

Non-erythematous lesions
Normal surface
Brown colour
Patches and plaques (>3cm size)
Appear after age 10 years

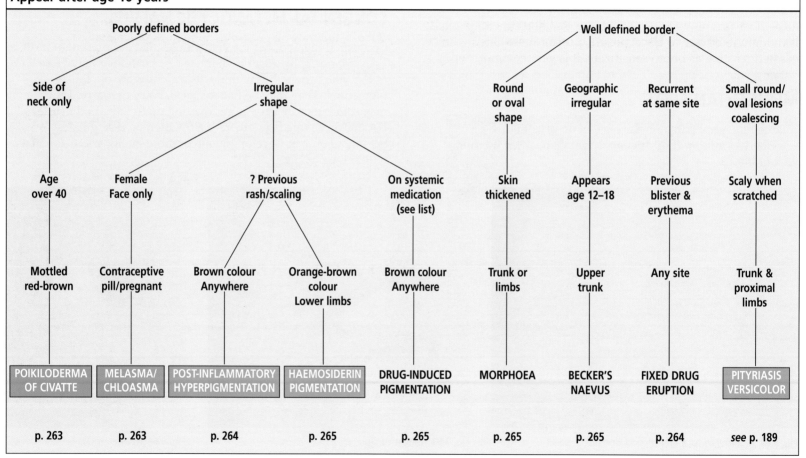

Poorly defined borders

- Side of neck only
  - Age over 40
    - Mottled red-brown
    - **POIKILODERMA OF CIVATTE**
    - p. 263
- Irregular shape
  - Female Face only
    - Contraceptive pill/pregnant
    - **MELASMA/ CHLOASMA**
    - p. 263
  - ? Previous rash/scaling
    - Brown colour Anywhere
    - **POST-INFLAMMATORY HYPERPIGMENTATION**
    - p. 264
    - Orange-brown colour Lower limbs
    - **HAEMOSIDERIN PIGMENTATION**
    - p. 265
  - On systemic medication (see list)
    - Brown colour Anywhere
    - **DRUG-INDUCED PIGMENTATION**
    - p. 265

Well defined border

- Round or oval shape
  - Skin thickened
    - Trunk or limbs
    - **MORPHOEA**
    - p. 265
- Geographic irregular
  - Appears age 12–18
    - Upper trunk
    - **BECKER'S NAEVUS**
    - p. 265
- Recurrent at same site
  - Previous blister & erythema
    - Any site
    - **FIXED DRUG ERUPTION**
    - p. 264
- Small round/ oval lesions coalescing
  - Scaly when scratched
    - Trunk & proximal limbs
    - **PITYRIASIS VERSICOLOR**
    - *see* p. 189

POIKILODERMA OF CIVATTE

Poikiloderma is identified by the combination of pigment, atrophy and telangiectasia. Poikiloderma of Civatte is the commonest type and occurs in middle aged and older patients on the sides of the neck. The skin becomes a mottled red-brown colour with atrophic areas. The area immediately under the chin and ears is spared. It is thought to be due to UV exposure, possibly associated with cosmetics acting as photo-sensitizers. It is very common and patients rarely bring it to the attention of their doctors. No treatment is available other than using a sunblock.

MELASMA (CHLOASMA)

Unsightly symmetrical pigmented patches occur in women on the forehead, cheeks and moustache area which darken after sun exposure. They occur most commonly during pregnancy or on taking the contraceptive pill. The pigmentation usually fades after delivery or on stopping the pill, but may be permanent. Identical pigmentation is sometimes seen in men, and in women who are not pregnant or on the pill.

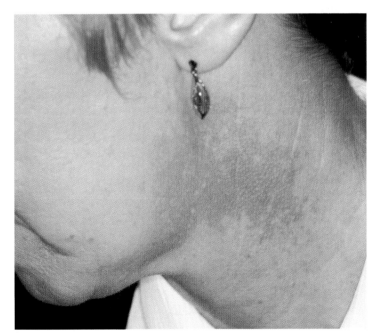

Fig. 9.65 Poikiloderma of Civatte.

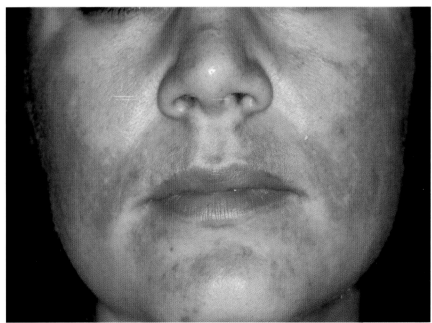

Fig. 9.66 Melasma.

TREATMENT MELASMA

If on the contraceptive pill stop taking it. Try 4% hydroquinone (*Eldoquin*[UK]/*Aldoquin*[USA]) cream b.i.d. for up to 6 months (not longer). A mixture of 0.05% tretinoin, 4% hydroquinone and 0.01% fluocinolone acetonide in a hydrophilic cream base (*Triluma*[USA]) applied b.i.d. for 8 weeks works much better. Once the pigment has gone, the patient must keep out of the sun and/or use a high factor (15+) sunscreen or it will reoccur.

POST-INFLAMMATORY HYPERPIGMENTATION

Macular melanin pigmentation may follow any inflammatory process in the epidermis (e.g. eczema, psoriasis, lichen planus). It is commoner in darker skinned individuals. There is usually a history of a rash before the pigment change. No treatment is available but it will improve with time. The inflammatory phase of a **fixed drug eruption** (*see* p. 160) can also be followed by a dark brown patch which remains for several months.

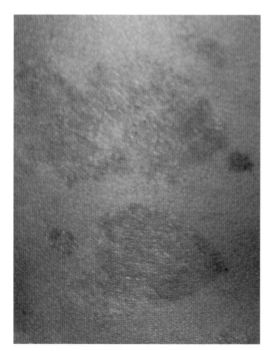

Fig. 9.67 Post inflammatory hyperpigmentation following psoriasis.

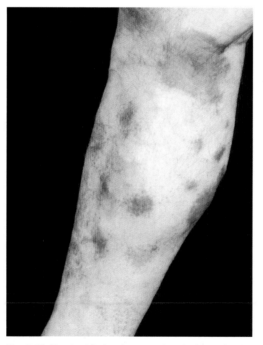

Fig. 9.68 Haemosiderin pigmentation on lower leg.

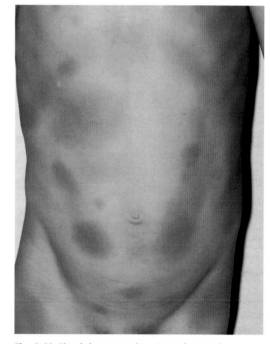

Fig. 9.69 Fixed drug eruption. Round or oval pigmented patches.

HAEMOSIDERIN PIGMENTATION

This is seen following purpura where haemoglobin is broken down to haemosiderin. The haemosiderin pigment looks similar to melanin except that it is a more rusty-brown colour (*see* p. 354).

HYPERPIGMENTATION DUE TO DRUGS

The following drugs can cause an increase in melanin in the skin: amiodarone, arsenic (raindrop pigmentation), busulphan, chloroquine, the contraceptive pill (on face) and phenytoin.

Non-melanin pigmentation can be caused by clofazimine (red-pink), β-carotene (orange), mepacrine (yellow), and dapsone, gold (Fig. 1.75, p. 15), minocycline (Fig. 1.74) and chlorpromazine (all blue-grey colour).

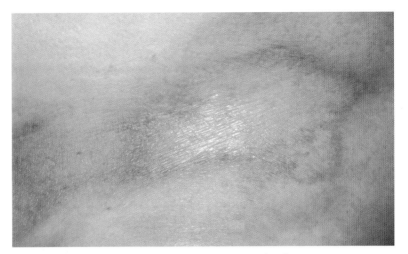

Fig. 9.70 Morphoea. Brown plaque with purple brown border.

MORPHOEA

Morphoea can present as a brown patch or plaque with a purple brown border, *see also* p. 248.

BECKER'S NAEVUS

This is a congenital harmatoma of the skin that is androgen-sensitive so appears in the mid-late teens and then persists for life. It is an irregularly shaped patch of hyperpigmentation containing more hairs than is normal. It most commonly occurs over the shoulder region but can occur anywhere. No treatment is available although the hair can be treated with a laser (Alexandrite, *see* p. 53) but this can make the hyperpigmentation worse.

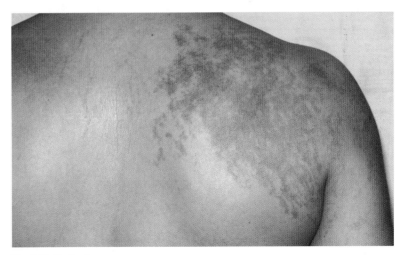

Fig. 9.71 Becker's naevus.

Non-erythematous lesions
Normal surface
Brown colour
Papules, plaques & nodules

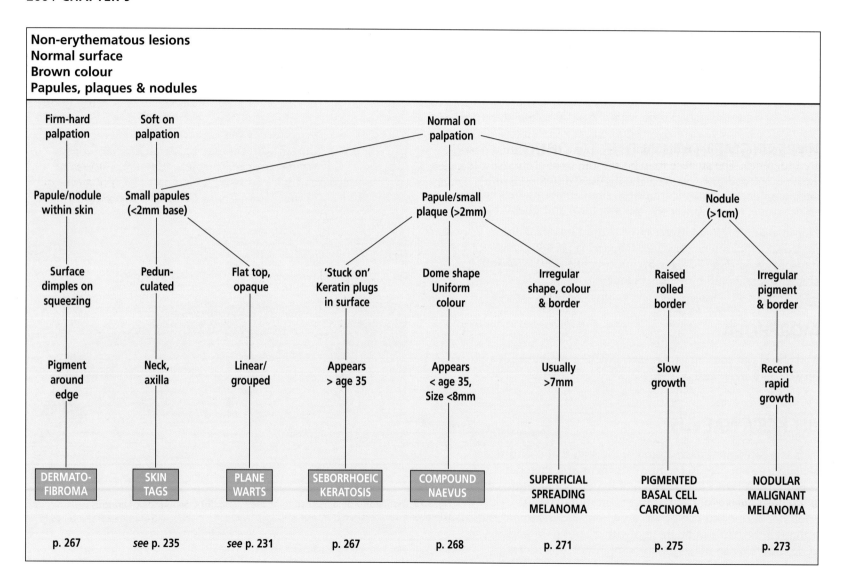

Firm-hard palpation	Soft on palpation		Normal on palpation				
Papule/nodule within skin	Small papules (<2mm base)		Papule/small plaque (>2mm)			Nodule (>1cm)	
Surface dimples on squeezing	Pedun-culated	Flat top, opaque	'Stuck on' Keratin plugs in surface	Dome shape Uniform colour	Irregular shape, colour & border	Raised rolled border	Irregular pigment & border
Pigment around edge	Neck, axilla	Linear/ grouped	Appears > age 35	Appears < age 35, Size <8mm	Usually >7mm	Slow growth	Recent rapid growth
DERMATO-FIBROMA	SKIN TAGS	PLANE WARTS	SEBORRHOEIC KERATOSIS	COMPOUND NAEVUS	SUPERFICIAL SPREADING MELANOMA	PIGMENTED BASAL CELL CARCINOMA	NODULAR MALIGNANT MELANOMA
p. 267	*see* p. 235	*see* p. 231	p. 267	p. 268	p. 271	p. 275	p. 273

DERMATOFIBROMA (Histiocytoma)

This is a firm-hard papule situated in the dermis and occurs anywhere on the body. It often follows an insect bite, so is most commonly found on the legs. It is usually small (<5mm), attached to the skin and mobile over deeper structures. Squeezing the lesion from the sides results in puckering of the skin since dermatofibromas are situated very high in the dermis. The colour ranges from skin coloured, to pink to brown, often with a darker circumference. The surface may be smooth or slightly scaly. It looks like a compound naevus but is distinguished by being much firmer on palpation.

SEBORRHOEIC KERATOSIS/WART

Seborrhoeic keratoses usually have a warty or keratotic surface (*see* p. 285). Occasionally they have a smooth surface and can be confused with compound naevi or even malignant melanoma if very heavily pigmented. If you look carefully at the surface you may see small keratin plugs which are specific to seborrhoeic keratoses. In addition the lesion will tend to be sitting on top of the skin and have no deep component at all.

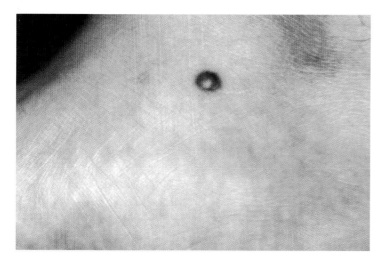

Fig. 9.72 Dermatofibroma.

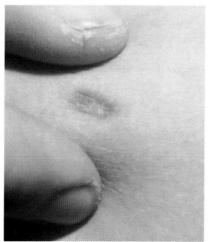

Fig. 9.73 Dermatofibroma. Puckering of the skin over it occurs when it is squeezed.

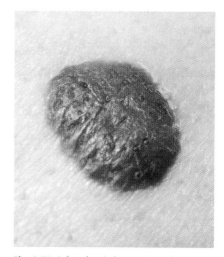

Fig. 9.74 Seborrhoeic keratosis with smooth surface. Note tiny keratin plugs in the surface.

COMPOUND NAEVUS

These are melanocytic naevi that are both raised and pigmented. On histology the melanocytes are both at the dermo-epidermal junction and within the dermis (hence compound). The melanocytes at the dermo-epidermal junction give moles their brown colour while the intradermal melanocytes result in elevation. The natural history of moles is a maturation from junctional naevi (flat & dark brown) to compound naevi (brown and dome-shaped or papillomatous) to intradermal naevi (skin coloured papules) (*see* Fig. 9.78).

Established benign moles change (see above) and new moles occur or get bigger after sun exposure, at around puberty and during pregnancy. Assuming that all moles that change are malignant is misleading. It is the type of change that is important. If a benign mole becomes more *elevated* and at the same time *lightens* in colour, this is the normal change from junctional to intradermal naevus. Sometimes moles can look irregular if part of the periphery of the mole is flat and brown (junctional) and the centre raised and lighter in colour (intradermal) (Fig. 9.77). Malignant change should be thought of if there is lateral spread of pigment (*see* Fig. 9.79, p. 270).

TREATMENT DERMATOFIBROMA & COMPOUND NAEVUS

Only remove if they are very unsightly or get caught on clothing. For compound naevi removal by shave biopsy will generally leave an acceptable scar which is flat and no bigger than the original lesion although recurrence of pigment may occur. Dermatofibromas need to be excised but in young people this can leave ugly scars. Always send the lesion off for histology.

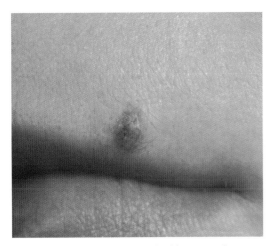

Fig. 9.75 Compound naevus: raised brown mole.

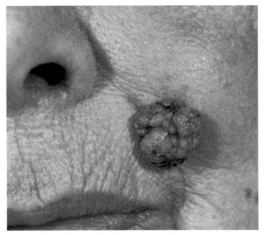

Fig. 9.76 Compound naevus with papillomatous surface.

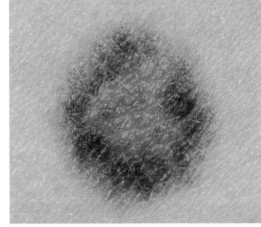

Fig. 9.77 Compound naevus with peripheral junctional area.

a. Junctional naevus (p. 257)

HISTOLOGICAL FEATURES:–
Naevus cells at dermo-epidermal junction

b. Compound naevus (p. 268)

Naevus cells at dermo-epidermal junction & within the dermis

c. Intradermal naevus (p. 233)

Naevus cells only within the dermis

d. Combined juctional & compound naevus

Intradermal naevus cells centrally, junctional cells at the edge

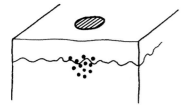
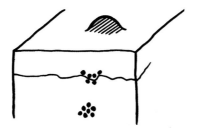
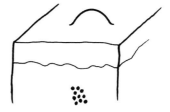
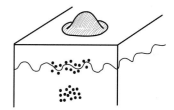

CLINICAL FEATURES:–

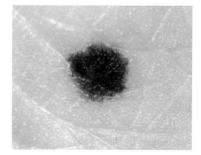
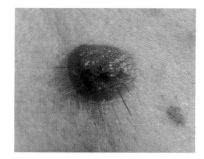
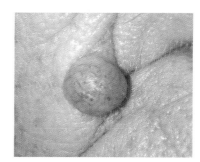
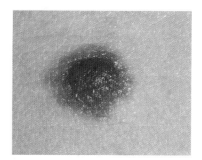

Flat & brown

Raised (dome shaped or papillomatous) & brown

Raised (dome shaped or papillomatous) & skin coloured

Periphery flat & brown, centre raised & brown

Fig. 9.78 Clinico-pathological correlation of melanocytic naevi (moles).

a. Lentigo maligna (p. 258)

HISTOLOGICAL FEATURES:–
Malignant melanocytes
restricted to epidermis only
Has an *excellent prognosis.*

**b. Superficial spreading
malignant melanoma** (p. 271)

Malignant melanocytes
migrating laterally along the
dermo-epidermal junction
Has a *good prognosis.*

**c. Superficial spreading
melanoma with nodule** (p. 271)

Malignant cells now growing
downwards as well as
laterally
Has a *worse progosis.*

d. Nodular malignant melanoma
(p. 273)

Malignant naevus cells
migrating vertically
downwards
Has a *poor prognosis.*

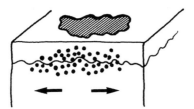 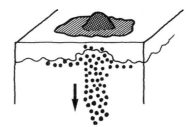 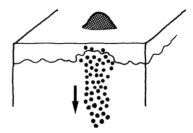

CLINICAL FEATURES:–

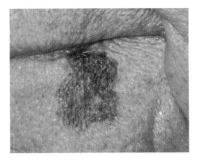 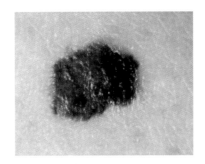 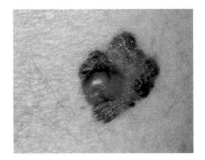 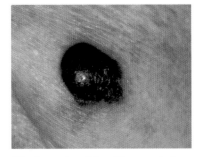

Large irregular brown patch
on sun exposed skin in the
elderly

Irregular shape & pigment;
↑ diameter; slightly elevated

Irregular shape & pigment;
nodule within pigmented area

Black, red or bleeding nodule.
No surrounding pigmentation

Fig. 9.79 Clinico-pathological correlation of malignant melanoma.

MALIGNANT MELANOMA

A malignant melanoma is a malignant tumour of melanocytes. Two-thirds arise from normal skin and one-third from a pre-existing mole. There are four clinical patterns of malignant melanoma.

1. **Lentigo maligna**. A large (1–3cm size) brown patch on sun exposed skin in an elderly patient. The tumour cells are confined to the epidermis (*see* p. 258). Later an invasive melanoma can develop with a lentigo maligna as a papule or nodule within the original patch (Fig. 9.55, p. 258).

2. **Superficial spreading malignant melanoma**. The initial growth phase of malignant melanocytes is along the dermo-epidermal junction (*radial growth phase*). This change is seen clinically as a flat brown patch enlarging in diameter. Because the radial growth is usually uneven, there will be variation in the degree of pigmentation and an irregular border, often with scalloped edges. There may also be evidence of inflammation, erythema and sometimes an altered sensation.

Tumour cells remain high in the dermis and are unlikely to invade blood vessels or lymphatics. As a result superficial spreading melanomas generally carry a good prognosis.

Superficial spreading melanoma with a nodular component. Eventually the malignant melanocytes grow downwards (*vertical growth phase*). A papule or nodule will appear within the flat irregular brown patch (*see* Fig. 9.82). Once this happens the prognosis becomes worse because tumour cells are more likely to have entered dermal blood vessels and lymphatics leading to metastases.

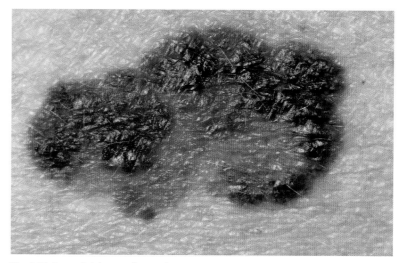

Fig. 9.80 Superficial spreading melanoma. Irregular in colour and shape.

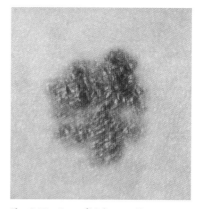

Fig. 9.81a Superficial spreading melanoma with background erythema.

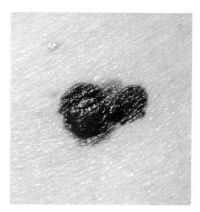

Fig. 9.81b Superficial spreading melanoma. Small early lesion.

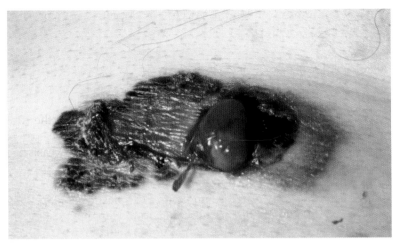

Fig. 9.82 Superficial spreading melanoma with amelanotic nodule.

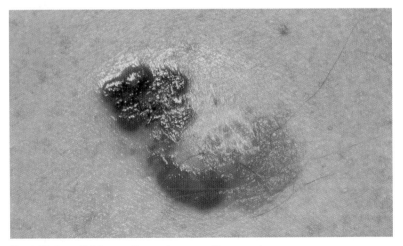

Fig. 9.83 Superficial spreading melanoma with regression.

Diagnosis of superficial spreading malignant melanoma

It is important to diagnose malignant melanomas while they are thin so that removal results in cure. In practice this means distinguishing them from junctional and compound naevi. Remember that benign moles can change (*see* Fig. 9.78, p. 269). To identify early superficial spreading melanomas there are two possible check lists that are helpful, the American ABCDE list or the Glasgow seven point checklist.

The **American ABCDE** list:–
  Asymmetry
  Border irregular
  Colour irregular
  Diameter over 1cm
  Erythema.

The **Glasgow** list:–
Major features (score 2 points)

1. Change in size (diameter)
2. Change or irregular shape
3. Change or irregular colour.

Minor features (score 1 point)

4. Diameter more than 6mm
5. Inflammation
6. Oozing or bleeding
7. Mild itch or altered sensation.

Suspect a melanoma if any major feature is present or there is a total score of 3 or more.

3. **Nodular malignant melanoma**. This type needs to be distinguished from the superficial spreading melanoma. Here there is no radial growth and the malignant melanocytes grow down vertically from the start. The lesion is a nodule without any surrounding irregular pigmentation. Neither the ABCDE nor the Glasgow rules help in making the diagnosis. A typical nodular melanoma is a black dome shaped nodule. The surface of the lesion will eventually break down to bleed, ooze and crust over. Sometimes nodules may be red (amelanotic – *see also* Fig. 8.22, p. 182) rather than brown.

The diagnosis can be delayed as there is no superficial spread to alert the patient, and prognosis is often poor as the lesion will be relatively thick before it has been diagnosed and removed.

4. **Acral lentiginous melanomas** occur on the palms, soles or under the nails (*see* p. 399).

Aetiology of malignant melanoma

Malignant melanoma is more likely to occur in:–

- Those with fair or red hair who burn rather than tan in the sun (skin types 1 & 2).
- Those who have been badly burnt on more than one occasion in childhood.
- Those who have a large number of moles (>50).
- Those with multiple atypical moles (*see* dysplastic naevi, p. 257).
- Those with a family history of malignant melanoma.
- Those who have already had a malignant melanoma.

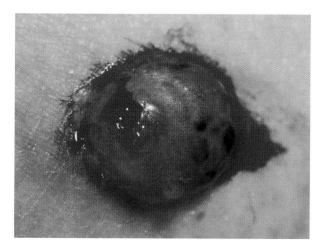

Fig. 9.84 Nodular melanoma with no horizontal growth phase.

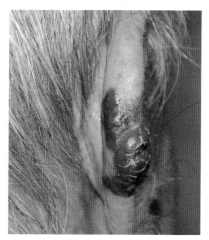

Fig. 9.85 Nodular melanoma on the ear.

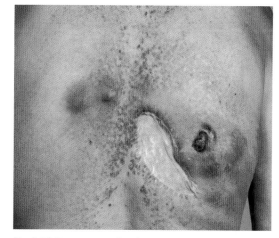

Fig. 9.86 Recurrence of melanoma around skin graft on the back.

Prognosis of malignant melanoma (*see* Table 9.01)

The following have been found to accurately predict prognosis:–
- Breslow's thickness (Fig. 9.87). This is the depth of the tumour in mm measured by the pathologist from the top of the granular cell layer of the epidermis to the deepest point of invasion. This is by far the most important prognostic indicator.
- Ulceration. For any given thickness this worsens the prognosis.
- Involvement of regional lymph nodes or satellite/in-transit metastases makes the prognosis worse (Stage III). The more nodes involved (>3) and if the metastases are clinically apparent (macroscopic), the worse the prognosis.
- Distant metastases and elevated levels of lactic dehydrogenase imply a very poor prognosis (Stage IV).

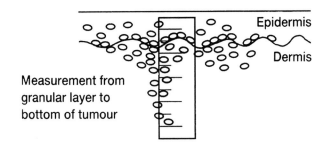

Fig. 9.87 Breslow's thickness. Measure in mm the depth of invasion from the granular layer to the deepest tumour cells.

PROGNOSIS OF MALIGNANT MELANOMA (% SURVIVAL RATES 1–15 YEARS)

No lymph node involvement or distant metastasis

Stage	Thickness	Ulceration	1 year	2 years	5 years	10 years	15 years
IA	<1mm	No	99.7	99.0	95	88	85
IB**	<1mm	Yes	99.8	98.7	91	83	72
	1–2mm	No	99.5	97.3	89	79	72
IIA	1–2mm	Yes	98.2	93	77	64	57
	2–4mm	No	98.7	94	79	64	57
IIB	2–4mm	Yes	95.1	85	63	51	44
	>4mm	No	95	89	67	54	44
IIC	>4mm	Yes	90	71	45	32	29

With lymph node involvement or distant metastasis – any thickness

Stage	Nodes	Ulceration	1 year	2 years	5 years	10 years	15 years
IIIA	1–3 micro	No	95	86	67	60	59
IIIB	1–3 micro	Yes	88	75	53	38	31
	1–3 macro	No	88	75	53	38	31
IIIC	1–3 macro	Yes	71	49	27	19	17
	>4 or in-transit	Yes/No	71	49	27	19	17
IV	Distant metastases		50	25	10	7	5

TREATMENT MALIGNANT MELANOMA

All suspicious lesions should be excised with a 2mm margin of normal skin and sent for histology. Having confirmed the diagnosis histologically, wider excision is carried out as follows (UK & Australian guidelines):–

   Confined to the epidermis – 0.5cm margin
   Tumours <1mm thick – excise with 1cm margin
   Tumours 1–2mm thick – excise with 1–2cm margin
   Tumours >2mm thick – excise with >2cm margin

Adjuvent therapy with interferon alpha-2b and vaccines are being trialled but there is no proven clinical benefit at present.

Table 9.01 (left) Prognosis of malignant melanoma showing % survival rates at up to 15 years (from Balch *et al. J. Clin. Oncol.* 2001;**19**:3635–3648).

** also Clark's level IV & V , depth <1mm with no ulceration

Sentinel node biopsy

Removal of the nearest lymph node (the sentinel node) to which the lymphatics at the site of the tumour drain may help predict the prognosis. It is found by injecting a radioactive tracer and a blue dye. If this node does not contain tumour, the prognosis is obviously better than if it does. Block dissection of the nodes is usually done if the sentinel node is positive. Otherwise lymph nodes are not removed unless clinically involved.

There is no evidence that sentinel node biopsy or removal of lymph nodes improves the prognosis. It should only be performed to give the patient or physician a better idea of prognosis.

Prevention of melanomas

Almost all melanomas are induced by sun exposure, particularly short sharp bursts leading to sunburn. Everyone should protect themselves from sunburn and in particular parents should protect their children from sunburn by using a high protective factor sunscreen (30+ SPF, broad spectrum, waterproof) on all exposed skin and covering as much skin as possible with clothes and a broad-brimmed hat.

There is no evidence that having a melanoma during pregnancy affects the prognosis; likewise taking the contraceptive pill or hormone replacement therapy do not alter the natural history of melanoma.

PIGMENTED BASAL CELL CARCINOMA

Occasionally basal cell carcinomas are heavily pigmented and they may then be confused with a nodular malignant melanoma. The typical rolled edge should suggest the diagnosis – *see* p. 242.

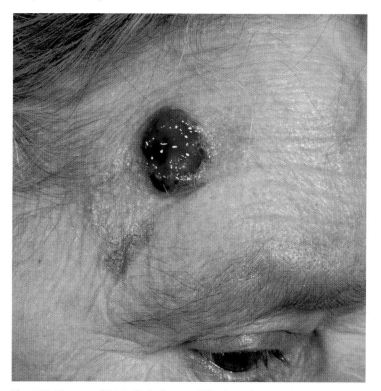

Fig. 9.88 Pigmented BCC. Clinically very difficult to distinguish this from a malignant melanoma but most of the pigment is in the rolled edge.

Non-erythematous lesions
Normal surface
Black/blue/purple colour
Macules, papules & nodules

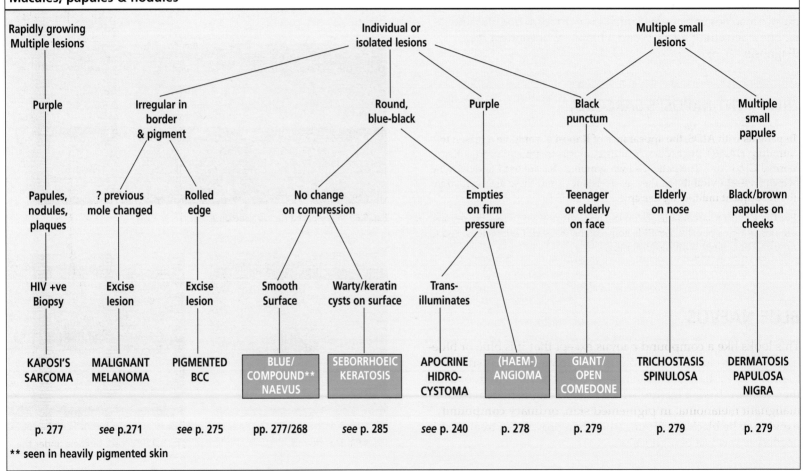

** seen in heavily pigmented skin

KAPOSI'S SARCOMA

This is a malignant growth of blood vessels caused by human herpes virus 8. It is seen mainly in patients with HIV/AIDS. The lesions begin as small reddish-purple, reddish-brown or purple macules or papules which grow to form nodules and plaques. Screening for HIV and a biopsy will confirm the diagnosis.

TREATMENT KAPOSI'S SARCOMA

In patients with AIDS, the appearance of Kaposi's would be a reason to introduce HAART (highly active anti-retrovirus treatment) even with a normal CD_4 count. The patient's own lymphocytes are used to determine which anti-retroviral drugs they are resistant to and these are avoided in the subsequent multi-drug therapy.

For the Kaposi's sarcoma itself, no treatment is needed unless the lesions are unsightly or painful. Small lesions can be excised. Lesions localised to a limb can be treated with radiotherapy.

BLUE NAEVUS

This looks like a compound naevus except that it is blue or blue-black rather than brown in colour. It is dome shaped, usually less than 10mm in diameter. Blue naevi appear during childhood and then remain fixed, a feature which will distinguish them from a malignant melanoma. In pigmented skin, ordinary **compound naevi** may be black in colour rather than brown. No treatment is needed as this is a benign lesion.

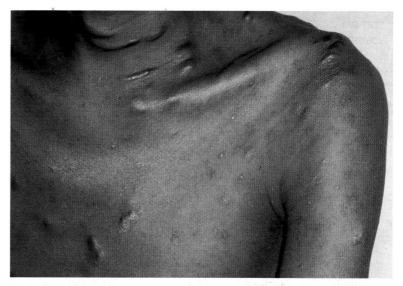

Fig. 9.89 Widespread Kaposi's sarcoma.

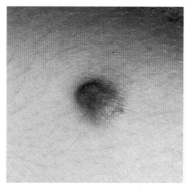

Fig. 9.90 Blue neavus.

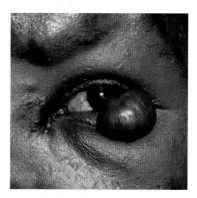

Fig. 9.91 Kaposi's sarcoma under the eye.

(HAEM)ANGIOMA & ANGIOKERATOMA

The terms angioma and haemangioma are interchangeable. Red or purple papules and plaques which have been present since childhood are due to a localised overgrowth of blood vessels. The stagnant blood within the lesion may be compressed partially, but the colour will never fade completely.

Those occurring in adult life may be very dark in colour and mimic an early melanoma. If you look carefully you will see a lobulated vascular pattern; this is easily seen using a dermatoscope (*see* p. 18).

Angiokeratomas are similar to angiomas but have a scaly surface. They may be almost black in colour.

TREATMENT ANGIOMA & HAEMANGIOMA

Small lesions can be excised or cauterised. Larger lesions are best left alone as the vascular malformation in the deeper tissues may be extensive.

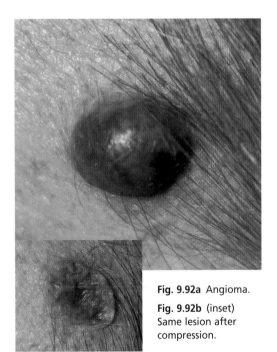

Fig. 9.92a Angioma.

Fig. 9.92b (inset) Same lesion after compression.

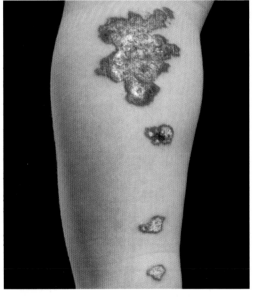

Fig. 9.93 Angiokeratoma differs from an ordinary angioma in having a scaly surface.

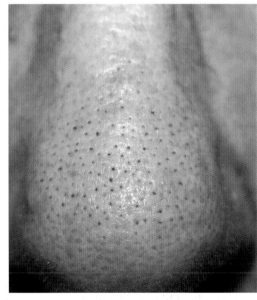

Fig. 9.94 Trichostasis spinulosa on the nose.

GIANT COMEDO

Single large comedones can occur on the trunk and face in the elderly. They are much larger than the blackheads associated with acne in teenagers, but the aetiology is basically the same, i.e. a single follicle with a keratin plug at its mouth, filling up with keratin and sebum behind it. Clinically it is a white/cream papule with a central black punctum.

TRICHOSTASIS SPINULOSA

Small blackheads on the nose in elderly patients are very common. They are due to the failure of shedding of vellus hairs in the hair follicles of the nose.

TREATMENT TRICHOSTASIS SPINULOSA

If the patient complains about the problem and wants treatment 0.025% tretinoin (*Retin-A*) cream or lotion applied at night for 6–8 weeks will give a fairly dramatic improvement. It can be kept clear by using it twice a week.

DERMATOSIS PAPULOSA NIGRA

Multiple small black or brown papules occur on the cheeks particularly of blacks. Histologically the lesions are seborrhoeic keratoses. They are inherited as an autosomal dominant trait. They are harmless and best left alone.

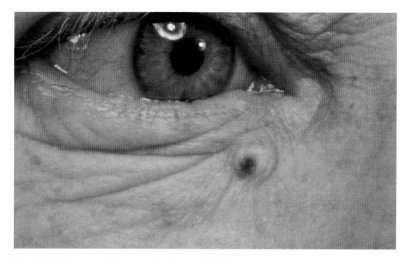

Fig. 9.95 Giant comedone on the lower eyelid.

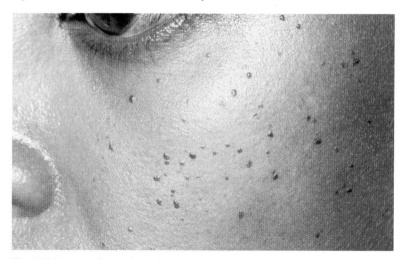

Fig. 9.96 Dermatosis papulosa nigra.

Non-erythematous lesions
Normal surface
Red/orange colour
Macules & papules (Nodules, *see* pp. 180 & 237)

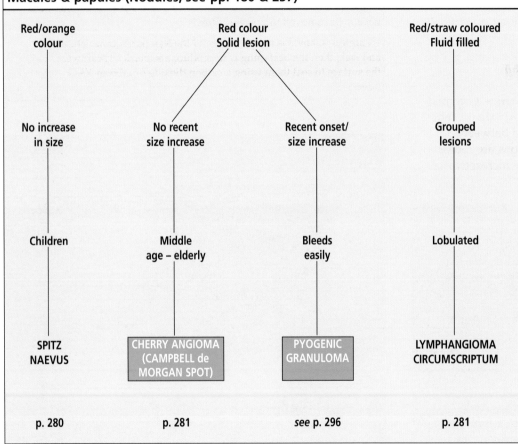

Red/orange colour	Red colour Solid lesion	Red/straw coloured Fluid filled

Red/orange colour → No increase in size → Children → **SPITZ NAEVUS** → p. 280

Red colour Solid lesion:
- No recent size increase → Middle age – elderly → **CHERRY ANGIOMA (CAMPBELL de MORGAN SPOT)** → p. 281
- Recent onset/ size increase → Bleeds easily → **PYOGENIC GRANULOMA** → *see* p. 296

Red/straw coloured Fluid filled → Grouped lesions → Lobulated → **LYMPHANGIOMA CIRCUMSCRIPTUM** → p. 281

SPITZ NAEVUS

These look like moles but they are red/orange in colour. They mainly occur in children. In adults they can be confused histologically with malignant melanoma. Reassurance that they are benign is all that is necessary.

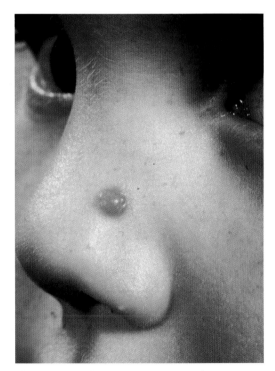

Fig. 9.97 Spitz naevus.

CHERRY ANGIOMA (Campbell de Morgan spot)

These small (1–4mm) bright red or purple papules appear on the trunk and proximal limbs in patients over the age of 35. Usually there are multiple lesions. They are a normal finding and do not need to be removed.

LYMPHANGIOMA CIRCUMSCRIPTUM

This is an uncommon malformation of the lymphatics. Grouped straw coloured papules which look like frog spawn are present in the skin. Usually there is some communication between lymphatics and blood vessels so some of the lesions are red or black. The lesions may remain static or gradually increase in extent over the years.

TREATMENT LYMPHANGIOMA CIRCUMSCRIPTUM

As well as the visible surface component, there is a deep component (muscular cistern) in the subcutaneous fat. If treatment is required, surgical excision is the treatment of choice but the deep component will have to be removed to prevent recurrence.

If surgical removal is not possible and the lesions get traumatised and leak, then the best thing is to produce a superficial scar over the surface to seal them using a carbon dioxide or erbium-YAG laser.

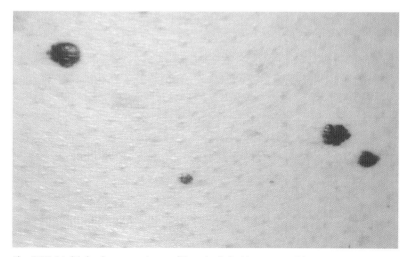

Fig. 9.98 Multiple cherry angiomas (Campbell de Morgan spots).

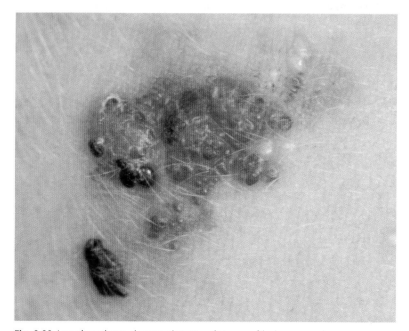

Fig. 9.99 Lymphangioma circumscriptum – close up of lesion on neck.

Non-erythematous lesions
Warty surface
Brown/skin colour
Papules & nodules

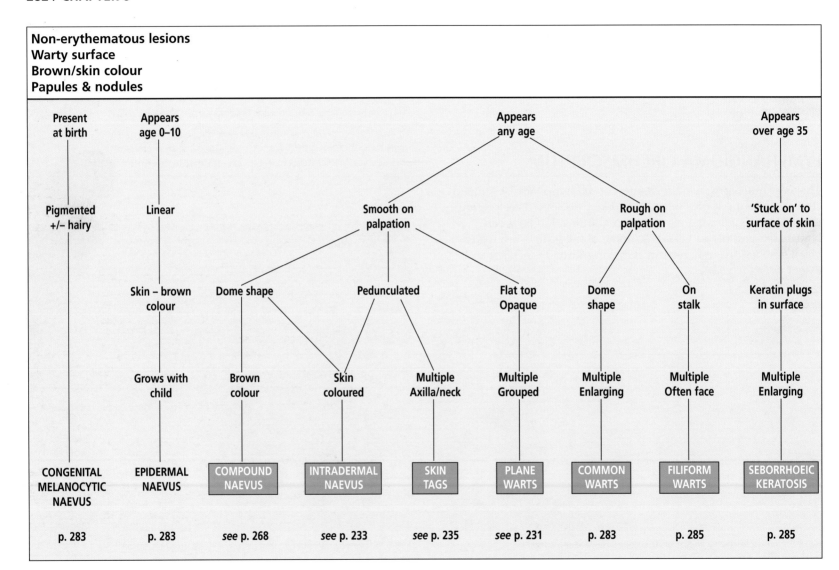

CONGENITAL MELANOCYTIC NAEVUS

Congenital melanocytic naevi unlike acquired moles are present at birth. They are usually >2cm in diameter and are brown with a warty and sometimes hairy surface (*see also* p. 261).

EPIDERMAL NAEVUS

An epidermal naevus is a developmental defect which presents as a skin coloured or brown linear warty plaque. It often looks like a line of viral warts, but it is present from birth or early childhood. It may be quite small (1–2cm long) or go down the length of an arm or leg, or in a line around one side of the trunk.

TREATMENT EPIDERMAL NAEVUS

None is usually needed. Surgical removal is difficult especially if the lesion is large. A compromise is to shave and cauterise the superficial component. There is a tendency for the warty papules to regrow but this may take several years.

COMMON WARTS

Warts are an infection of the epidermis with one of the numerous human papilloma viruses. They are transmitted from one individual to another through broken skin (cuts, grazes etc.). They disappear spontaneously without scarring after weeks to years (average about 2 years) when the body has built up enough cell mediated immunity. Unfortunately immunity to one type of wart virus does not confer immunity to any of the others,

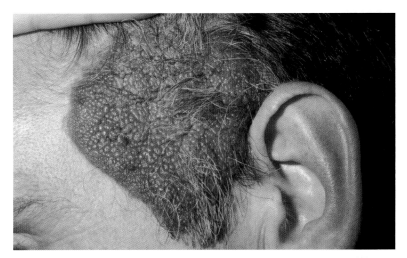

Fig. 9.100 Congenital melanocytic naevus with a papillomatous surface.

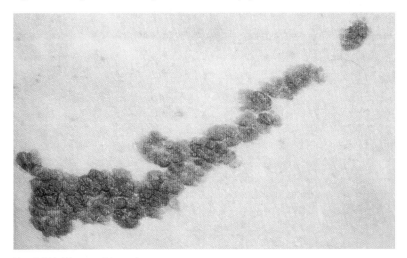

Fig. 9.101 Warty epidermal naevus.

i.e. having had an infection with the common wart virus does not prevent infection with the plantar wart or plane wart virus.

Common warts are easily recognised as firm, rough, skin coloured or brown papules with black pin point dots on the surface.

TREATMENT COMMON WARTS

Treatment of warts depends on the age of the patient and how many are present.

In **young children** the best treatment is to leave alone. You will need to explain to parents that they are a viral infection which will resolve spontaneously.

For **older children** and **adults**

If there is a *single wart or only a few warts* the options are:–

- Cryotherapy. First pare down any hyperkeratosis on the surface and then freeze with liquid nitrogen until the wart and a halo of normal skin go white (10–30secs). The patient should get a blister at the site within 48 hours as the epidermis which contains the wart lifts off. It is important that the treatment is repeated every 2–3 weeks until they go. Do not use several freeze-thaw cycles as you may get necrosis of the underlying skin. Large warts (>5mm diameter) do *not* respond well to cryotherapy.

- Curettage and cautery under local anaesthetic is very effective and should result in clearance immediately. This is a very good treatment for single warts on the face and elsewhere.

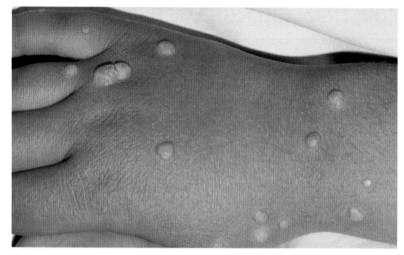

Fig. 9.102 Multiple warts on the dorsum of the hand of a child.

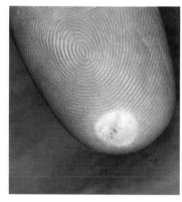

Fig. 9.103 Wart treated with liquid nitrogen, showing halo of frozen normal skin.

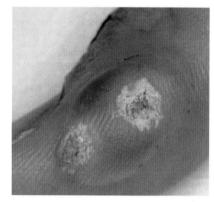

Fig. 9.104 Blister after treating with liquid nitrogen.

For *multiple warts* the options are:–

- Leave alone and await natural resolution.
- A keratolytic agent (salicyclic ± lactic acid) or 20% podophylline. Apply at night before going to bed. First the excess keratin should be paired down, and the agent applied. The area can be covered with a plaster unless it contains a collodian gel that sets. You should remind the patient that keratolytic agents do not cure warts themselves. Any effect is probably as an adjunct to the development of natural immunity.
- 5% Imiquimod cream applied 3× week for 12 weeks. Use a keratolytic agent first (*see* p. 31) to reduce surface keratin to allow better penetration of the imiquimod.
- Pulse dye laser. This results in coagulation of the blood vessels within the wart. A single shot of 8 joules/cm^2 is given to each wart. Treatment is expensive but in many cases 2–3 treatments will be effective.

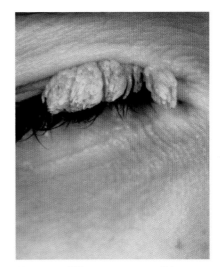

Fig. 9.105 Filiform warts on eyelid.

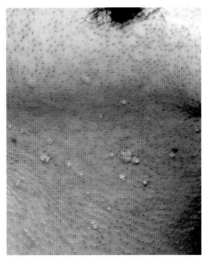

Fig. 9.106 Filiform warts on beard area.

FILIFORM WARTS

These are warts with long finger-like protrusions. They occur around the eyelids, on the nose, lips and beard area.

TREATMENT FILIFORM WARTS

For single or few lesions curettage and cautery under local anaesthetic is the treatment of choice. Cryotherapy is also effective. For multiple warts in the beard area, frizzle them up with a hyfrecator.

SEBORRHOEIC KERATOSIS/WART (Basal cell papilloma)

These very common lesions have a flat but warty surface, and typically look as if they are 'stuck on' to the skin. Sometimes small keratin cysts can be seen in the surface (these can be black or white in colour). Initially they are skin coloured and not very noticeable, but gradually become more prominent and deepen in colour from light brown to jet black. They are usually multiple and occur most commonly on the face and trunk of middle aged or elderly people. They are usually easy to diagnose but their appearance late in life, the black or brown colour and the increase in size are all features that cause alarm to the patient. Occasionally they may become inflamed, particularly if they have been caught in clothing and partly torn off (*see* Fig. 9.124, p. 296).

They need to be distinguished from moles, solar keratoses, and occasionally from pigmented basal cell carcinomas and malignant melanomas. Moles (melanocytic naevi) are more dome shaped and do not have the 'stuck on' appearance, while solar keratoses are rough to palpation, being felt more easily than seen. Basal cell carcinoma has a more shiny surface and a rolled edge with surface telangiectasia, while a malignant melanoma has an irregular edge, colour variation and does not look as if it is 'stuck on' to the surface.

TREATMENT SEBORRHOEIC WART

Most lesions require no treatment. Unsightly lesions on the face and trunk can be removed by curettage and cautery under local anaesthesia or by freezing with liquid nitrogen.

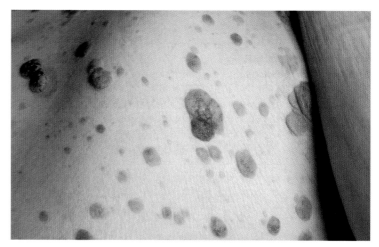

Fig. 9.108 Multiple seborrhoeic keratoses on the trunk of an elderly lady.

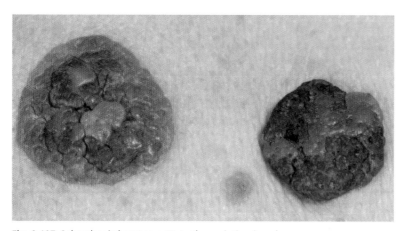

Fig. 9.107 Seborrhoeic keratoses. Note the variation in colour.

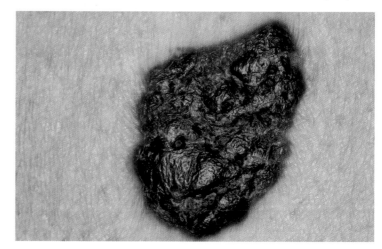

Fig. 9.109 Seborrhoeic keratosis. This lesion could be easily confused with a malignant melanoma but note the keratin cysts and 'stuck on' appearance.

Non-erythematous lesions
Scaly/keratin/rough surface
Papules, plaques & nodules
Single/few (1–5) lesions

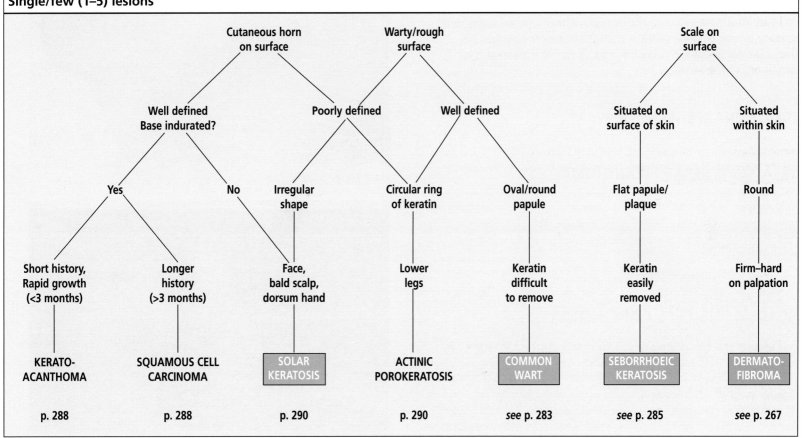

KERATOACANTHOMA

A rapidly growing benign tumour occurring on sun exposed skin. It grows fast for about 3 months reaching a size of up to 3cm in diameter. It then regresses spontaneously and should have disappeared within 6 months. It has a symmetrical configuration with an erythematous or translucent circumference and a horny volcano-like centre. It looks a bit like a basal cell carcinoma but it grows too quickly, and a BCC has crust rather than keratin in the centre. A well differentiated squamous cell carcinoma tends to be more irregular in shape, slower growing and does not regress spontaneously.

TREATMENT KERATOACANTHOMA

If the patient is prepared to wait, the lesion will resolve spontaneously. In most instances it is best removed either by excision or curettage and cautery as it is not always possible to be certain that it is not a squamous cell carcinoma.

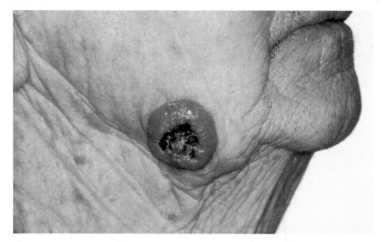

Fig. 9.110 Keratoacanthoma.

SQUAMOUS CELL CARCINOMA

Squamous cell carcinoma is less common on the skin than a basal cell carcinoma. It arises from previously normal skin or from a pre-existing lesion such as a solar keratosis or Bowen's disease. Squamous cell carcinomas (SCCs) occur at sites of maximum sun exposure, i.e. on a bald head, the lower lip, cheeks, nose, top of ear lobes and dorsum of hands. There is always other evidence of sun damage such as solar elastosis (*see* p. 251) and solar keratoses (*see* p. 290). Well differentiated tumours produce keratin so the

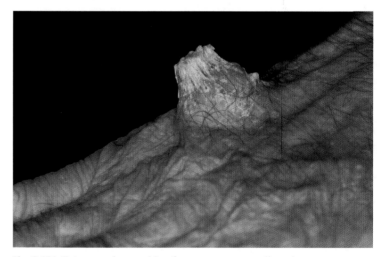

Fig. 9.111 Cutaneous horn arising from a squamous cell carcinoma.

surface will be scaly or horny (Fig. 9.111). SCCs are differentiated from solar keratoses by being larger and indurated at the base and are often painful to touch. Later tumours may ulcerate and be covered with crust. The edge of an ulcer is craggy and indurated, while the base bleeds easily. An SCC can be distinguished from a basal cell carcinoma (*see* p. 242) by the production of keratin and its faster growth (it may grow to 1–2cm in diameter over a few months).

Squamous cell carcinomas can also occur on non-sun exposed skin – at sites of previous radiotherapy, or in chronic scars such as in old burn scars, osteomyelitis, lupus vulgaris or leg ulcers.

TREATMENT SQUAMOUS CELL CARCINOMA

Excise the lesion with a 4mm margin of normal skin around it. Lesions in patients under 70 years age around the central face should have their margins checked by frozen section (Mohs surgery, *see* p. 242). Most cutaneous lesions do not spread so the prognosis is excellent, but always check the regional lymph nodes.

Radiotherapy is a possibility for primary lesions in the very elderly who cannot tolerate surgery, or when the lesion is too large to remove surgically. 10 daily fractions of 3.75Gy work well. Electrons rather than superficial X-rays are useful on the ear and nose as they are less likely to damage the cartilage.

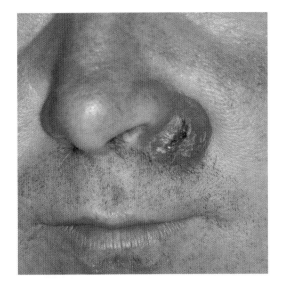

Fig. 9.112 Squamous cell carcinoma. A rapidly growing indurated ulcer in a patient aged 40 which needed Mohs surgery to remove.

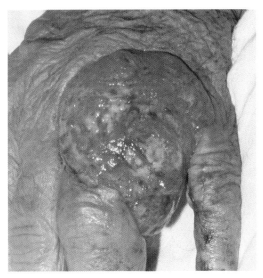

Fig. 9.113 Squamous cell carcinoma on the dorsum of the hand.

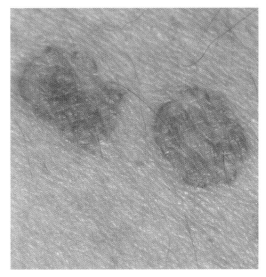

Fig. 9.114 Actinic porokeratosis. Close up of lesions, note thread-like scale around the edge.

ACTINIC POROKERATOSIS

This is a common problem on the lower legs and forearms mainly in women. Numerous small (5mm) round, slightly scaly macules are seen. All have a raised edge like a thread of cotton stretched around which can be more easily seen if illuminated from the side (*see* Fig. 9.114). The lesions are caused by chronic sun exposure. Usually the patient only notices the lesions when they itch or become erythematous in the sun.

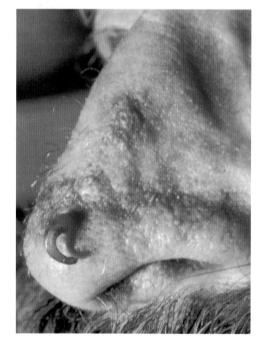

Fig. 9.115 Cutaneous horn arising from a solar keratosis and multiple other solar keratoses on the nose.

TREATMENT ACTINIC POROKERATOSIS

If they are symptomless it is best to leave them alone although the patient should be encouraged to wear long sleeved shirts and trousers to prevent further sun exposure. Treatment options include cryotherapy, 5-FU cream, retinoic acid cream or a vitamin D_3 analogue, but none are particularly effective.

CUTANEOUS HORN

This term is used to describe a horny outgrowth from the skin. At its base will be a solar keratosis, Bowen's disease or a squamous cell carcinoma.

SOLAR (Actinic) KERATOSES

These are rough, scaly papules on chronically sun-exposed skin. They are most commonly seen on the bald scalp, face and dorsum of the hands and forearms in patients over the age of 50 who have fair skin and other evidence of sun damage (*see* p. 251). Generally they are more easily felt than seen due to the roughness of the abnormal keratin. The surrounding skin may be normal or pink/red. Sometimes scaling is not present and the lesion is just a fixed pink macule (*see* p. 94). Seborrhoeic warts look similar but are not so rough to the touch, and are generally more easily seen than felt.

TREATMENT SOLAR KERATOSES

For a **single or a few lesions** the treatment of choice is cryotherapy. You should freeze them just enough to cause a blister at the dermo-epidermal junction. This is done by freezing the lesion until a 2mm halo of normal skin goes white around it (5–10 seconds). Warn the patient that they will develop a blister and that it will crust and drop off after 7–10 days. If there is any doubt over the diagnosis or you suspect an SCC, remove the lesion by excision and send for histology.

Large numbers of solar keratoses can be treated with:–

- **5% 5-fluorouracil** (*Efudix*) cream. This is applied b.i.d. daily for 4 weeks. You can treat just local areas or the whole of the bald scalp and/or face. Not a lot will be seen for the first 2 weeks, but over the second 2 weeks the area will become inflamed and sore. At the end of 4 weeks all the solar keratoses (even ones not clinically apparent) will be red and eroded (*see* Fig. 9.116). 1% hydrocortisone cream can then be applied for a further week to settle the inflammatory reaction down (Fig. 9.117). The effectiveness of 5-FU therapy may be increased by using 0.01% tretinoin cream for the first 1–2 weeks as well as the 5-FU. Patients who cannot cope with the severe reaction to 5-FU can use it b.i.d. on one day/week for 12 weeks instead. This produces less inflammation but is also less effective.

- **Photodynamic therapy**. 5% methyl aminolaevulinate (*Metvix*) is applied to affected skin and irradiated 3 hours later with a red light source for 12 minutes. The *Metvix* is preferentially taken up by solar keratoses (*see* p. 51).

- **5% imiquimod** (*Aldara*) cream applied 3 times a week for 12 weeks. The skin will look inflamed but does not hurt as it does after 5-FU cream (*see* Fig. 9.57a, p. 258).

- **3% diclofenac** (*Solaraze*) gel applied b.i.d. for 2–3 months. This results in less of a reaction than 5-FU but it is also less effective.

- **Chemical peels** using glycolic or trichloracetic acid (TCA). A single application of 35% TCA (Jessner's solution) produces a severe reaction like 5-FU.

- **Carbon dioxide** or **Erbium YAG laser** (2–3 passes) will remove the epidermis and allow regeneration from the residual follicles.

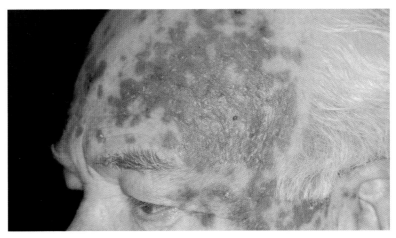

Fig. 9.116 Solar keratoses treated with 5-fluorouracil cream for four weeks. This is the type of reaction to expect at the end of the treatment.

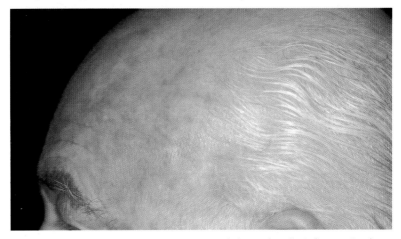

Fig. 9.117 Same patient as Fig. 9.116, one month later after the inflammation has settled.

Non-erythematous lesions
Scaly/keratin/rough surface
Multiple papules/patches/plaques
Multiple lesions/rash

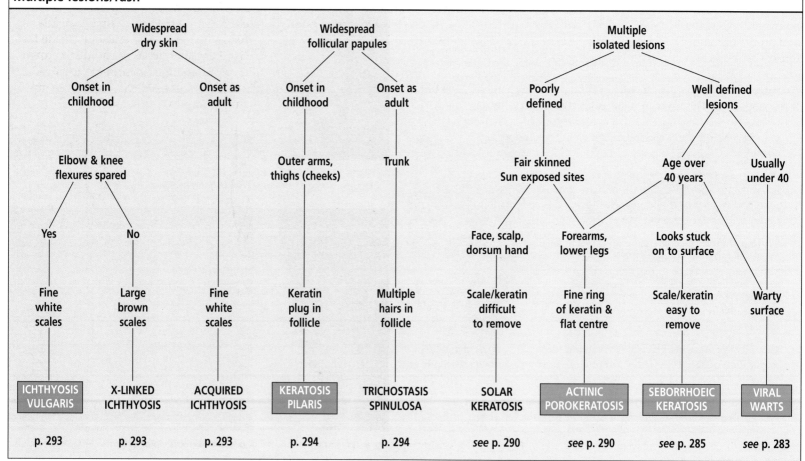

ICHTHYOSIS VULGARIS	X-LINKED ICHTHYOSIS	ACQUIRED ICHTHYOSIS	KERATOSIS PILARIS	TRICHOSTASIS SPINULOSA	SOLAR KERATOSIS	ACTINIC POROKERATOSIS	SEBORRHOEIC KERATOSIS	VIRAL WARTS
p. 293	p. 293	p. 293	p. 294	p. 294	*see* p. 290	*see* p. 290	*see* p. 285	*see* p. 283

Widespread dry skin
- Onset in childhood
  - Elbow & knee flexures spared
    - Yes → Fine white scales → ICHTHYOSIS VULGARIS
    - No → Large brown scales → X-LINKED ICHTHYOSIS
- Onset as adult → Fine white scales → ACQUIRED ICHTHYOSIS

Widespread follicular papules
- Onset in childhood → Outer arms, thighs (cheeks) → Keratin plug in follicle → KERATOSIS PILARIS
- Onset as adult → Trunk → Multiple hairs in follicle → TRICHOSTASIS SPINULOSA

Multiple isolated lesions
- Poorly defined → Fair skinned Sun exposed sites
  - Face, scalp, dorsum hand → Scale/keratin difficult to remove → SOLAR KERATOSIS
  - Forearms, lower legs → Fine ring of keratin & flat centre → ACTINIC POROKERATOSIS
- Well defined lesions
  - Age over 40 years → Looks stuck on to surface → Scale/keratin easy to remove → SEBORRHOEIC KERATOSIS
  - Usually under 40 → Warty surface → VIRAL WARTS

ICHTHYOSIS VULGARIS

This is a genetic disorder transmitted as an autosomal dominant trait. It is first noticed at or soon after birth. The skin is dry with small fine white scales, affecting the whole of the skin except the antecubital and popliteal fossae. There are increased skin markings on the palms and soles (*see* Fig. 8.73, p. 207), and some individuals will also have keratosis pilaris and atopic eczema. The main complaint is of the appearance and the itching. It often improves in the sun and with increasing age.

Acquired ichthyosis is clinically similar to ichthyosis vulgaris but occurs later in life. It may be idiopathic or due to an underlying lymphoma.

X-LINKED ICHTHYOSIS

This is transmitted by an X-linked recessive gene, so appears in boys but is transmitted though females. It is much less common than ichthyosis vulgaris from which it is distinguished by the fact that the scales are large and dirty brown in colour and the flexures are involved. Sunshine does not help and it does not usually improve with age.

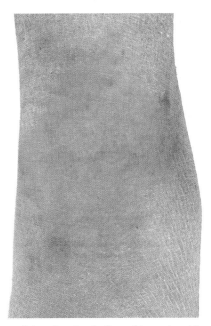

Fig. 9.118 Ichthyosis vulgaris: fine white scale with sparing of the popliteal fossa.

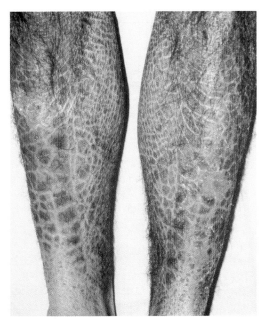

Fig. 9.119 X-linked ichthyosis: large dark scales.

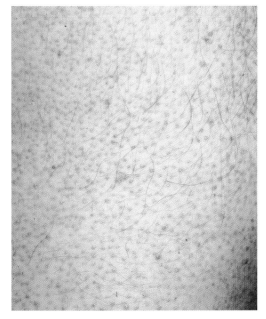

Fig. 9.120 Keratosis pilaris.

TREATMENT ICHTHYOSIS

Since central heating tends to dry out the skin, this should be kept to a minimum and if the weather is cold and the humidity low, then this needs to be increased with a humidifier.

Add a capful of one of the proprietary dispersible bath oils such as *Alpha-keri*[USA], *Balneum*, *Dermol 500*[UK], *Emulsiderm*[UK], *Oilatum* to the bath water and stay in the bath for 15 minutes/day. Wash with aqueous cream or *Epaderm*[UK] ointment instead of soap because soap removes the natural grease and makes the skin even drier.

After getting out of the bath while the skin is moist and warm apply a greasy moisturiser. A wide range is available. Some contain keratolytic agents such as urea (*Aquadrate*[UK], *Calmurid*[UK], *Calmol*[USA]), salicylic or lactic acid which also help remove the excess keratin.

Severe cases may be improved by systemic retinoids such as acitretin 10–25mg day (*see* p. 41). These are available only from a dermatologist.

KERATOSIS PILARIS

This is such a common condition in childhood and adolescence that it can be regarded as one end of the normal spectrum of skin changes. Many patients will not notice it or complain about it. It often improves spontaneously in the summer. Skin coloured follicular papules develop on the cheeks, the upper arms and thighs (*see* Fig. 9.120). Sometimes the papules are red rather than skin coloured. It may be associated with ichthyosis vulgaris or atopic eczema, and is often familial (*see also* p. 97).

TREATMENT KERATOSIS PILARIS

If treatment is required a topical keratolytic agent can be applied. 10% urea cream (*Calmurid*), 2% salicylic acid ointment or 0.025% tretinoin cream (*Retin-A*) put on once or twice a day will not cure it but will remove the rough surface temporarily and make it feel more comfortable.

TRICHOSTASIS SPINULOSA

Multiple hairs which for some reason are not shed can block the hair follicles on the trunk. The result is an itchy follicular rash over the chest and back. The hairs can be extracted and visualised under a microscope. The best treatment is to remove all the hairs by waxing or sugaring which is best done by a beautician. Tretinoin cream may also help.

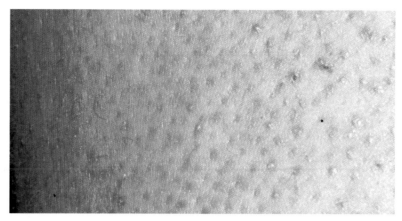

Fig. 9.121 Trichostasis spinulosa on the trunk.

Non-erythematous (& erythematous) lesions
Crusted, ulcerated or bleeding surface
Papules, plaques & nodules
Single/few (1–5) lesions: fixed in site (Multiple lesions, variable in site & time – see p. 223)

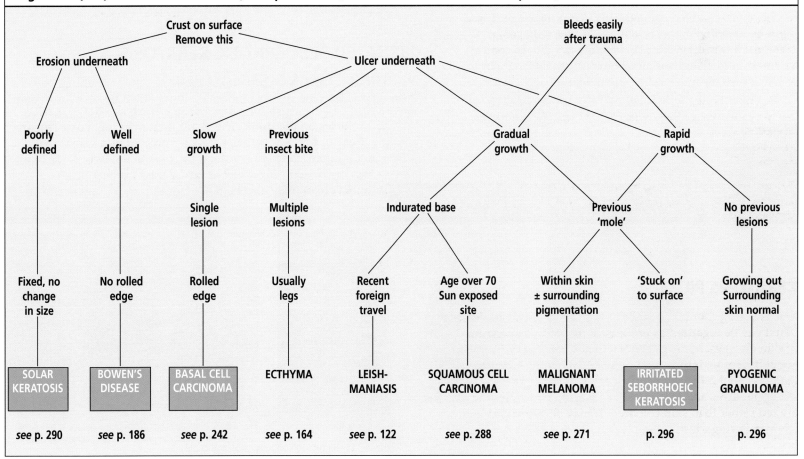

PYOGENIC GRANULOMA

This is due to a localised overgrowth of blood vessels in response to trauma, often a graze or a prick. There is very rapid growth over a few weeks, and usually a history of the lesion having bled spontaneously at some stage. The lesion is round in shape, bright red or purple in colour, and the surrounding skin will be quite normal. In contrast an amelanotic malignant melanoma is usually irregular in shape, has some surrounding pigmentation and grows over a period of months rather than days or weeks. Kaposi's sarcoma can also ulcerate but there will be other lesions elsewhere.

TREATMENT PYOGENIC GRANULOMA

The best treatment is curettage and cautery under local anaesthetic. Sometimes there is quite a large blood vessel at the base but cautery will eventually seal this. **Always send the lesion for histology**.

IRRITATED SEBORRHOEIC KERATOSIS

A seborrhoeic keratosis (*see* p. 267) may be caught in clothing, half torn off and become red and inflamed. It may then be easily mistaken for a melanoma. The lesion usually has the 'stuck on' appearance of the original lesion, but will have surrounding erythema rather than pigmentation. If the diagnosis is in doubt, it should be removed for histological examination.

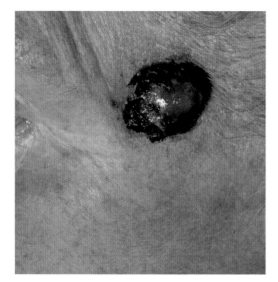

Fig. 9.122 Nodular malignant melanoma. There is evidence of pigmentation at the base.

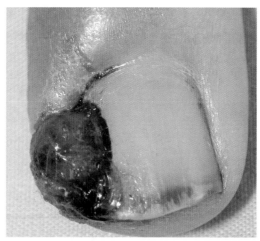

Fig. 9.123 Pyogenic granuloma. Rapidly growing red papule which bleeds easily after trauma.

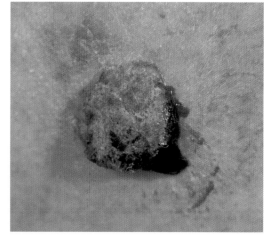

Fig. 9.124 Irritated seborrhoeic keratosis. It has been caught in the patient's clothing and partly torn off – hence the bleeding.

Flexures: axillae, groins, natal cleft, submammary area

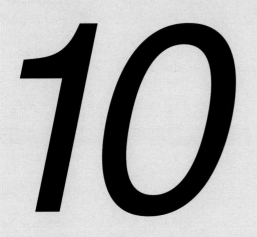

Erythematous lesions/rash

Non-erythematous lesions

Flexures
Erythematous lesions
Papules, patches & plaques

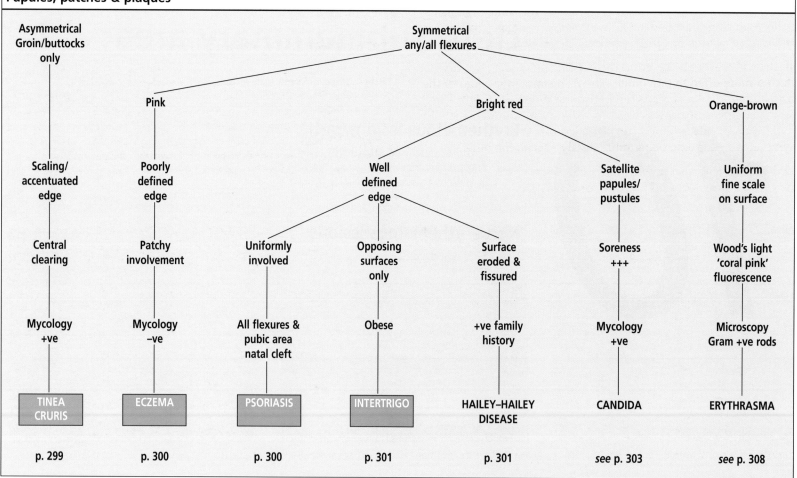

Asymmetrical Groin/buttocks only		Symmetrical any/all flexures

Asymmetrical
Groin/buttocks
only

Symmetrical
any/all flexures

Pink

Bright red

Orange-brown

Scaling/
accentuated
edge

Poorly
defined
edge

Well
defined
edge

Satellite
papules/
pustules

Uniform
fine scale
on surface

Central
clearing

Patchy
involvement

Uniformly
involved

Opposing
surfaces
only

Surface
eroded &
fissured

Soreness
+++

Wood's light
'coral pink'
fluorescence

Mycology
+ve

Mycology
−ve

All flexures &
pubic area
natal cleft

Obese

+ve family
history

Mycology
+ve

Microscopy
Gram +ve rods

TINEA CRURIS

ECZEMA

PSORIASIS

INTERTRIGO

HAILEY–HAILEY
DISEASE

CANDIDA

ERYTHRASMA

p. 299

p. 300

p. 300

p. 301

p. 301

see p. 303

see p. 308

TINEA CRURIS

Flexural tinea only occurs in the groin; it does not involve the axillae or submammary folds. It is caused by the same organisms as those causing tinea pedis, i.e. *Trichophyton mentagrophytes*, *Trichophyton rubrum* or *Epidermophyton floccosum*.

Infection is nearly always from the patient's own feet and men are affected more often than women. The rash starts in the fold of the groin and gradually spreads outwards and down the thigh. The leading edge is scaly unless treated with topical steroids when the whole area may become red (tinea incognito). The rash is usually asymmetrical, one side being more involved than the other.

The infection may also involve the buttocks and back of thighs. The genitalia are never involved. In practice eczema and tinea involving the groin may be difficult to differentiate, especially if partially treated. Mycological examination (p. 19) is therefore necessary in all groin rashes to establish whether fungus is present.

TREATMENT TINEA CRURIS

An imidazole (clotrimazole, econazole, ketaconazole, miconazole, oxiconazole[USA] or sulconazole) cream should be applied to the affected area of the groin (and buttock) and to the toewebs twice a day for 2–3 weeks or until it is clear. Alternatively use one of the allylamine creams (butenafine [*Mentax*[USA]], naftifine [*Naflin*[USA]] or terbinafine [*Lamisil*]) for 7–10 days. Almost all groin infections have been acquired from the patient's own feet, so they must always be examined and treated at the same time if they are involved.

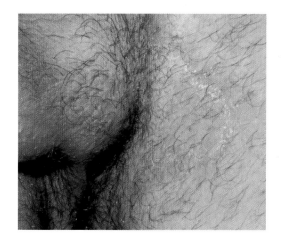

Fig. 10.01 Tinea cruris. Note the scaly edge.

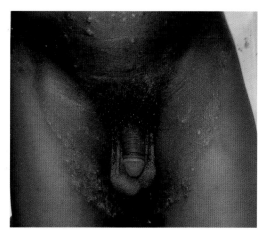

Fig. 10.02 Extensive tinea cruris in a patient with HIV infection.

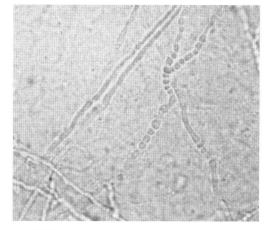

Fig. 10.03 Fungal hyphae on direct microscopy.

FLEXURAL ECZEMA

Eczema in the flexures is seen as symmetrical poorly defined pink patches or plaques. The eczema may be localised to one or more flexures only or be part of seborrhoeic eczema elsewhere. Contact dermatitis in the axillae may be due to irritants (depilatories, deodorants) or allergens (deodorants, dyes or resins in clothes). Patch testing will distinguish between these. Eczema in the groin usually also involves the genitalia.

PSORIASIS

Psoriasis of the flexures (any flexure) is distinguished from all other rashes by its bright red colour and well defined edge. Silvery scaling will not be seen on the moist skin of the flexure, but may be seen at the very edge of the plaque. Often psoriasis is present elsewhere to confirm the diagnosis. Characteristically the pubic area and natal cleft are involved.

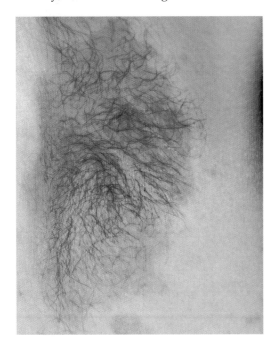

Fig. 10.04 Seborrhoeic eczema in the axilla.

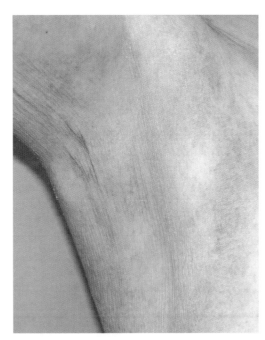

Fig. 10.05 Eczema around the axilla due to an allergic contact dermatitis to dye in clothing.

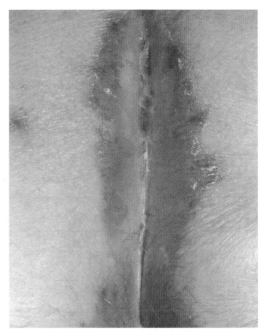

Fig. 10.06 Psoriasis in natal cleft with uniform erythema and a well demarcated edge but no scale.

INTERTRIGO

The word intertrigo comes from the latin verb *'intertrere'* meaning to rub together. Intertrigo therefore describes painful red skin due to two moist surfaces rubbing together. It occurs in the summer months in the flexures of individuals who are too fat. It can be distinguished from psoriasis since non-flexural sites are never involved. In the summer it is impossible to prevent intertrigo from developing in patients who are overweight because the sweaty skin surfaces will rub together.

TREATMENT FLEXURAL ECZEMA & INTERTRIGO

Use a weak[UK]/group 7[USA] topical steroid such as 1% hydrocortisone cream b.i.d. The occlusion that naturally occurs in the flexures will increase the potency of the steroid so avoid stronger steroids as they are likely to cause atrophy and striae. Loss of weight is the only real answer for persistent intertrigo.

TREATMENT FLEXURAL PSORIASIS

Tar, dithranol and retinoids are likely to make the skin sore in the flexures and on the genitalia, so they should not be used. The vitamin D_3 analogues calcitriol (*Silkis*) and tacalcitol (*Curatoderm*) are non-irritant and can be used in the flexures b.i.d. and should be tried first. If they do not help then you can use a topical steroid. The weakest possible steroid to clear the skin is required, but 1% hydrocortisone is ineffective and is not worth trying. Use a moderate[UK]/group 4–5[USA] topical steroid such as 0.05% clobetasone butyrate (*Eumovate*) or 0.1% hydrocortisone 17-butyrate (*Locoid*) cream or ointment applied twice a day. Do not use topical steroids in the flexures for long periods of time as steroid atrophy and striae are likely.

HAILEY–HAILEY DISEASE

Also termed chronic benign familial pemphigus, this rare condition is inherited as an autosomal dominant trait. The patient complains of soreness in any of the flexures, and on examination the surface is red and finely fissured (Fig. 10.08). As in pemphigus vulgaris (*see* p. 225) there is an abnormality of cohesion of epidermal cells. This disease typically remits and relapses. It is exacerbated by friction, heat, secondary infection with *Staphylococcus aureus*, *Candida albicans*, or herpes simplex and by stress. The patient complains of itching, pain and smell. There may be long periods when the patient is entirely asymptomatic, especially in the winter.

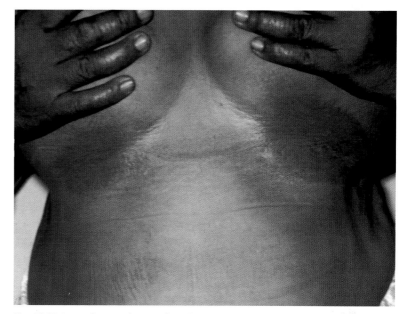

Fig. 10.07 Intertrigo. Erythema where breasts are in contact with the chest skin.

TREATMENT HAILEY–HAILEY DISEASE

If the skin is weeping wet dressings of aluminium acetate (Burow's solution) or dilute potassium permanganate solution (*see* p. 26) can be applied to the affected areas once or several times a day. Topical steroids are often helpful. Use the weakest possible steroid which is effective so as to reduce the risk of skin atrophy in the flexures. Start with a moderate[UK]/group 5–6[USA] topical steroid b.i.d., and increase the strength when required. Secondary infection should be treated early. Rarely patients may need systemic steroids, methotrexate or superficial X-ray treatment.

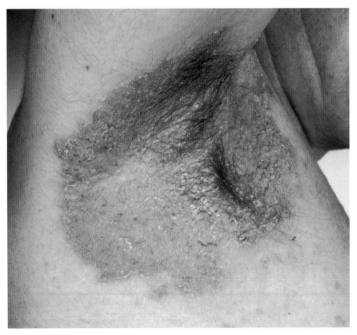

Fig. 10.08 Hailey–Hailey disease.

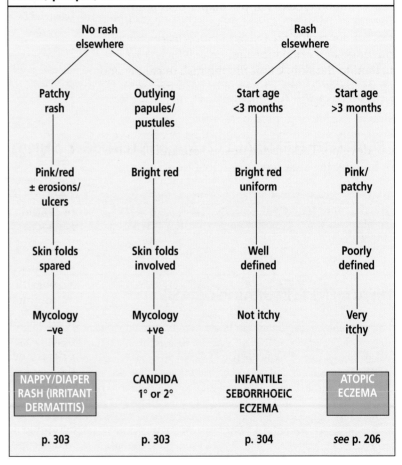

Flexures – under nappy/diaper
Erythematous lesions
Patch, plaque, erosions

No rash elsewhere		Rash elsewhere	
Patchy rash	Outlying papules/pustules	Start age <3 months	Start age >3 months
Pink/red ± erosions/ulcers	Bright red	Bright red uniform	Pink/patchy
Skin folds spared	Skin folds involved	Well defined	Poorly defined
Mycology –ve	Mycology +ve	Not itchy	Very itchy
NAPPY/DIAPER RASH (IRRITANT DERMATITIS)	**CANDIDA 1° or 2°**	**INFANTILE SEBORRHOEIC ECZEMA**	**ATOPIC ECZEMA**
p. 303	p. 303	p. 304	*see* p. 206

NAPPY/DIAPER RASH
(Irritant contact dermatitis)

The common type of nappy/diaper rash is an irritant reaction to urine and faeces held next to the skin under occlusion. Bacteria in the faeces break down urea in urine into ammonia, which is very irritant to the skin. Clinically the rash is patchy and tends to involve the convex skin in contact with the nappy (buttocks, genitalia, thighs) rather than the skin in the folds. In mild cases there is just erythema, but when severe, erosions or even ulcers can develop. The affected area is sore and cleaning or bathing the area produces a lot of discomfort.

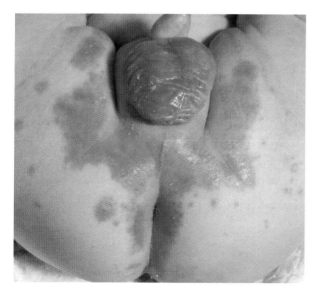

Fig. 10.09 Nappy/diaper rash.

TREATMENT NAPPY/DIAPER RASH

Nappies/diapers should be changed as soon as they are wet or soiled and the skin cleaned and dried. A moisturiser such as zinc and castor oil cream is then applied to the area which is covered by the nappy. Disposable nappies/diapers are much better than towelling ones as they draw the fluid away from the skin. Avoid plastic pants.

If the rash is very bad and does not improve after taking the simple measures outlined above, a weak[UK]/group 7[USA] topical steroid such as 1% hydrocortisone ointment can be applied b.i.d. for few days to speed things up.

CANDIDIASIS

Candida usually affects patients at the extremes of life; babies and old people. There is always a reason for the presence of the pathogenic form of candida and this should be looked for and treated. The commonest causes are:–

- broad spectrum antibiotics
- diabetes
- obesity
- contraceptive pill
- iron deficiency
- pregnancy
- immunosuppression–AIDS, systemic steroids, cytotoxic drugs, cancer.

It affects all the flexures (axillae, groins, submammary area, toe webs) and is usually symmetrical. Infection of the napkin area with candida can occur as a primary event or secondary to an irritant dermatitis. The rash is bright red, and the key feature is that outlying satellite papules or pustules occur around the main rash (Fig. 10.10). In addition the skin is sore rather than itchy, a feature that may help distinguish it from psoriasis or tinea cruris.

Scrapings taken from the edge of the lesions can be examined under the microscope (*see* Fig. 10.12) for spores and hyphae, or cultured to prove the diagnosis. It is important to do this because so often flexural rashes are assumed to be 'fungal' without any evidence.

TREATMENT CANDIDIASIS

An imidazole cream twice daily is most convenient for the patient. In women if the pubic area or groin is involved also treat the vagina with a single 500mg clotrimazole pessary. Involvement of the perianal skin will necessitate oral treatment with nystatin tablets 100,000 units q.d.s. for 5 days to clear the gut.

Itraconazole 200mg for 7 days or fluconazole 50mg daily for 2 weeks are useful but expensive alternative treatments.

INFANTILE SEBORRHOEIC ECZEMA
(Napkin psoriasis)

Infants under 3 months of age may develop an eruption that starts in the napkin area but later spreads to involve the scalp, face and trunk. It looks like psoriasis consisting of well demarcated bright red plaques. In the nappy/diaper area involvement extends into the flexures (unlike the usual nappy/diaper rash). There is no itching and the infant remains unaffected by the rash. The condition goes away by itself after a few months. This rash is distinct from adult seborrhoeic eczema and has nothing to do with atopic eczema or psoriasis but is a type of nappy rash secondarily infected with *Candida albicans*. Once it disappears it does not recur; it is good to reassure the parents on this score from the beginning.

TREATMENT INFANTILE SEBORRHOEIC DERMATITIS

Parents are usually very distressed because it looks unsightly. 1% hydrocortisone ointment applied to the affected areas 2 or 3 times a day will clear it up fairly speedily. Usually there is secondary infection with candida or bacteria so use a cream containing both hydrocortisone and an imidazole, nystatin, or clioquinol, e.g. *Daktacort*, *Nystaform* or *Vioform HC*.

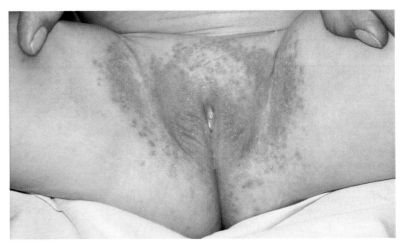

Fig. 10.10 Candida in nappy/diaper area: note satellite lesions.

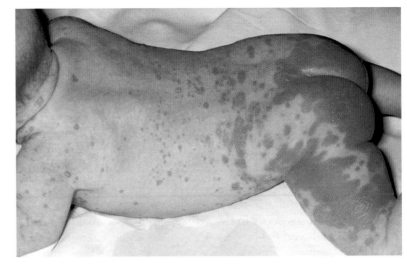

Fig. 10.11 Infantile seborrhoeic eczema.

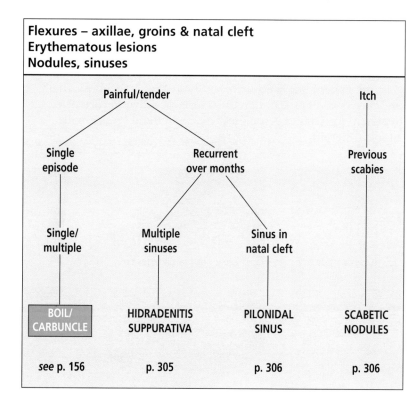

Flexures – axillae, groins & natal cleft
Erythematous lesions
Nodules, sinuses

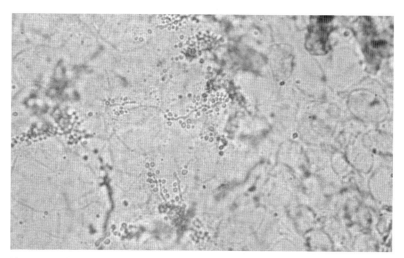

Fig. 10.12 Microscopy of *Candida albicans* (spores and short hyphae).

TREATMENT HIDRADENITIS SUPPURATIVA

Minor degrees of hidradenitis can be controlled by long-term, low dose antibiotics as for acne. Erythromycin or clindamycin 250mg twice daily, or co-trimoxazole 1–2 tablets twice a day, given over a period of years will keep some patients free of disease. If they do not work a combination of rifampicin 600mg/day plus doxycline 100mg/day may work better. Systemic retinoids such as acitretin 10–50mg daily may also be of benefit and in severe cases they can be combined with antibiotics (clindamycin) and steroids (prednisolone). Surgery is really the last resort. All the apocrine glands in the affected area need to be removed. Excision of the abnormal skin together with the underlying sinuses and abscesses is a major undertaking. In the axillae it is often possible to excise the affected area and close the defect as a primary procedure. In the perineum that is not usually possible, so the patient will be left with a large open wound which is left to granulate up on its own, which may take many months.

HIDRADENITIS SUPPURATIVA

This is a disease of the apocrine sweat glands which are found in the axillae and perineum. Tender papules, nodules and discharging sinuses occur in the axillae, groins, perianal area and very occasionally on the breasts. They heal leaving scars. It is thought to be due to an infection with *Streptococcus milleri*, but does not always respond to antibiotics.

PILONIDAL SINUS

A tender papule or nodule in the midline of the natal cleft may be due to pilonidal sinus where hairs become buried within the skin. Usually the patient has a sedentary occupation and has hairy skin. The sinus needs to be opened up, laid open and allowed to granulate up from the base. This is best done by a surgeon under a general anaesthetic.

SCABETIC NODULES

A few patients with scabies develop persistent itchy papules especially around the axillae. These may last for weeks or months after the patient has been successfully treated for scabies. Their presence does not mean that the scabies is active so further treatment for scabies is unnecessary. Treat these lesions with a topical steroid.

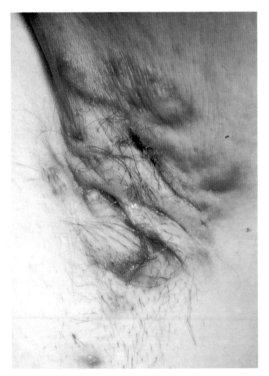

Fig. 10.13 Hidradenitis suppurativa in the axilla.

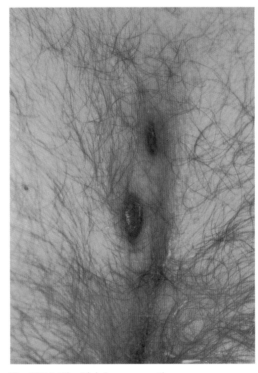

Fig. 10.14 Pilonidal sinuses over the sacrum.

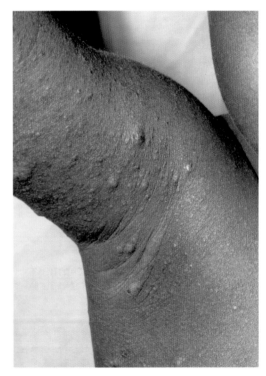

Fig. 10.15 Scabetic nodules.

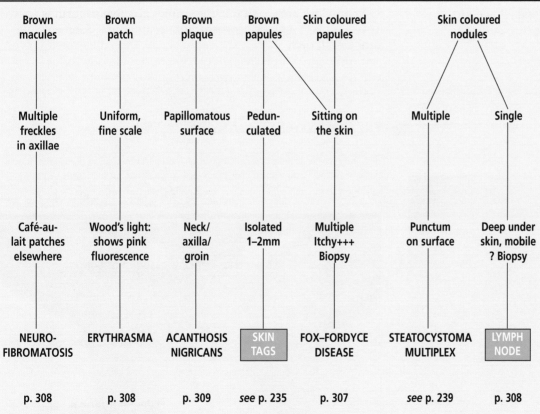

Flexures
Non-erythematous lesions
Macules, patches, papules, plaques, nodules
Skin coloured, brown (*see also* Chapter 9)

Brown macules	Brown patch	Brown plaque	Brown papules	Skin coloured papules		Skin coloured nodules	
Multiple freckles in axillae	Uniform, fine scale	Papillomatous surface	Pedunculated	Sitting on the skin		Multiple	Single
Café-au-lait patches elsewhere	Wood's light: shows pink fluorescence	Neck/ axilla/ groin	Isolated 1–2mm	Multiple Itchy+++ Biopsy		Punctum on surface	Deep under skin, mobile ? Biopsy
NEURO-FIBROMATOSIS	ERYTHRASMA	ACANTHOSIS NIGRICANS	SKIN TAGS	FOX–FORDYCE DISEASE		STEATOCYSTOMA MULTIPLEX	LYMPH NODE
p. 308	p. 308	p. 309	*see* p. 235	p. 307		*see* p. 239	p. 308

FOX–FORDYCE DISEASE

Very itchy skin coloured or yellowish papules occur in the axillae due to blockage of the apocrine ducts. The itching may be precipitated by the emotional stimuli which can cause axillary sweating. It mainly occurs in young women. Treatment is unsatisfactory.

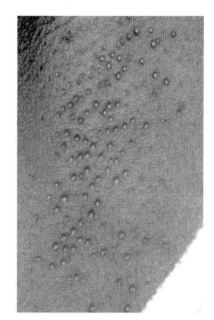

Fig. 10.16 Fox–Fordyce disease in the axilla.

NEUROFIBROMATOSIS

'Axillary freckles' or light brown macules are pathognomic of neurofibromatosis. In children this sign may pre-date the development of the neurofibromas (p. 234), but there will be café-au-lait patches present on the trunk (p. 260).

LYMPH NODES

Lymph node enlargement may be reactive to a local infection, or due to malignancy, either a lymphoma or a secondary carcinoma. If in doubt do a fine needle aspiration for cytology or refer to a surgeon for biopsy.

ERYTHRASMA

Erythrasma is caused by *Corynebacterium minutissimum* infection of the flexures. Symmetrical orange-brown scaly plaques spread across the folds. Usually all flexures are involved – axillae, groins, submammary areas and toe webs although the natal cleft is spared. This condition may be confused with tinea cruris, but the colour is different, there is no scaly leading edge, the axillae are involved and mycology will be negative. A Gram stain on the scales will reveal Gram-positive cocci, and on Wood's light (UVA) examination there is a bright pink fluorescence (*see* Fig. 1.91, p. 18).

TREATMENT ERYTHRASMA

Erythromycin 250mg orally four times a day for 14 days will clear it at any site. Nothing needs to be applied to the skin although topical imidazoles are effective.

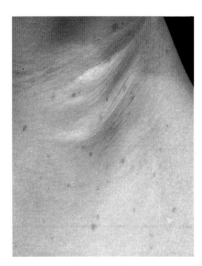

Fig. 10.17 Axillary freckling.

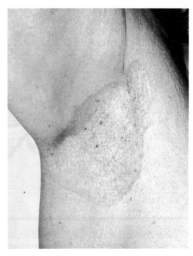

Fig. 10.18 Erythrasma.

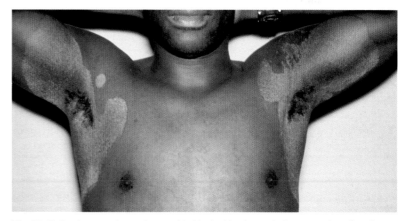

Fig. 10.19 Erythrasma. In patients with black skin the scale is grey rather than brown.

ACANTHOSIS NIGRICANS

This is a rare condition but it is important because when it occurs in patients over the age of 40, you should look for an underlying malignancy – carcinoma of the lung, stomach or ovary. In younger patients it is usually associated with obesity and insulin resistance. It is then called **pseudoacanthosis nigricans**. The skin of the flexures becomes dark brown, dry, and thickened with a papillomatous velvety surface. In the malignant form the skin changes are often associated with marked itching, and there may be widespread lesions that look like viral warts. Treatment involves finding the cause and treating this. Weight loss is necessary for pseudoacanthosis nigricans.

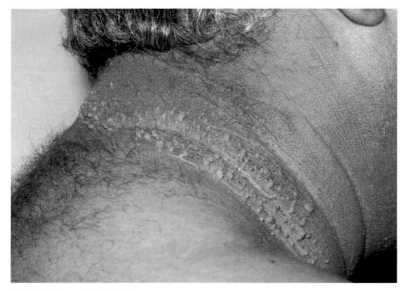

Fig. 10.20 Acanthosis nigricans.

ABNORMALITIES OF SWEATING

PHYSIOLOGY OF SWEATING

Eccrine sweat glands are distributed all over the body surface but they are most numerous on the palms and soles and in the axillae. The secretory coil (sweat gland) is situated deep in the dermis and is linked to the skin surface by a straight duct. It produces an isotonic secretion which can be modified as it passes up the duct. Secretion of sweat is controlled by the sympathetic nervous system but the mediator is acetylcholine not adrenaline or noradrenaline (epinephrine/norepinephrine).

AXILLARY HYPERHIDROSIS

Hyperhidrosis is excessive production of sweat. In the axillae it causes embarrassment because of staining of clothes, the need to change clothes frequently and the rotting of clothes.

BROMHIDROSIS (Body odour)

Smelly armpits is not due to smelly apocrine sweat but breakdown of the sweat by bacteria on the skin. It can also be caused by secretion of smelly substances in the sweat such as garlic.

CHROMHIDROSIS (Coloured sweat)

Apocrine sweat may be coloured yellow, blue or green when it is secreted. More commonly colourless apocrine sweat is broken down to different colours by bacteria on the skin surface or on axillary or pubic hair. The main problem is staining of the clothes.

TREATMENT AXILLARY HYPERHIDROSIS

The options available for treatment are:–

1. 20% **aluminium chloride hexahydrate** in absolute (or 95%) alcohol. This is available commercially as *Anhydrol forte*[UK], *Drichlor*[UK], *Drysol*[USA]. It works by the aluminium ions migrating down the sweat ducts and blocking them. If applied to a sweaty axilla it will combine with the water in sweat to form hydrochloric acid which will make the skin sore. It should be applied before going to bed after washing and drying the axillae carefully. It can be applied every night for about a week to control the sweating, and thereafter applied only when the sweating reoccurs (usually every 7–21 days). Mild irritation of the axilla can be relieved by applying 1% hydrocortisone cream in the morning.

Commercially available antiperspirants contain aluminium hypochlorite. These work well for normal individuals but are ineffective for excessive sweating.

2. **Botulinum toxin.** Up to 50 units of *Botox* or 125 units of *Drysport* dissolved in 2ml saline is injected intradermally into each axilla. The hairy axillary vault is divided into 1cm squares and about 0.05ml injected into each square. This will abolish sweating for any time from a few weeks to a year. It is very effective and safe, but expensive and needs to be repeated when sweating reoccurs. It is the treatment of choice for severe disabling hyperhidrosis.

3. **Surgery.** Removal of the axillary vault will remove most of the eccrine sweat glands and so stop sweating.

TREATMENT BROMHIDROSIS

Frequent washing of the axilla with soap and water is all that is needed. Control of excessive sweating does not help. Avoid spicy foods.

TRICHOMYCOSIS AXILLARIS

This is a very common superficial infection of axillary or pubic hairs with a variety of corynebacteria. White or coloured concretions are fixed to the hair. Most people do not notice this but occasionally some complain of it.

TREATMENT TRICHOMYCOSIS AXILLARIS

The axillary hair can be shaved off and the patient told to wash the axilla with soap and water at least once a day.

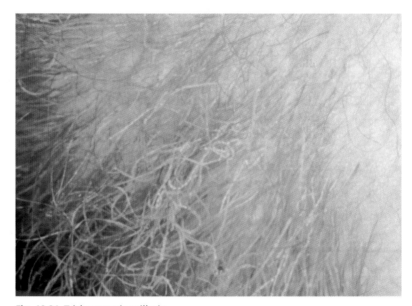

Fig. 10.21 Trichomycosis axillaris.

Genitalia

including pubic, perianal & perineal areas

11

Genitalia
Ulcers and erosions

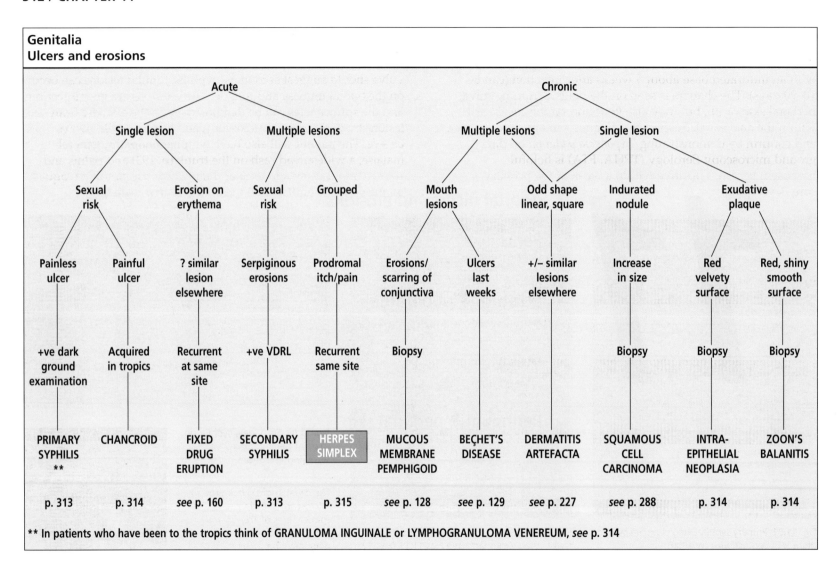

Acute

- Single lesion
  - Sexual risk
    - Painless ulcer
      - +ve dark ground examination
        - PRIMARY SYPHILIS **
        - p. 313
    - Painful ulcer
      - Acquired in tropics
        - CHANCROID
        - p. 314
  - Erosion on erythema
    - ? similar lesion elsewhere
      - Recurrent at same site
        - FIXED DRUG ERUPTION
        - see p. 160
- Multiple lesions
  - Sexual risk
    - Serpiginous erosions
      - +ve VDRL
        - SECONDARY SYPHILIS
        - p. 313
  - Grouped
    - Prodromal itch/pain
      - Recurrent same site
        - HERPES SIMPLEX
        - p. 315

Chronic

- Multiple lesions
  - Mouth lesions
    - Erosions/ scarring of conjunctiva
      - Biopsy
        - MUCOUS MEMBRANE PEMPHIGOID
        - see p. 128
    - Ulcers last weeks
      - BEÇHET'S DISEASE
      - see p. 129
  - Odd shape linear, square
    - +/– similar lesions elsewhere
      - DERMATITIS ARTEFACTA
      - see p. 227
- Single lesion
  - Indurated nodule
    - Increase in size
      - Biopsy
        - SQUAMOUS CELL CARCINOMA
        - see p. 288
  - Exudative plaque
    - Red velvety surface
      - Biopsy
        - INTRA-EPITHELIAL NEOPLASIA
        - p. 314
    - Red, shiny smooth surface
      - Biopsy
        - ZOON'S BALANITIS
        - p. 314

** In patients who have been to the tropics think of GRANULOMA INGUINALE or LYMPHOGRANULOMA VENEREUM, *see* p. 314

PRIMARY SYPHILIS

Primary syphilis presents as a round painless ulcer (1° chancre) with an indurated base about 3 weeks after infection (can be 10–90 days). The chancre is seen on the penis, scrotum, vulva, perianal skin or lip, but may also be found on the cervix or within the anal canal. Suspect the diagnosis in any genital ulcer, and confirm by demonstrating *Treponema pallidum* on dark ground microscopy. Serology (TPHA, FTA) is helpful because it becomes positive within a week of the primary sore developing.

SECONDARY SYPHILIS

Irregular shallow serpiginous erosions on the penis, scrotum or vulva should suggest secondary syphilis. Similar lesions can occur on the buccal mucosa and tongue. These lesions are very infectious and the spirochaetes can be demonstrated in the exudate from such lesions by dark ground microscopy, and serology will always be +ve. The patient will also have lymphadenopathy, general malaise, a widespread rash on the trunk (p. 193) and palms and soles, a 'moth-eaten' alopecia and flat warty papules and plaques on the genitalia and around the anus (condylomata lata).

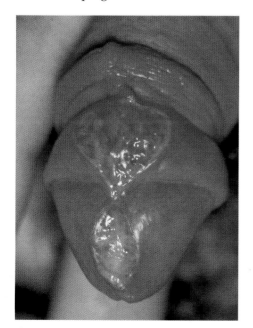

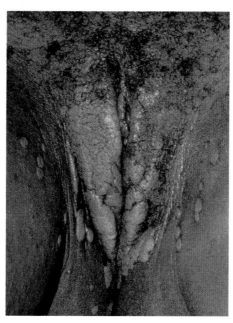

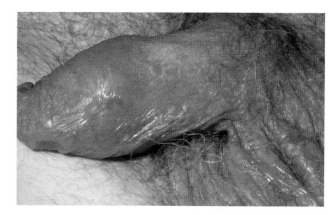

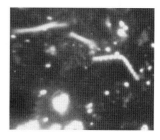

Fig. 11.01 Primary syphilis. Two chancres where glans is in contact with foreskin.

Fig. 11.02 Condylomata lata. These are much flatter than viral warts (*see* Figs 11.11 & 11.12).

Fig. 11.03 Secondary syphilis on shaft of penis and scrotum – serpiginous erosions.

Fig. 11.04 (right) Dark ground microscopy showing spirochaetes of *Treponema pallidum* (use 100× magnification).

TREATMENT SYPHILIS

All patients with syphilis should be seen in a department of genito-urinary medicine so that other sexually transmitted diseases can also be screened for and the patient's sexual contacts traced. A single dose of benzathine penicillin, 2.4 megaunits by intramuscular injection is all that is needed. If the patient is allergic to penicillin, the treatment is doxycycline 100mg b.d. for 14 days or erythromycin 250mg every 4 hours (6 times a day) for 21 days.

OTHER SINGLE/MULTIPLE GENITAL ULCERS

If the patient has multiple ulcers and has been to the tropics consider **granuloma inguinale** (due to *Chlamydia granulomatis*), **lympho-granuloma venereum** (due to *Chlamydia trachomatis*), or **chancroid** (due to *Haemophilus ducrei*). The latter two are usually associated with marked local lymphadenopathy. All such patients should be referred to a department of genito-urinary medicine where the diagnosis can be confirmed.

Any indurated ulcer on the genitalia which is negative on dark ground microscopy should be biopsied to exclude a **squamous cell carcinoma** or **intra-epithelial neoplasia.** These conditions should be managed by genito-urinary surgeons. An ulcer which has an odd shape should make you think of **dermatitis artefacta** (*see* p. 227).

ZOON'S BALANITIS

Zoon's plasma cell balanitis is uncommon. It usually occurs as a single shiny red plaque on the glans penis of a middle aged or elderly man. Biopsy and histology are required to reach a correct diagnosis. Circumcision is usually curative.

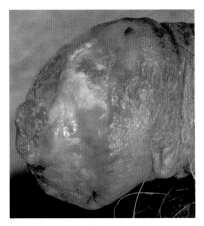

Fig. 11.05 Squamous cell carcinoma.

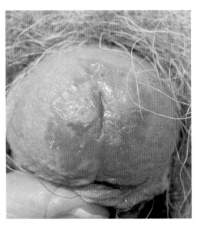

Fig. 11.06 Intra-epithelial neoplasia.

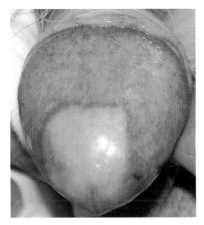

Fig. 11.07 Zoon's balanitis.

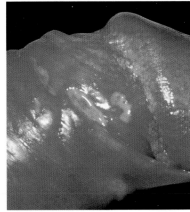

Fig. 11.08 Herpes simplex.

GENITAL HERPES SIMPLEX

This is by far the commonest cause of genital ulceration and is usually due to infection with *Herpes simplex type 2* (HSV-2). About 50% of **primary infections** with HSV-1 or 2 are asymptomatic. The rest present with localized burning, itching or soreness of the penis, vulva, anus or thighs together with grouped vesicles which break down to form erosions/ulcers. These heal in 7–10 days. Pain may be severe and there may be associated fever, malaise, headache and pain in the back and buttocks. In women there may be dysuria if there are ulcerated lesions on the vulva, and in patients of either sex there can be proctitis with anal infections.

Recurrent episodes of herpes simplex are common and can be precipitated by fever, stress and sexual trauma. Not all patients who have had a primary infection with HSV-2 will get recurrent episodes. For those who do, it is usually a lot less severe than the primary episode. It consists of painful grouped vesicles that break down to form erosions/ulcers. Ulcers in patients with HIV infection may last for months. Patients should be seen at the local genito-urinary medicine clinic. Here the diagnosis can be confirmed and the presence or absence of other sexually transmitted diseases checked for.

Herpes simplex type 2 infections in pregnancy
A primary infection with HSV-2 in the first 3 months of pregnancy can cause infection in the foetus and lead to spontaneous abortion. If there is active infection with HSV-2 at the time of birth, the child should be delivered by Caesarean section to prevent encephalitis.

Association of herpes simplex type 2 with carcinoma of the cervix
There is a considerable body of evidence to suggest that genital infection with HSV-2 is one of the causative factors in the development of carcinoma of the cervix. Other factors include early age of first coitus, multiple sexual partners and infection with genital warts.

TREATMENT GENITAL HERPES SIMPLEX

Primary infection with *Herpes simplex type 1 or 2*
In both men and women provided that they present within 48 hours of the appearance of the vesicles treat with one of the following for 5 days:–

- aciclovir 200mg 5 times/day
- famciclovir 250mg t.d.s.
- valaciclovir 500mg b.i.d.

This will relieve the pain and cut the attack short; it will also decrease the time that the virus is shed and therefore the time that the patient is infectious.

The following may be useful to bring symptomatic relief to patients of either sex:–

- Take aspirin or paracetamol for the pain.
- Apply lignocaine gel to the erosions/ulcers.
- Urinate in a warm bath if there is dysuria.
- Leave the affected area open if possible to avoid clothes rubbing.
- Avoid sexual intercourse until the ulcers have healed.

Recurrent infection with *Herpes simplex type 1 or 2*
In some patients recurrent episodes cause a lot of pain and this may ruin their sex life by causing dyspareunia, frigidity and impotence. Such patients should have a 5 day supply of oral aciclovir (or alternatives, see above) at home to take at the first sign of recurrence. If they are getting frequent recurrences long-term prophylaxis with oral aciclovir, 400mg twice daily, can be used.

The use of aciclovir during pregnancy and lactation. Aciclovir is not teratogenic or mutagenic in animals, so it is probably safe to give during pregnancy. Given during lactation, aciclovir will be present in the mother's breast milk; since it is not harmful to babies this probably does not matter.

Penis
Papules & plaques
(note list is not exhaustive – *see* other Chapters if necessary)

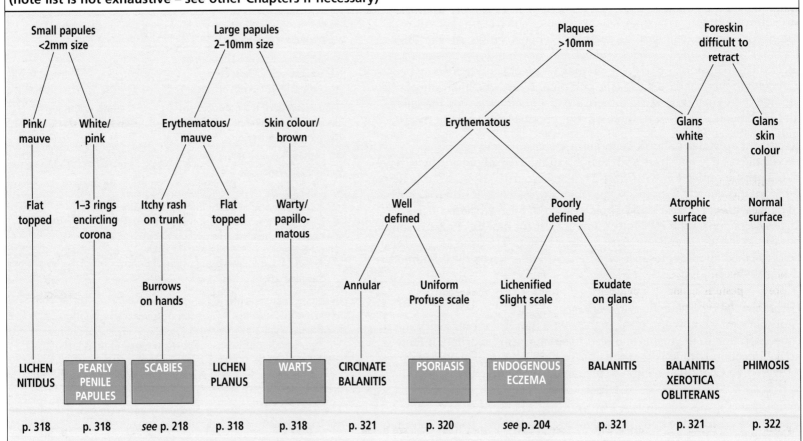

| Small papules <2mm size | | Large papules 2–10mm size | | Plaques >10mm | | Foreskin difficult to retract | |

| Pink/ mauve | White/ pink | Erythematous/ mauve | Skin colour/ brown | Erythematous | | Glans white | Glans skin colour |

| Flat topped | 1–3 rings encircling corona | Itchy rash on trunk | Flat topped | Warty/ papillo-matous | Well defined | Poorly defined | Atrophic surface | Normal surface |

| | | Burrows on hands | | | Annular | Uniform Profuse scale | Lichenified Slight scale | Exudate on glans |

| LICHEN NITIDUS | PEARLY PENILE PAPULES | SCABIES | LICHEN PLANUS | WARTS | CIRCINATE BALANITIS | PSORIASIS | ENDOGENOUS ECZEMA | BALANITIS | BALANITIS XEROTICA OBLITERANS | PHIMOSIS |

| p. 318 | p. 318 | *see* p. 218 | p. 318 | p. 318 | p. 321 | p. 320 | *see* p. 204 | p. 321 | p. 321 | p. 322 |

Scrotum & pubic area
Papules, plaques & nodules
(note list is not exhaustive – *see* other Chapters if necessary)

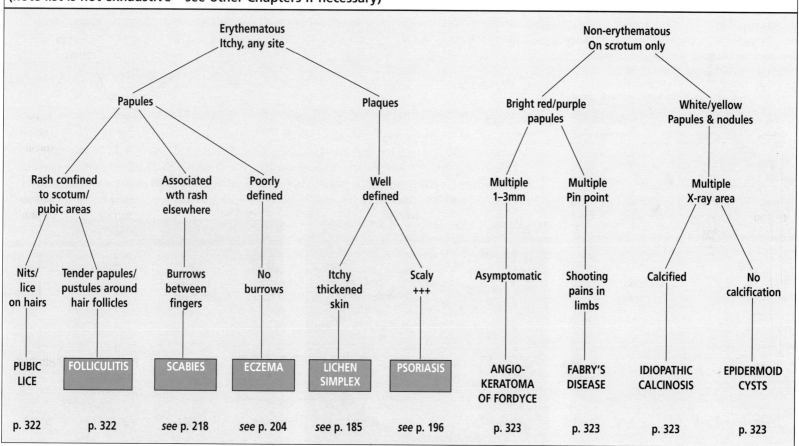

see p. 218 · see p. 204 · see p. 185 · see p. 196

Erythematous
Itchy, any site

Papules — Plaques

Rash confined to scotum/ pubic areas · Associated wth rash elsewhere · Poorly defined

Well defined

Nits/ lice on hairs · Tender papules/ pustules around hair follicles · Burrows between fingers · No burrows · Itchy thickened skin · Scaly +++

PUBIC LICE · FOLLICULITIS · SCABIES · ECZEMA · LICHEN SIMPLEX · PSORIASIS

p. 322 · p. 322 · *see* p. 218 · *see* p. 204 · *see* p. 185 · *see* p. 196

Non-erythematous
On scrotum only

Bright red/purple papules · White/yellow Papules & nodules

Multiple 1–3mm · Multiple Pin point · Multiple X-ray area

Asymptomatic · Shooting pains in limbs · Calcified · No calcification

ANGIO-KERATOMA OF FORDYCE · FABRY'S DISEASE · IDIOPATHIC CALCINOSIS · EPIDERMOID CYSTS

p. 323 · p. 323 · p. 323 · p. 323

LICHEN NITIDUS/LICHEN PLANUS

Lichen planus nearly always affects the genital area. The lesions are identical to those elsewhere, i.e. flat topped, shiny, mauve polygonal papules. If the papules are very small they are called lichen nitidus. For treatment *see* p. 171.

PEARLY PENILE PAPULES

Small skin coloured, pink or pearly papules 1–3mm across, occur around the corona in about 10% of males after puberty. Many young men go to their doctor when they first notice them thinking that they are abnormal. Reassurance that they are normal is all that is needed.

WARTS

Warty lesions on the penis, scrotum, vulva or perianal skin may be due to:–

1. **Genital warts (condyloma accuminata)** These are due to one of the human papilloma viruses (HPV 6,11,16,18) and are spread by sexual contact. These single or multiple, skin coloured, pink or brown warty papules with a moist rather than rough surface can occur anywhere on the genitalia or perianal skin. The patient's sexual partner should also be checked and other sexually transmitted diseases should also be looked for and excluded.

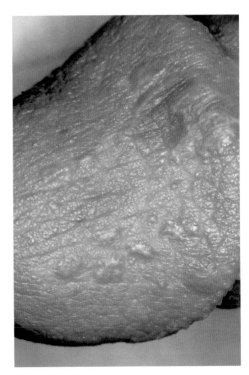

Fig. 11.09 Lichen planus on glans. Flat shiny mauve papules with Wickham's striae on surface.

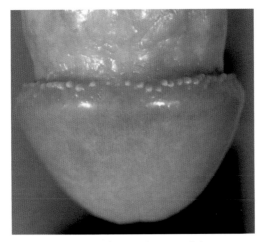

Fig. 11.10 Pearly penile papules around the corona of the glans.

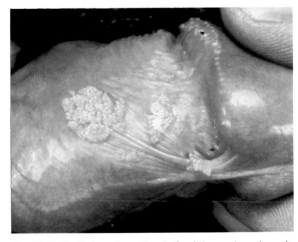

Fig. 11.11 Genital warts on the shaft of the penis and pearly penile papules on the corona.

2. **Common warts** (*see* p. 283).
3. **Plane warts** (*see* p. 231).
4. **Seborrhoeic warts** (*see* p. 285).
5. **Condylomata lata**. Lesions that look like flat viral warts (*see* Fig. 11.02, p. 313) may occur in secondary syphilis. They are teeming with spirochaetes which can be demonstrated by dark ground microscopy (*see* Fig. 11.04). Think of this if the patient is unwell and check the VDRL.

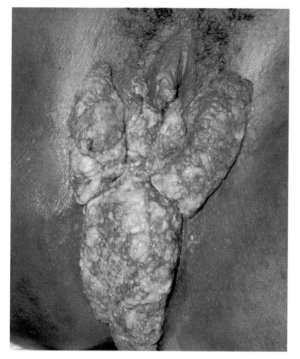

Fig. 11.12 Genital warts on the vulva.

TREATMENT GENITAL AND PERIANAL WARTS

The most important part of the treatment for genital warts is to screen the patient for other sexually transmitted diseases so referral to the local genito-urinary medicine department is required.

Modalities of treatment that are commonly used:–

1. **Imiquimod** (*Aldara*) **cream**. This has replaced podophyllin as the treatment of choice. It is applied 3× a week for up to 12 weeks (*see* p. 29). Each application is left on for 12 hours and then washed off with soap and water. It should be washed off before sexual intercourse as it can produce a lot of irritation, inflammation and swelling.

2. **0.5% Podophyllotoxin** in an alcohol base is applied to each wart twice a day for 3 consecutive days. It can be done by the patient himself but he needs to be able to see the warts so that it is applied carefully to the wart and not the surrounding skin, otherwise it can cause erythema, oedema and erosions.

3. **Freezing with liquid nitrogen** is a suitable treatment if there is a single wart or only a few warts present. The skin around the wart is put on the stretch so that the liquid nitrogen can be applied accurately to the wart and not to the adjacent normal skin. It is applied with a hand made cotton wool bud (so that it can be the same size as the wart) until the whole wart goes white. Treatment can be repeated every 3 weeks until the wart has gone.

   If you have a **nitrous oxide cryoprobe**, this is very suitable for genital warts. The end of the probe is dipped in KY jelly and then applied to the wart. The probe is switched on and the wart frozen until a 1mm white halo appears around it. Cryoprobes come with varying sized ends, so one that is the same size as the wart can be used.

4. **Surgical removal** under a general anaesthetic is a useful treatment if there are very extensive warts, particularly if the anal canal is involved as well as the skin. 50–75ml of 1:30,000 adrenaline in physiological saline is injected subcutaneously underneath the warts. This causes the skin to swell up like a balloon so that the warts are separated from each other and stick out like fingers. Taking hold of the warts with a pair of fine toothed forceps they are then snipped off with a pair of sharp pointed scissors. The presence of adrenaline means that there will be very little bleeding; any persistent bleeding points can be diathermied.

PSORIASIS

The diagnosis of psoriasis on the glans or shaft of the penis is not usually difficult since the bright red colour is just like psoriasis elsewhere. On the glans scaling will be absent, but on the shaft the plaques often have the typical silvery scaling. In boys between the ages of 5 and 15 psoriasis may first appear on the penis and cause considerable anxiety to their parents. In adults it often is a problem because of pain and embarrassment during sexual intercourse.

TREATMENT PSORIASIS OF THE GENITALIA

Tar, dithranol and calcipotriol are likely to make the skin sore in the flexures and on the genitalia, so they should not be used. Calcitriol (*Silkis*) is the treatment of choice at these sites since it produces less irritation than other vitamin D_3 analogues. Topical steroids can also be used to clear the skin, but 1% hydrocortisone is ineffective and is not worth trying. Start with a moderately potent[UK]/group 4–5[USA] topical steroid cream or ointment applied twice a day. Whether the patient will prefer a cream or ointment you will have to discover by trial and error.

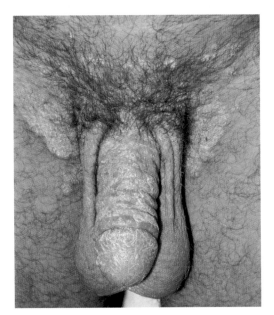

Fig. 11.13 Psoriasis on penis, pubic area and groins.

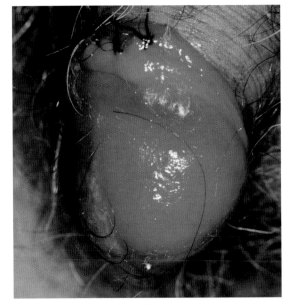

Fig. 11.14 Balanitis with no obvious cause.

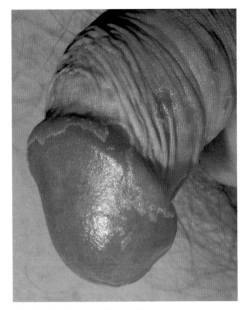

Fig. 11.15 Circinate balantitis.

BALANITIS

Balanitis means inflammation of the glans penis. It is uncommon in those who have been circumcised. It may be due to poor hygiene (particularly if the foreskin is tight and difficult to retract), urethral discharge or trauma. Always check for *Candida albicans*, which may not have the typical appearance with outlying pustules as it does in the groin. If candida is present, test the urine for sugar since this may be a presenting sign of diabetes mellitus in middle or old age. If it occurs very acutely consider an allergic contact dermatitis due to latex condoms, spermicidal foams or applied medicaments.

TREATMENT BALANITIS

If *Candida* is not present and the patient is not diabetic, soaking the penis in normal saline (1 tablespoon of salt in one pint of water) for 10 minutes twice a day for a week will clear the problem in 80–90% of patients. If it recurs this can be repeated.

If the patient is diabetic or *Candida* is present, after soaking in saline, the patient should apply topical nystatin cream or ointment or one of the imidazole creams (e.g. miconazole cream) two or three times a day until it clears.

If neither of these measures work, a urethral swab should be taken looking for anaerobes. If they are not found, the patient's sexual partner should also be examined. If anaerobes are found in the patient or his sexual partner, treatment is with oral metronidazole 400mg three times a day for 10 days.

If none of the above methods help, 1% hydrocortisone cream can be tried. In some patients the cause is never found.

CIRCINATE BALANITIS

This occurs in some patients with Reiter's disease (HLA B27 +ve arthritis [sacro-ilitis +/– polyarthritis], urethritis or dysentery and conjunctivitis). A red scaly or eroded area occurs on the glans which spreads outwards in phases with a grey circinate edge.

BALANITIS XEROTICA OBLITERANS (BXO)

(Lichen Sclerosus et Atrophicus)

This is the same condition which in females is called lichen sclerosus et atrophicus (p. 327). It most commonly affects young adults. It can present in a number of ways. The patient may notice white discolouration of the glans or prepuce, blistering or haemorrhage, difficulty in retracting the foreskin (*see* Fig. 11.16) or the urine spraying out uncontrollably during micturation. On examination ivory white macules, papules or plaques are present on the glans with or without obvious atrophy. Blisters or haemorrhage may also be seen (Fig. 11.17).

TREATMENT BALANTITIS XEROTICA OBLITERANS

If the man has not been circumcised, circumcision is probably the treatment of choice. If the problem is itching or soreness, a topical steroid in the form of 1% hydrocortisone cream applied twice daily is all that is needed. If that does not work, or if there is a problem with urethral stenosis, a very potent[UK]/group 1[USA] topical steroid cream will be required. It is applied twice a day to the affected area (and to the urethra if necessary) and produces a very rapid and dramatic improvement. This should not be continued for more than 2–3 weeks. Once the disease is under control, a weaker topical steroid usually works just as well.

PHIMOSIS

Difficulty in retracting the foreskin in a young adult without any clinical signs may be due to a congenitally tight foreskin, repeated trauma or underlying balanitis xerotica obliterans (*see* p. 321).

TREATMENT PHIMOSIS

If there is no obvious infection present the patient will need to be circumcised; he should be referred to a surgeon.

If you suspect that there is an underlying infection present, of which the commonest are *Chlamydia trachomatis*, *Gardnerella vaginalis* and *Candida albicans*, the patient should be referred to a genito-urinary medicine department so that the diagnosis can be confirmed. Sometimes the penis is so tender that it is impossible to take urethral swabs. In that case the patient's sexual partner should be examined and the diagnosis confirmed from her. If no infection is found, ice or 1% hydrocortisone cream applied twice a day can be helpful.

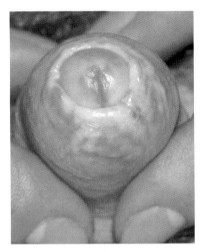

Fig. 11.16 Phimosis due to BXO.

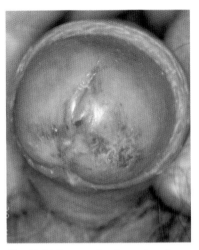

Fig. 11.17 Haemorrhagic erosions in balanitis xerotica obliterans.

PUBIC LICE

Itching confined to the pubic area may be due to lice. Pubic lice (crab lice) like other lice live on human blood. They grip the pubic hair and feed on blood through the pubic skin. The eggs are laid on the pubic hairs. These look identical to the nits which are found in the scalp; oval white shiny capsules 1–2mm long firmly attached to the pubic hairs. If no nits are present look for other evidence of eczema or scabies to confirm the diagnosis of these. In individuals who are very hairy, pubic lice can also be found in the axillae, on the body hair and in the eyelashes.

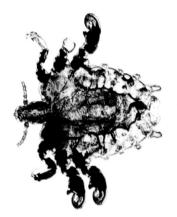

Fig. 11.18 Crab louse (×25).

FOLLICULITIS/BOIL

Small red papules around a hair follicle, some of which have pus in the centre are due to folliculitis. Larger nodules are boils. Both are caused by infection with *Staphylococcus aureus* (*see* pp. 162, 164). With both there may be painful lymphadenopathy in the groin. Bacteriology culture will confirm the diagnosis.

TREATMENT PUBIC LICE

Shaving the pubic hair is the simplest solution.

0.5% malathion lotion (*Derbac-M*), 0.5% phenothrin lotion or 5% permethrin cream are applied to the pubic hair and washed off 12 hours later. Treatment is repeated after 7 days to kill any adults that have hatched since the first application. Alcoholic solutions are not suitable for applying to the pubic area.

In individuals who are very hairy pubic lice can also be found in the axillae, on the body hair and in the eyelashes. These areas should always be checked and if involved the whole body treated as above.

Lice and nits on the eyelashes should be picked off with the fingers and *Vaseline* applied 3 or 4 times a day so that the lice cannot hold on!

All sexual contacts must also be treated.

ANGIOKERATOMA OF FORDYCE

Numerous small bright red or purple non-itchy papules on the scrotum are quite common particularly in the elderly. They are usually asymptomatic, but occasionally bleed. The diagnosis can be confirmed by skin biopsy. They are quite harmless.

FABRY'S DISEASE
(Angiokeratoma corporis diffusum)

This is a very rare X-linked disorder in which tiny angiokeratomas occur on the skin in the area usually covered by the underpants. They occur just before puberty and are associated with excruciating pains in the limbs and with renal failure. If this diagnosis is suspected, a specialist opinion should be sought.

EPIDERMOID CYSTS & IDIOPATHIC CALCINOSIS

Single or multiple white papules confined to the scrotal skin (*see* Fig. 1.36 on p. 10) are most commonly due to epidermoid cysts. In women similar cysts occur on the labia majora. Histologically they are identical to epidermoid cysts elsewhere, with a lining that looks like normal epidermis and the centre filled with keratin.

Sometimes lesions that look exactly the same as epidermoid cysts are found not to be cysts histologically but lumps of calcium lying in the dermis. There is no capsule around them and there is no indication of why they are there. They are not associated with hypercalcaemia or deposition of calcium elsewhere. If the diagnosis is thought of before excision, the calcification can be shown on X-ray. Both conditions are completely harmless.

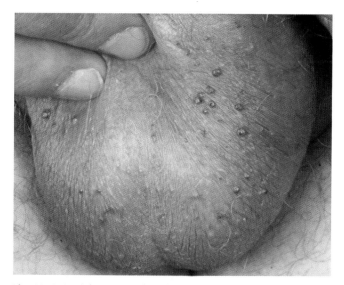

Fig. 11.19 Angiokeratoma of Fordyce.

Vulva, perianal & perineal skin
Papules, plaques & nodules

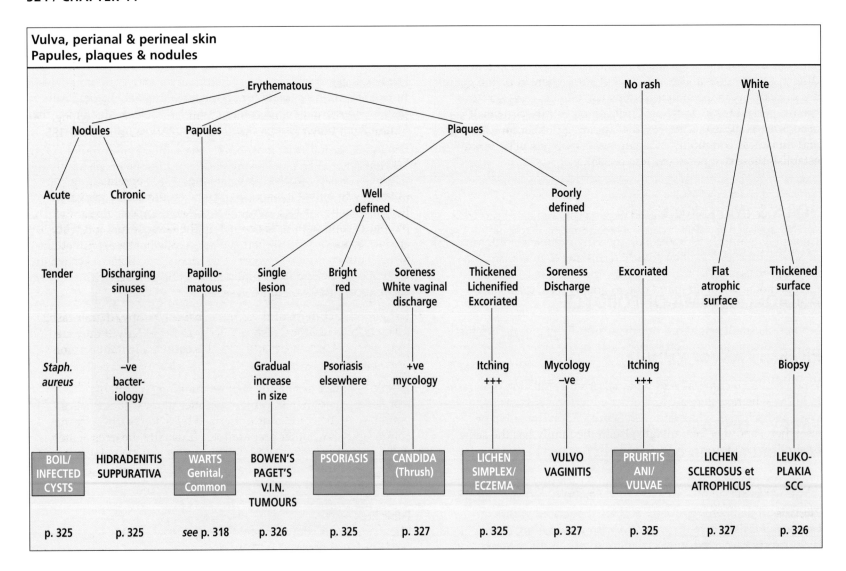

HIDRADENITIS SUPPURATIVA

This is an uncommon condition where painful papules, nodules, discharging sinuses and scars occur at sites where apocrine glands are present, i.e. in the axillae, pubic area, labia majora, scrotum, groins, perianal skin, buttocks or the areolae of the breasts. If such lesions are confined to the perianal skin think of Crohn's disease and much less commonly tuberculosis. A biopsy will be needed to establish these diagnoses (*see also* p. 305).

BOILS & INFECTED CYSTS

An acutely painful red nodule on the vulva, pubic area or scrotum may be an abscess of a hair follicle (boil) due to infection with *Staphylococcus aureus* or in women a similar lesion can be an infection of a Bartholin gland due to gonorrhoea, *Chlamydia trachomatis* or *Gardnerella vaginalis*.

PRURITIS ANI or VULVAE

When a patient complains of perianal or vulval itching, you need to know whether there are any other symptoms such as pain or vaginal discharge, whether a rash is present on the vulva or elsewhere, and whether anyone else in the family has the same or similar symptoms.

RASHES PRESENTING WITH PERIANAL, SCROTAL OR VULVAL ITCHING

Psoriasis
When psoriasis is itchy the diagnosis is often missed. If the plaque is bright red rather than pink or mauve, whether scaly or not, it is probably psoriasis. Look at the natal cleft, the rest of the skin, the scalp and the finger nails for other signs of psoriasis.

Lichen simplex
Lichen simplex is a single lichenified plaque with or without obvious excoriations caused by continual rubbing or scratching. The scrotum and vulva are common sites for this condition, *see* p. 185.

Eczema
Atopic eczema or unclassifiable **endogeneous eczema** may present with vulval itching. In the former intolerable genital itching may be the final straw that makes it impossible for the patient to cope with their eczema. In the latter sexual infidelity or anxiety about possible venereal disease may be the precipitating factor. Both conditions are clinically identical to eczema elsewhere with poorly defined itchy pink papules and plaques with excoriations, scaling and no vesicles.

Irritant contact dermatitis occurs in babies (nappy/diaper rash, *see* p. 303); an identical rash can occur in the elderly if they are incontinent. Applied irritants can also cause an irritant eczema or an acute vulvitis.

Allergic contact dermatitis is often due to medicaments (containing lanolin, parabens, antibiotics or local anaesthetics bought over the counter or prescribed by a doctor), deodorants, contraceptives or other preparations. It usually presents acutely with vesicles, weeping and crusting, and it may be extremely sore rather than itchy. Patch testing once the acute reaction has settled down will sort out the cause.

Pubic lice
The diagnosis is confirmed by finding nits or adult lice on the pubic or labial hair (*see* p. 322).

Scabies

There should be an itchy rash all over the body except on the face, and the tell-tale burrows will be found between the fingers. Other members of the family or sexual contacts may also be itching (*see* p. 218).

Herpes simplex

This often causes pain as well as itching. Patients should be referred to the local department of genito-urinary medicine so that other sexually acquired diseases can be excluded.

Vaginal intra-epithelial neoplasia (VIN)

White plaques on the vulva which are thickened rather than atrophic may be due to VIN (leukoplakia). If in doubt histology will distinguish between leukoplakia and lichen sclerosus et atrophicus.

Tumours

A single red scaly plaque unresponsive to treatment should be biopsied to exclude **Bowen's disease**, **extramammary Paget's disease** or a **squamous cell carcinoma**.

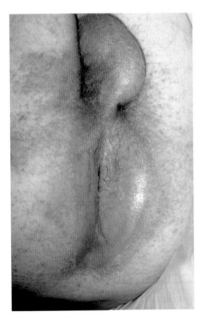

Fig. 11.20 Allergic contact dermatitis to a local anaesthetic cream.

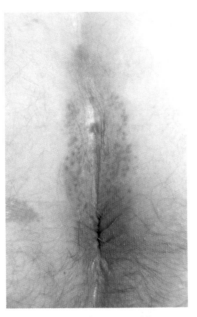

Fig. 11.21 Perianal eczema with erythema and excoriations.

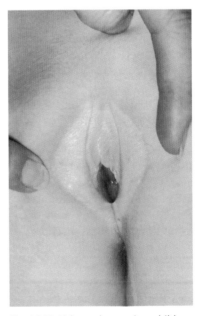

Fig. 11.22 Lichen sclerosus in a child.

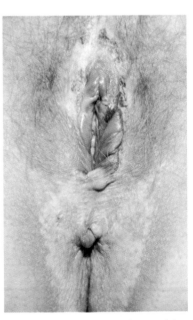

Fig. 11.23 Lichen sclerosus in an adult.

Lichen sclerosus et atrophicus

This is a very itchy condition which principally occurs on the vulva or perianal skin. It occurs in little girls or in middle-aged women. In children itching, soreness or blisters are the presenting symptoms; it gets better spontaneously at puberty. In older women intolerable itching, soreness or dyspareunia are the reasons for seeking help. White atrophic papules and plaques with or without follicular plugging or haemorrhagic blisters are seen on the vulva and/or perianal skin. Occasionally lesions may occur elsewhere on the skin where they are very similar to lichen planus with flat topped, shiny, polygonal papules, but white in colour rather than mauve and with a wrinkled atrophic surface (*see* Fig. 9.40, p. 250).

Vulvo-vaginitis

This is inflammation of the vagina primarily with secondary involvement of the vulva. It can be caused by:–

- *Candida albicans*. Soreness rather than itching is usually the presenting symptom on the vulva. An acute vulvitis with a red glazed appearance is characteristic and there may be an associated thick white vaginal discharge. The diagnosis can be confirmed by direct microscopy (*see* Fig. 10.12, p. 305), or culture of the discharge. Remember to test the urine for sugar. If negative, think of:–
- An infection with *Gardnerella vaginalis* (a vaginal discharge with a fishy smell). Wet smears of the discharge show clue cells – multiple organisms stuck to the epithelial cells. Gram staining shows Gram-negative rods.
- An infection with *Trichomonas vaginalis* (a frothy greenish-white vaginal discharge). Direct microscopy of the discharge will show the protozoae.
- A **retained foreign body** in the vagina.

WHEN NO RASH IS PRESENT consider the following diagnoses:–

Threadworms

These usually cause pruritis ani in children, but in females may wander forward to the vulva causing itching there too. Scratching leads to the ova being transferred to the patient's fingers and fingernails and thence to the mouth (directly, or indirectly on food eaten with unwashed hands). Inside the patient's large bowel the ova mature and the cycle starts again. The diagnosis is made by seeing the worms wriggling out of the faeces (tell the patient or the mother to look), by seeing them on the perineum, or by the Sellotape test (apply some sticky transparent tape to the perianal skin, place on a glass slide and look for the eggs).

Anal discharge

A discharge or liquid faeces can cause itching due to the perianal area being continually wet. Mucous discharge, bleeding or diarrhoea can all cause problems and a rectal examination is essential to exclude haemorrhoids, a fistula-in-ano or carcinoma of the rectum. Patients with poor perianal hygiene, particularly if they have diarrhoea or soft stools, may itch because faeces are left on the skin after defecation. You can check for this by looking; if it is not obvious, try wiping the perianal skin with a gauze swab – any trace of brown or yellow indicates that the hygiene of the area is not ideal.

Psychological

In adults the cause of vulval itching when there is nothing to see may be due to a psycho/sexual problem, particularly if symptoms follow intercourse.

Idiopathic

Perianal and vulval itching are quite common and a specific cause may not be found.

TREATMENT PRURITIS ANI or VULVAE

Any coexisting disease should be treated:–

1 **Psoriasis** *see* p. 197

2 **Eczema** *see* p. 208

3 **Lichen planus** *see* p. 171

4 **Scabies** *see* p. 218

5 **Pubic lice** *see* p. 323

6 **Genital warts** *see* p. 319

7 **Herpes simplex** *see* p. 315

8 **Lichen sclerosis et atrophicus.** In little girls 1% hydrocortisone cream or ointment applied twice a day is usually sufficient. In adult women a very potent[UK]/group 1[USA] topical steroid cream will be required to dramatically improve the symptoms and make the patient believe that there is some hope for the future. It is applied twice a day to the affected area and produces a very rapid and dramatic improvement. This should not be continued for more than 2–3 weeks. Once the disease is under control, the weakest topical steroid that controls the disease should be used, as the condition does not remit spontaneously. Trial and error may be needed to find which preparation is most suitable for any particular patient and how frequently it needs to be used. Control of the disease is also important to prevent the development of squamous cell carcinoma in the atrophic skin.

9 **Candidiasis.** An imidazole pessary placed high in the vagina at night, clotrimazole (500mg) single dose or miconazole (1200mg) single dose.

10 *Trichomonas vaginalis* infection. Both the patient and her sexual partner should be given metronidazole 200mg orally three times a day for 7 days (alcohol must be avoided while taking metronidazole).

11 *Gardnerella vaginalis* infection. Both the patient and her sexual partner should be given metronidazole 400mg orally three times a day for 7 days (alcohol must be avoided while taking metronidazole).

12 **Surgical problems.** Haemorrhoids, fistula-in-ano, or carcinoma of the rectum can all present with pruritis ani and will need dealing with surgically.

13 **Threadworms.** The whole family should be treated with mebendazole 100mg orally as a single dose (except for pregnant women and children under the age of 2). If re-infection occurs treatment can be repeated after 2–3 weeks. Children under the age of 2 are treated with piperazine 50mg/kg body weight daily for 7 days. As well as the drug treatment, the patient should be told to wash the perianal skin first thing in the morning to remove any ova laid during the night, and to wash his hands and scrub under his fingernails with a nail brush after going to the toilet and before meals.

14 **Idiopathic group.** There remain a large number of patients with **pruritis ani** for whom no physical cause can be found. 1% hydrocortisone cream applied twice a day is often helpful in breaking the itch–scratch cycle. Whatever the original cause of the itching, scratching damages the skin and makes it itch more. Wearing loose fitting cotton underpants to keep the area as cool as possible is often helpful and it is important to pay particular attention to keeping the perianal skin clean and dry. He should wash his bottom with soap and water after defaecation. A bidet is very helpful in this respect and if the patient does not have one, he might find it helpful to buy a plastic one (from a boat shop or a surgical appliance department) which can be placed over the toilet.

If these simple measures do not work he should be referred to a dermatologist so that any other diagnosis can be ruled out and patch testing carried out. Very often such patients become allergic to the numerous ointments and creams that they have used to treat the condition (especially local anaesthetics).

15 **Pruritis vulvae** like pruritis ani may be due to some psychosexual problem. It is a mistake to think that it is just a question of finding the right cream or ointment to use. It is worth exploring with the patient whether there is some anxiety at the bottom of it (guilt about her own or her partner's adultery or impotence, a previous abortion or sexual abuse in childhood) and if possible sort this out. Meanwhile the application of 1% hydrocortisone ointment twice a day is likely to be helpful in stopping the itching.

Lower legs

Lower legs
Acute erythematous lesions
Normal/exudate/crust surface
Patches, papules, plaques, blisters

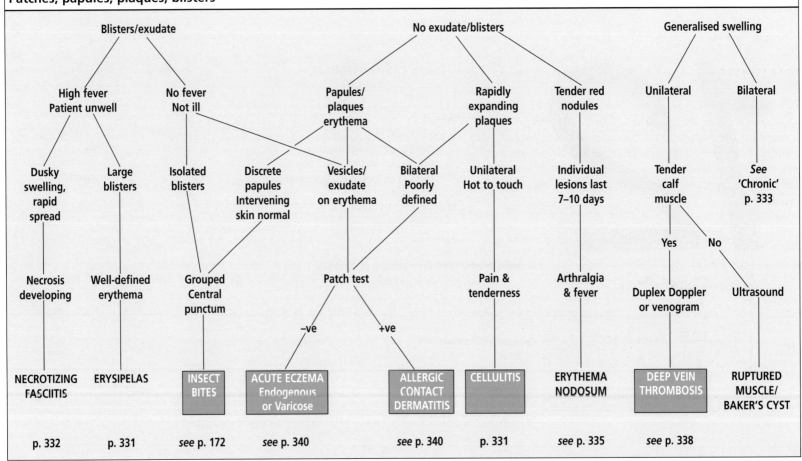

see p. 172   see p. 340   see p. 340   see p. 335   see p. 338

p. 332   p. 331   p. 331

ERYSIPELAS

This is an infection of the upper half of the dermis with a group A β-haemolytic streptococcus (*Streptococcus pyogenes, see also* p. 88). There is a well-defined red swollen area with central blistering. No obvious portal of entry for the bacteria is seen which distinguishes it from cellulitis.

CELLULITIS

This is an infection of the lower half of the dermis by a group A, C or G β-haemolytic streptococcus. There is usually an obvious portal of entry for the organism such as a leg ulcer, tinea between the toes or eczema on the feet or legs. It looks like erysipelas but the area of erythema is less well defined, and there is associated lymphangitis and lymphadenopathy. There are no blisters and the patient is less unwell.

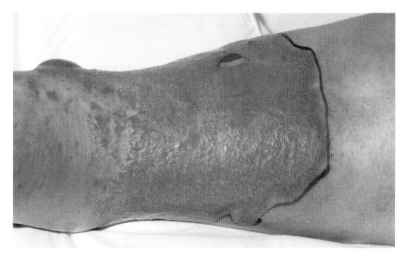

Fig. 12.02 Erysipelas. Blisters and a well-demarcated edge.

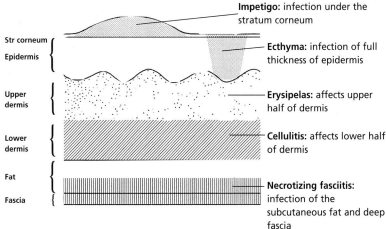

Impetigo: infection under the stratum corneum

Ecthyma: infection of full thickness of epidermis

Erysipelas: affects upper half of dermis

Cellulitis: affects lower half of dermis

Necrotizing fasciitis: infection of the subcutaneous fat and deep fascia

Str corneum
Epidermis
Upper dermis
Lower dermis
Fat
Fascia

Fig. 12.01 Sites of infection with a group A beta-haemolytic streptococcus.

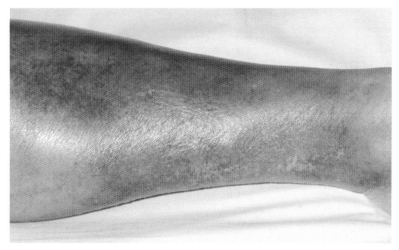

Fig. 12.03 Cellulitis. Erythema less well defined, no blisters.

TREATMENT CELLULITIS & ERYSIPELAS

> β-haemolytic streptococci are always sensitive to penicillin so intramuscular or intravenous benzyl penicillin, 600mg every 6 hours, is the treatment of choice. Treat epysipelas for 7 days and cellulitis for at least 2 weeks otherwise relapse is likely. For patients who are allergic to penicillin, oral erythromycin 500mg six hourly can be used instead. Do not use flucloxacillin or ampicillin because they do not work. If the infection is slow to settle, check that the patient is not diabetic. Cellulitis is always slower to resolve than erysipelas, which usually responds within 24 hours.
>
> As well as treating the cellulitis, you must also treat any co-existing eczema, tinea pedis or leg ulcer which has allowed entry of the streptococcus into the skin. Otherwise recurrent cellulitis will occur and this leads to chronic lymphoedema. If there have been more than two epidsodes of cellulitis within 6 months, long-term prophylactic penicillin is needed. You can use oral phenoxymethyl-penicillin (penicillin V) 250mg twice daily or monthly i.m. injections of benzathine penicillin 2.4 megaunits.

NECROTIZING FASCIITIS

This is an acute fulminant infection of the subcutaneous fat and deep fascia by a group A β-haemolytic streptococcus or *Staphylococcus aureus*. A toxin released from the organism causes thrombosis of the blood vessels in the skin and thence necrosis. Initially it looks like cellulitis or erysipelas but purple areas followed by frank necrosis occur within 2–3 days. The most important thing here is to think of the diagnosis in any patient who has what looks like erysipelas or cellulitis which does not begin to improve with penicillin or erythromycin after 24–48 hours, or who has dusky purple areas appearing within the larger red swollen area. The diagnosis can be confirmed by finding a high level of anti-DNAase B in the patient's serum, if your local microbiology department can measure it.

It can be an acute fulminant illness with the patient dying almost before you can think of the diagnosis or it can be a much slower process with the necrotic tissue gradually separating from the surrounding normal skin.

TREATMENT NECROTIZING FASCIITIS

> Patients should be admitted urgently to hospital so that wide surgical debridement of the affected skin can be carried out. Antibiotics alone are not sufficient treatment. This is because the streptococci produce a toxin which causes the blood vessels in the affected area to thrombose. This not only causes the necrosis of the skin, which is the hallmark of the disease, but also prevents the antibiotics from getting to where they are needed. Without surgery some patients with necrotising fasciitis will die and others will spend many months in hospital.

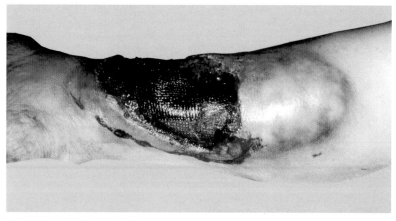

Fig. 12.04 Necrotizing fasciitis.

Lower legs
Chronic erythematous rash/lesions
Normal surface
Patches, papules, pustules, plaques, nodules & swelling

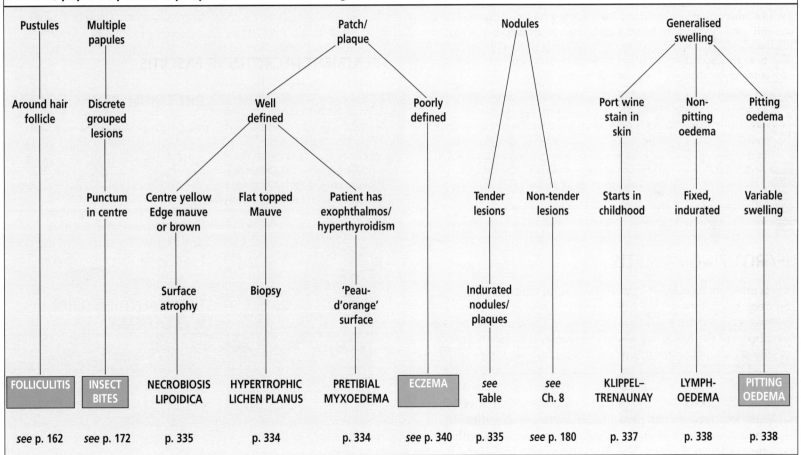

FOLLICULITIS	**INSECT BITES**	**NECROBIOSIS LIPOIDICA**	**HYPERTROPHIC LICHEN PLANUS**	**PRETIBIAL MYXOEDEMA**	**ECZEMA**	*see* Table	*see* Ch. 8	**KLIPPEL–TRENAUNAY**	**LYMPH-OEDEMA**	**PITTING OEDEMA**
see p. 162	*see* p. 172	p. 335	p. 334	p. 334	*see* p. 340	p. 335	*see* p. 180	p. 337	p. 338	p. 338

HYPERTROPHIC LICHEN PLANUS

Multiple itchy, thickened, pink-purple, violaceous or hyper-pigmented plaques on the lower legs may be due to lichen planus. The surface may be slightly scaly or warty. The presence of typical lichen planus elsewhere will suggest the diagnosis, but an isolated plaque needs to be distinguished from lichen simplex by skin biopsy.

TREATMENT HYPERTROPHIC LICHEN PLANUS

Hypertrophic lichen planus on the legs may last for years rather than months and is often extremely itchy. A very potent[UK]/group 1[USA] topical steroid cream or ointment, such as 0.05% clobetasol propionate (*Dermovate*[UK]/*Temovate*[USA]), will frequently be effective when less potent topical steroids have not helped. Occasionally steroids will have to be injected intralesionally in order to be effective (triamcinolone 10mg/ml).

PRETIBIAL MYXOEDEMA

Pink, skin-coloured or yellow waxy plaques or nodules are seen on the anterior shins of around 10% of patients with hyper-thryoidism associated with diffuse thyroid enlargement, exophthalmos, and thyroid acropachy. The surface of the skin has a 'peau-d'orange' effect.

TREATMENT PRETIBIAL MYXOEDEMA

Treat the skin with a very potent[UK]/group 1[USA] topical steroid under occlusion. The thyroid disease will need to be treated with anti-thyroid drugs or thyroidectomy.

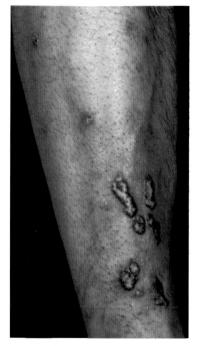

Fig. 12.05 Hypertrophic lichen planus in pigmented skin.

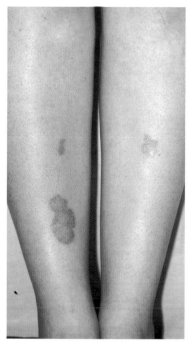

Fig. 12.06 Necrobiosis lipoidica.

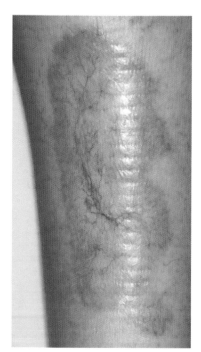

Fig. 12.07 Necrobiosis lipoidica.

NECROBIOSIS LIPOIDICA

Well-defined round or oval plaques on the front of the shins are characteristic. The plaques have a raised mauve or brown edge while the centre is yellow in colour with obvious telangiectasia. 70% of patients with this condition are diabetic but there seems to be no relationship between the appearance or spread of the skin disease and control of the diabetes. The affected areas of skin are atrophic and occasionally may ulcerate after trauma (usually obvious trauma like being kicked or knocked with a supermarket trolley).

TREATMENT NECROBIOSIS LIPOIDICA

Always check for underlying diabetes mellitus. Treatment is aimed at stopping the plaques from enlarging. If the disease is active (raised mauve border) treat with a potent[UK]/group 2–3[USA] topical steroid cream twice a day until the edge has flattened off. The patient should be warned that the treatment will not get rid of the marks altogether. If the edge is not raised, and the area of skin merely discoloured, treatment with topical steroids will not help. Cosmetic camouflage may be necessary at this stage in ladies.

It can be very difficult to get ulceration to heal. The legs should be carefully protected from further trauma, and a non-stick hydrocolloid or foam dressing applied (see Tables 2.03 & 2.06, pp. 35 & 38). The dressings can be changed twice a week until the ulcer(s) heal. Systemic steroids such as prednisolone 30mg/day for a few weeks may induce healing. Alternatively a skin graft may be required.

If an area of necrobiosis lipoidica has been ulcerated in the past, the patient should take every care to protect the legs from further injury in the future. This may involve wearing shin pads under the trousers and avoiding trauma.

TENDER RED NODULES ON LOWER LEGS

One or several tender red nodules or indurated plaques on the lower legs are distinguished by a careful history, examination and a biopsy (see Table below). A referral to a specialist is usually necessary.

Erythema nodosum	Tender red nodules on front of shins. Individual lesions only last 7–14 days. Associated fever & arthralgia.
Panniculitis	Single or multiple red nodules, mainly on lower legs but can be any area of subcutaneous fat. Lesions last weeks or months. Heal with scarring.
Nodular vasculitis	Impossible to distinguish from panniculitis except on biopsy of an early lesion. Mainly lower legs, lesions last weeks or months.
Polyarteritis nodosa	**Benign cutaneous form** associated with livedo reticularis and/or ulceration on lower legs. **Generalised form**: Patient unwell with involvement of lungs and kidneys. High ESR.
Superficial thrombophlebitis	Red papules over superficial veins. No deep involvement.

ERYTHEMA NODOSUM

Tender red nodules appear on the front of the shins mainly in young women. Individual lesions are 1–10cm in diameter initially bright red in colour, but fading through the colour changes of a bruise over 7–10 days. Lesions come in crops for 3–6 weeks. There may be associated general malaise, fever and arthralgia.

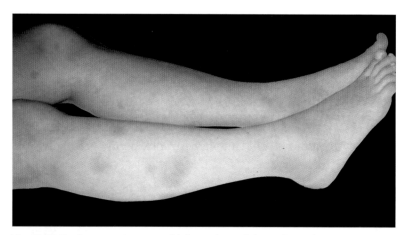

Fig. 12.08 Erythema nodosum: multiple tender nodules on lower legs.

Common causes of erythema nodosum:–

- Drugs, e.g. sulphonamides and the oral contraceptive pill
- Pregnancy
- Streptococcal sore throat
- Ulcerative colitis and Crohn's disease
- Numerous other viral, bacterial and fungal infections
- Sarcoidosis
- Tuberculosis

TREATMENT ERYTHEMA NODOSUM

First treat the underlying cause. Give regular oral analgesics for the pain (paracetamol, co-proxamol or one of the non-steroidal anti-inflammatory drugs). Tell the patient to rest with the feet up as much as possible, and to wear elastic support stockings when walking around.

NODULAR VASCULITIS/PANNICULITIS

One or several red nodules/indurated plaques on the lower legs which persist(s) for weeks or months is due to a nodular vasculitis (inflammation around the blood vessels in the deep dermis or subcutaneous fat) or a panniculitis (inflammation in the subcutaneous fat itself). These can be distinguished by a deep biopsy of an early lesion.

Panniculitis can be caused by:–

- Cold, especially in the newborn.
- Trauma to heavy breasts and buttocks.
- Release of enzymes by pancreatic disease (e.g. Ca pancreas).
- Discoid lupus erythematosus (**lupus profundus**).
- Artefact from self injection of oily liquids (look for the needle mark in the centre!).

In nodular vasculitis look for a focus of infection such as tuberculosis.

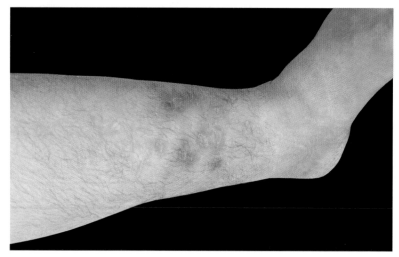

Fig. 12.09 Nodular vasculitis in patient with tuberculosis.

TREATMENT NODULAR VASCULITIS/PANNICULITIS

Look for the cause and treat that. Where none is found, treatment is symptomatic with analgesics or NSAIDs and compression stockings. Systemic steroids may be needed starting with prednisolone 30mg daily and gradually reducing as soon as the disease comes under control to a maintenance dose of 7.5–10mg daily. Ciclosporin, azathioprine or cyclophosphamide can be tried as steroid sparing agents. It is often a case of trial and error to find something that will work for a particular individual.

KLIPPEL–TRENAUNAY SYNDROME

Limb enlargement is associated with congenital vascular abnormalities such as a port wine stain, deeper cavernous vessels, arterio-venous fistulae or venous-lymphatic malformations. The limb enlargement is due to increased blood flow resulting in soft tissue and sometimes bone overgrowth. Typically a port wine stain is obvious at birth or in early childhood. The limb hypertrophy occurs gradually later on.

Fig. 12.10 Klippel–Trenaunay syndrome.

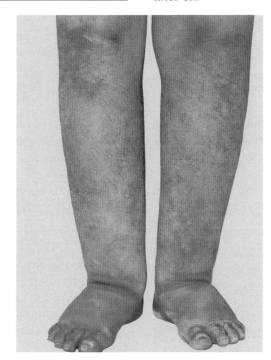

Fig. 12.11 Congenital lymphoedema.

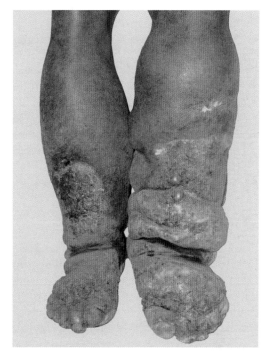

Fig. 12.12 Chronic lymphoedema in filariasis.

PITTING OEDEMA

Oedema is due to accumulation of fluid in the dermis and is demonstrated clinically by firm pressure producing a depression in the surface which only slowly fills in again. Pitting oedema is seen in the most dependent areas – ankles in someone who is ambulant and over the sacrum in someone who is bed-ridden. It will resolve with diuretics or if the affected area is elevated.

Unilateral oedema can be due to:–

- A deep vein thrombosis.
- Chronic venous disease, *see* p. 343.
- Severe skin disease, e.g. eczema, psoriasis, cellulitis, erysipelas.

Bilateral oedema can be due to:–

- Cardiac failure
- Hypoproteinaemia
- Obesity
- Renal disease
- Early lymphoedema
- Immobility
- Drugs causing salt and water retention, e.g. hormones, anti-hypertensives, calcium-channel blockers, monoamine oxidase inhibitors, systemic steroids
- Venous outflow obstruction in pregnancy & abdominal masses.

LYMPHOEDEMA

Damage to lymphatics results in retention of protein-rich interstitial fluid in the affected limb leading to swelling (Fig. 12.11) and fibrosis so that the oedema becomes non-pitting and non-dependent (i.e. will not improve with diuretics or on elevation of the limb). The skin becomes thickened (you will not be able to pinch a fold of skin over the base of the second toe) with accentuated skin creases. Hyperkeratosis and papillomatosis occur after a few years. Secondary complications of lymphoedema include discomfort and 'heaviness' in the limb, reduced mobility, leakage of fluid from breaks in the skin, secondary streptococcal infection (cellulitis) and tinea pedis between the toes.

The cause of primary lymphoedema is absent or hypoplastic lymphatics. The age the lymphoedema becomes apparent is determined by other factors such as infection and venous insufficiency.

Causes of secondary lymphoedema

- Infection – recurrent streptococcal infections.
- **Filariasis**. Microfilariae transmitted by mosquitoes mature into adult worms which obstruct the lymphatics (Fig. 12.12).
- Inflammation – chronic eczema or psoriasis.
- Neoplasia – cancer infiltrating lymph nodes.
- Trauma – surgical removal of lymph nodes
  – radiotherapy to lymph nodes
  – artefact, e.g. restrictive band applied to leg.

TREATMENT OF LYMPHOEDEMA

Because the lymphatics are permanently absent or damaged, the condition is incurable. Simple hygiene measures such as washing with soap and water and moisturising the skin can prevent recurrent bacterial infections. Deep breathing for 10 minutes before getting out of bed in the morning helps to empty the lymphatics in the chest and abdomen. Once this is done massaging the limb and applying a compression bandage will be helpful (*see* p. 345). It is important to keep the limb moving and when seated to elevate the limb. Complications should be prevented by the use of prophylactic penicillin V (250mg b.i.d.) and anti-fungals (½ strength Whitfield's ointment applied every night between the toes). Hyperkeratosis can be treated with 5% salicylic acid ointment and excessive papillomatosis can be removed by curettage.

Lower legs
Chronic erythematous rash/lesions
Scale, crust or exudate on surface
Large patches & plaques (>2cm diameter)   For lesions <2cm size *see* Chapter 8, pp. 188 & 215

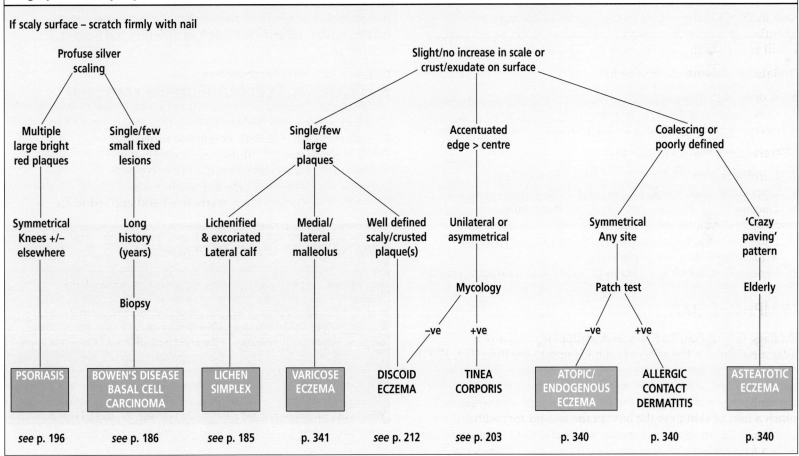

If scaly surface – scratch firmly with nail

Profuse silver scaling

Slight/no increase in scale or crust/exudate on surface

Multiple large bright red plaques

Single/few small fixed lesions

Single/few large plaques

Accentuated edge > centre

Coalescing or poorly defined

Symmetrical Knees +/– elsewhere

Long history (years)

Lichenified & excoriated Lateral calf

Medial/ lateral malleolus

Well defined scaly/crusted plaque(s)

Unilateral or asymmetrical

Symmetrical Any site

'Crazy paving' pattern

Biopsy

Mycology

Patch test

Elderly

–ve   +ve

–ve   +ve

| PSORIASIS | BOWEN'S DISEASE BASAL CELL CARCINOMA | LICHEN SIMPLEX | VARICOSE ECZEMA | DISCOID ECZEMA | TINEA CORPORIS | ATOPIC/ ENDOGENOUS ECZEMA | ALLERGIC CONTACT DERMATITIS | ASTEATOTIC ECZEMA |

| *see* p. 196 | *see* p. 186 | *see* p. 185 | p. 341 | *see* p. 212 | *see* p. 203 | p. 340 | p. 340 | p. 340 |

ECZEMA ON THE LOWER LEGS

Poorly defined papules or plaques on the lower legs are likely to be due to eczema. It may be possible to classify the eczema by the distribution and appearance:–

- Acute weeping exudate suggests an allergic contact dermatitis.
- Varicose eczema occurs around the malleoli in patients with other evidence of venous disease.
- Eczema craquelé is seen in elderly patients where the skin has been allowed to dry out.
- Atopic eczema elsewhere (previous or present flexural eczema in the antecubital or popliteal fossae or on the front of wrists).
- Symmetrical eczema which does not fit any of the above is an unclassifiable endogenous eczema.

Well defined plaques may be due to:–

- Varicose eczema around the medial or lateral malleoli.
- Discoid eczema – either the wet type if surface exudate and crust is present or the dry type if scaly.
- Lichen simplex if situated on the lateral calf or ankle and associated with itching and excessive scratching.

These will need to be distinguished from psoriasis (scratching the surface leads to profuse silver scaling).

ALLERGIC CONTACT DERMATITIS

Allergic contact dermatitis on the lower legs is usually due to medicaments applied in the treatment of varicose eczema or ulcers. The common sensitizers are various antibiotics (neomycin, soframycin, fucidin), lanolin in various ointments, parabens in creams and paste bandages, and occasionally the rubber in elastic support bandages.

TREATMENT ACUTE ALLERGIC CONTACT DERMATITIS

Dry up the exudate with potasssium permanganate[UK] or aluminium acetate[USA] soaks (*see* p. 26). Treat the eczema with a potent[UK]/group 2–3[USA] topical steroid ointment b.i.d. (not a cream as the preservative in a cream can itself be the causative allergen). Once the rash is better identify the allergen by patch testing so that it can be avoided in the future.

ASTEATOTIC ECZEMA (Eczema craquelé)

This condition is due to drying out of the skin especially in the elderly. It occurs in winter or when patients are hospitalized and made to bathe more frequently than they are used to. The skin is dry or scaly with irregular erythematous fissures like 'crazy paving'. The associated itching usually brings it to the attention of the doctor.

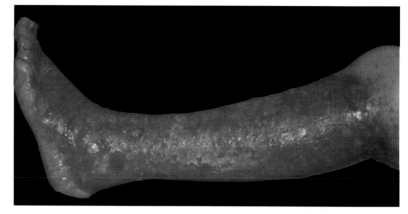

Fig. 12.13 Acute allergic contact dermatitis from bandages. Erosions and exudate but no ulceration.

TREATMENT ASTEATOTIC ECZEMA

The patient should either bathe less often or use one of the dispersible bath oils in the bath water each day and a greasy (water-in-oil) emollient (*see* p. 24) can then be applied to the dry scaly skin twice a day. Occasionally a weak [UK]/group 7[USA] topical steroid such as 1% hydrocortisone ointment may be needed.

VARICOSE/STASIS ECZEMA

Eczema may occur in patients with venous hypertension (*see* p. 343). It is distinguished from other types of eczema by being confined to the lower legs in a patient with other signs of venous disease. Acute-on-chronic varicose eczema should suggest a superadded allergic contact dermatitis rather than cellulitis, which is unilateral and feels hot.

TREATMENT VARICOSE ECZEMA

More important than what is put onto the eczema itself, is treatment of the underlying problem (chronic venous stasis due to incompetent valves in the deep veins of the calf) with proper elastic support. It is probably best to use bandages (p. 345) until the eczema is better and then change to elastic stockings because the treatment for the eczema may otherwise ruin the stockings.

For the eczema itself, a moderately potent[UK]/group 4–5[USA] topical steroid ointment can be applied twice a day. The patient may prefer a cream to an ointment, particularly since that will make less of a mess of their bandages. This should be resisted because many patients are allergic to parabens (from the use of creams or paste bandages). All patients with varicose eczema should be patch tested to make sure that you do not make things worse by applying ointments, dressings and bandages that they are allergic to.

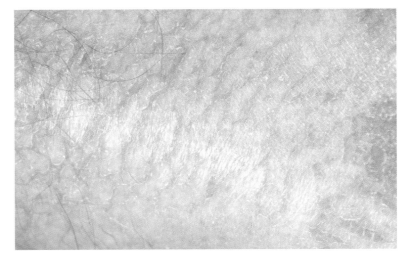

Fig. 12.14 Asteatotic eczema close up.

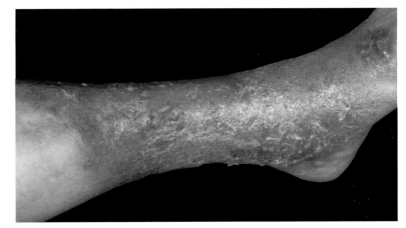

Fig. 12.15 Chronic varicose eczema which will require topical steroids and compression bandages.

Lower legs
Chronic erythematous rash/lesions
Ulcerated surface
Commoner causes

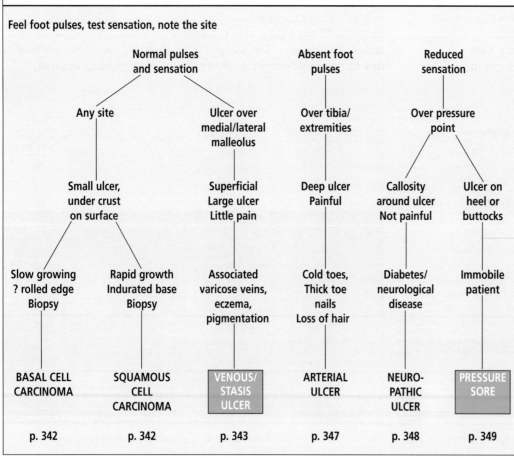

Feel foot pulses, test sensation, note the site

Normal pulses and sensation		Absent foot pulses	Reduced sensation	
Any site	Ulcer over medial/lateral malleolus	Over tibia/ extremities	Over pressure point	
Small ulcer, under crust on surface	Superficial Large ulcer Little pain	Deep ulcer Painful	Callosity around ulcer Not painful	Ulcer on heel or buttocks
Slow growing ? rolled edge Biopsy	Rapid growth Indurated base Biopsy	Associated varicose veins, eczema, pigmentation	Cold toes, Thick toe nails Loss of hair	Diabetes/ neurological disease	Immobile patient
BASAL CELL CARCINOMA	SQUAMOUS CELL CARCINOMA	VENOUS/ STASIS ULCER	ARTERIAL ULCER	NEURO-PATHIC ULCER	PRESSURE SORE
p. 342	p. 342	p. 343	p. 347	p. 348	p. 349

SKIN NEOPLASM

Squamous cell carcinoma (p. 288) and basal cell carcinoma (p. 242) are uncommon causes of leg ulcers in the elderly with fair skin. They are usually small, slow growing and can be anywhere on the lower legs. Rarely a squamous cell carcinoma can arise in a chronic venous ulcer or a chronic burn scar. Occasionally a tumour around the ankles can be misdiagnosed as a venous ulcer. Any chronic non-healing ulcer should be biopsied. Any red or pigmented lesion which ulcerates needs to be biopsied to exclude a malignant melanoma.

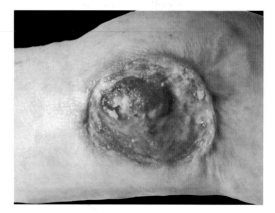

Fig. 12.16 Ulcer on side of knee. Any ulcer which does not fit the features of a venous, arterial or neuropathic ulcer should be biopsied.

VENOUS ULCERS

The cause of venous ulceration is loss of the valves in the deep or perforating veins. The venous blood returns from the lower legs back to the heart by the calf muscle pump. Compression of the calf muscles (by walking or running) squeezes blood up the legs. Blood is drawn from the superficial veins and pushed upwards by valves which prevent back flow. Loss or incompetence of these valves results in enormous pressure (venous hypertension) in the superficial veins which is transmitted back to the capillaries resulting in venous disease and ulceration.

Venous ulcers occur on the lower third of the leg either over the medial or lateral malleolus. They are large, superficial and painless. There will be other evidence of venous disease such as oedema, varicose veins, venous flare, pigmentation (orangy-brown due to haemosiderin or dark brown due to melanin), eczema,

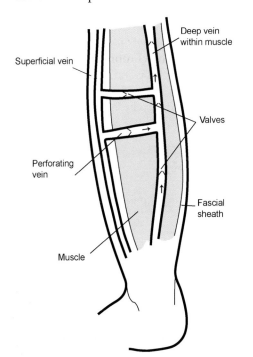

Fig. 12.17 Anatomy of veins in lower leg showing deep, superficial and perforating veins with one way valves.

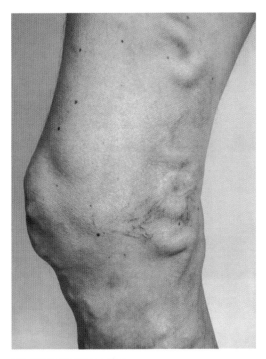

Fig. 12.18 Varicose veins.

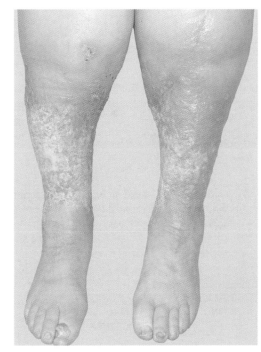

Fig. 12.19 Lipodermatosclerosis (inverted champagne bottle legs).

atrophie blanche (white scars with telangiectasia on the surface) and fibrosis around the ankle (lipodermatosclerosis).

Complications of venous ulceration are relatively rare, and include cellulitis, haemorrhage, soft tissue calcification and malignant change. Infection of the ulcer itself is of little consequence and mixed organisms are often present. Taking swabs for bacteriology should be discouraged as this tempts the physician to treat with potentially sensitising topical antibiotics. Cellulitis should be treated promptly, but this diagnosis is made on clinical grounds (*see* p. 331). Venous ulcers may be complicated by arterial insufficiency, and this is suggested by pain and poor healing with compression bandages.

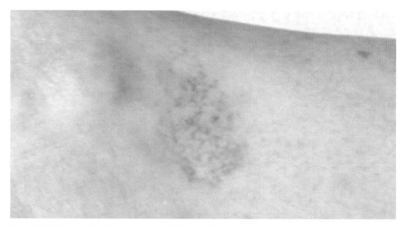

Fig. 12.21 Atrophie blanche around the ankle.

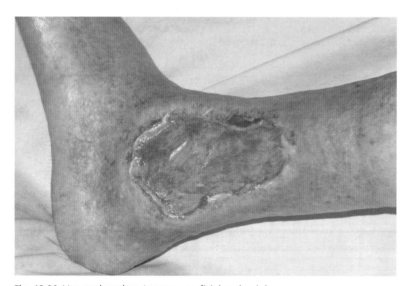

Fig. 12.20 Venous leg ulcer. Large, superficial and painless.

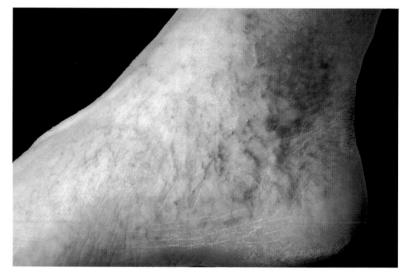

Fig. 12.22 Venous flare.

TREATMENT VENOUS LEG ULCERS

- Clean and debride the ulcer, *see* Table 2.03, p. 35.
- Apply a dressing to absorb any exudate (Table 2.05, p. 37) and protect the ulcer during healing (Table 2.06, p. 38).
- Assess arterial blood flow to leg (feel pulses and do Dopplers (p. 348)).
- Compression bandaging or stockings – see below.
- Treat any associated complications and consider skin grafting.

Compression bandaging

The only effective way of treating venous hypertension is by external compression of the leg by bandaging or support stockings. This compresses the superficial veins so that blood must flow in the deep veins (*see* Fig. 12.17, p. 343).

Four layer compression bandaging has been shown to be the most effective method of achieving this. The ulcer is covered with a non-adherent dressing and the leg skin is protected by tubigauze stockinette. The four layer bandage consists of the following:–

1. Orthopaedic wool (*Softban*) as a spiral with 50% overlap. This is absorbent and pads out any bony protuberances.
2. Crepe bandage as spiral at mid-stretch with 50% overlap.
3. High compression long stretch bandage:–
   - *Litepress/KPlus* as a figure of 8 (ankle circumference <25cm).
   - *Tensopress* as spiral with 50% overlap (ankle circumference >25cm).
4. Cohesive lightweight elastic bandage (*Co-plus/Coban*) with 50% overlap. These are available as a pack (*Hospifour, K-four, Profore, System4, Ultra 4*) or as separate components.

The disadvantages of the four layer bandage are that the pack is expensive, it may be difficult to wear normal shoes over it and it needs to be applied by a nurse who has had some training in applying bandages (this may be an advantage as the bandage will be applied properly). It is also less likely to slip down the leg and will remain in place and be effective for a full week.

Instructions for bandaging. Layered compression bandages should be applied by a nurse and changed weekly. Continue until the ulcer is healed (the average time is 12 weeks). To work, the patient must be using their calf muscles, so they need to be mobile and to walk about. While sitting the feet should be raised on a stool and the foot dorsiflexed frequently.

Two layer bandaging is an alternative which is less expensive and patients can wear normal footwear improving compliance. A tubular stockinette is applied over the skin and any ulcer dressings and then the two layers are:–

1. Orthopaedic wool (*Softban*) is applied as a spiral with 50% overlap.
2. Compression bandage. You can use either a **long stretch** where the bandage is pulled to 50% stretch (e.g. *Tensopress, Setopress, Surepress*) – used on mobile or non-mobile patients, or **short stretch** where the bandage is pulled to full stretch (e.g. *Actiban, Actico, Comprilan*). This is easier for patients to apply themselves but should be used only in mobile patients.

Compression stockings. Once the ulcer has healed, elastic support is necessary for the rest of the patient's life since the missing leg valves cannot be replaced. Support is achieved by wearing a Class II elastic stocking.

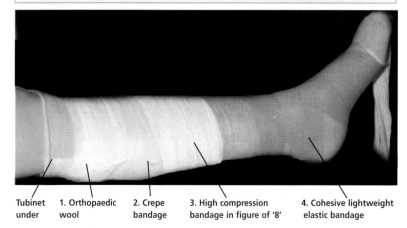

| Tubinet under | 1. Orthopaedic wool | 2. Crepe bandage | 3. High compression bandage in figure of '8' | 4. Cohesive lightweight elastic bandage |

Fig. 12.23 Four layer compression bandaging.

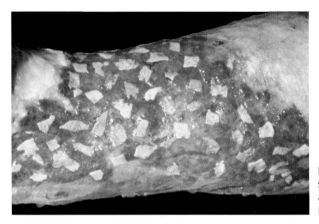

Fig. 12.24 Split skin grafts applied to large leg ulcer.

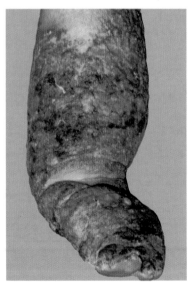

Fig. 12.25 Nodular polypoid hyperplasia.

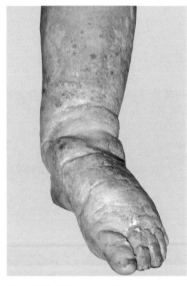

Fig. 12.26 After excess tissue removed by curettage.

Skin grafting

Pinch grafts or partial thickness skin grafts can be used to hasten the healing process. Small islands of skin are placed on the clean ulcer bed, and the area covered with a non-adherent dressing. The patient will need to remain on bed rest for two weeks with leg elevation to allow the graft to take.

Treatment of complications

1. Associated arterial disease, *see* p. 347.
2. Overgranulation of the ulcer. Too much granulation tissue will delay healing. This can be removed by applying a silver nitrate stick to the area before applying compression. Some patients find this extremely painful, and if this is the case apply a gauze swab soaked in 0.25% silver nitrate solution instead. Alternatively granulation tissue can be curetted off.
3. Secondary infection of the ulcer. Only two infections in leg ulcers matter.
    a. Pseudomonas infection causes an unpleasant smell. This can be eradicated with 5% acetic acid (use ordinary household vinegar). Cut a piece of gauze to the size of the ulcer and soak it in the vinegar. Apply the gauze daily to the ulcer until the smell goes. Alternatively a 0.25% solution of silver nitrate can be used (Table 2.04, p. 36). These are much more effective than intravenous piperacillin or ticarcillin!
    b. Group A beta haemolytic streptococci in an ulcer cause cellulitis. This is diagnosed clinically. Taking swabs from leg ulcers is to be discouraged. Treat with IV benzyl penicillin (p. 331).
4. Eczema around the ulcer – *see* p. 341.
5. Nodular polypoid hyperplasia. The excess tissue can be scraped off using a curette. No anaesthetic is needed. It will not reoccur if the patient wears compression bandages.

ARTERIAL ULCERS

These are due to a reduction in arterial blood supply to the lower limb usually due to atherosclerosis. They are typically painful, punched out and relatively deep (sometimes revealing the underlying tendons). They occur where the arterial supply is poorest – on the tips of toes, the dorsum of the foot, the heel and the front of the shin. The absence of peripheral pulses and a history of intermittent claudication will confirm the diagnosis. Other signs to look for are cold feet, blotchy erythema of the feet, loss of hair and thickened toenails. Untreated, gangrene will eventually follow. The patient may have evidence of more widespread arterial disease, e.g. a past history of coronary thrombosis or stroke.

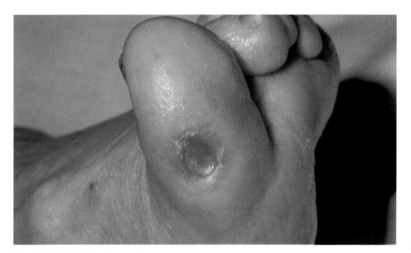

Fig. 12.27 Arterial ulcer on toe.

TREATMENT ARTERIAL LEG ULCERS

A patient with an arterial ulcer should be referred to a vascular surgeon. If it is not possible to improve the arterial blood supply, it is very unlikely that the ulcer will heal and gangrene will eventually occur. Early rather than late amputation is advised before the pain becomes intolerable.

Treatment of the ulcer itself. If there is any slough present, it should be removed either with a pair of sharp scissors or a scalpel or with a desloughing agent such as Varidase (for other desloughing agents *see* p. 35). Once the ulcer is clean it should be covered with a non-adhesive dressing (p. 38). This can be left in place for a week at a time so that any new epithelial cells will not be removed as soon as they have formed.
The dressing is covered with a light bandage simply to keep it in place. Do not apply tight bandages or any kind of elastic support because they can impede the arterial supply further. Adequate analgesics must also be given during the healing process since these ulcers are always painful.

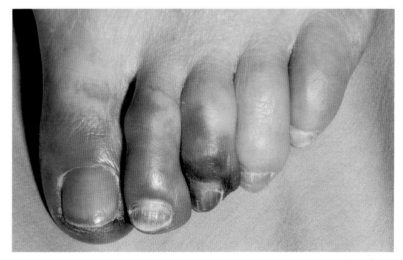

Fig. 12.28 Gangrene of toes due to arterial disease.

Investigations to determine the extent of arterial disease include:–

1. Feeling the pulses and listening for bruits.

2. Measurement of the blood pressure in the arm and at the ankle with a Doppler probe.

$$\frac{\text{Systolic blood pressure ankle}}{\text{Systolic blood pressure arm}} = \text{Resting ankle/brachial pressure index}$$

If it is > 0.9 there is no arterial disease.

If it is < 0.9 there is arterial disease.

If it is < 0.7 there is clinically significant arterial disease.

If it is < 0.5 the patient will be getting rest pain.

3. Duplex imaging Doppler. This combines the hand held continuous wave Doppler together with real time B-mode imaging to give picture images of the blood flow and measurement of blood flow.

4. Arteriogram to find out where the problem is, how extensive it is and whether the disease is amenable to surgery.

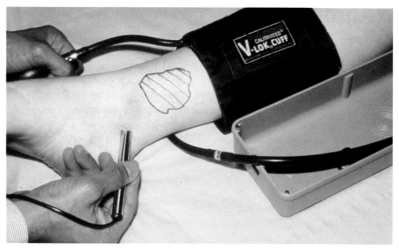

Fig. 12.29 Measurement of the systolic blood pressure at the ankle using a Doppler probe. Shaded area is the usual site for venous ulcers. Place cuff above this on calf.

NEUROPATHIC ULCERS

These ulcers result from trauma to anaesthetic feet, so occur over bony prominences, particularly the first metatarsophalangeal joint, the metatarsal heads or the heel, or at any other site of injury. Classically they are deep, painless, and often covered with thick callous. The diagnosis is confirmed by finding sensory loss and some associated disorder that has caused it, e.g. diabetes, leprosy, paraplegia, peripheral nerve injury, polyneuropathy, syringomyelia etc.

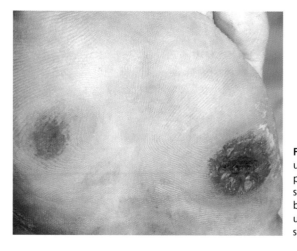

Fig. 12.30 Neuropathic ulcers over bony prominences on the sole. Hyperkeratosis builds up over the ulcer making it look smaller than it really is.

TREATMENT NEUROPATHIC ULCERS

Loss of sensation means that patients may not notice an injury to their anaesthetic feet or legs. Rubbing from shoes, treading on a nail, being bumped into by a supermarket trolley, having the toes accidentally trodden on, or burning by a hot water bottle are some of the common sources of injury. If the patient does not notice what has happened and does not protect the area from further damage an ulcer can form. On the sole of the foot callous often builds up around the injury making an ulcer seem smaller than it really is or sometimes completely covering it. It is essential to remove the callous with a scalpel to see how big the ulcer is. If nothing is done at this stage repeated trauma will cause the ulcer to enlarge and secondary infection is likely to occur (sometimes leading to osteomyelitis). The foot should be X-rayed and bacteriology swabs taken. If osteomyelitis is present the patient should be admitted to hospital so that high doses of intravenous antibiotics can be given.

To get the ulcers healed further injury/friction must be avoided. The simplest way of achieving this is by the patient resting in bed but this is not usually practical. An alternative is to apply a below knee walking plaster for 2 months at a time. This removes any friction and allows the ulcer to heal. After 2 months when the plaster is removed the ulcer is usually healed; if it is not, it is put back on for a further 2 months. If the ulcer is very dirty and there is a lot of exudate, the plaster can have a window cut in it to allow the ulcer to be cleaned regularly and to minimise the unpleasant smell for the patient.

Removing the slough (p. 35) and applying non-adherent dressings (p. 38) are the same as for venous ulcers. There is no need for elastic support. The idea is simply to keep the ulcer clean and free of friction while it heals.

The same principles apply to the treatment of **pressure sores**. Pressure on bony areas should be minimised by frequent changes of position and the use of a wool fleece or ripple bed.

ULCERS IN A DIABETIC PATIENT

Patients with diabetes mellitus can have both arterial and neuropathic ulcers. It is important to sort out which of the two is the main culprit and treat accordingly. The arterial disease can be due to atherosclerosis of the major limb vessels or small vessel disease (in which case the treatment options may be limited). Either type of ulcer (or both) can be complicated by bacterial infection. It is important to deal with this promptly with systemic antibiotics. Necrobiosis lipoidica (p. 335) can also ulcerate.

PRESSURE SORES

Sustained pressure over pressure points in immobile patients leads to localised ischaemia and eventual ulceration.

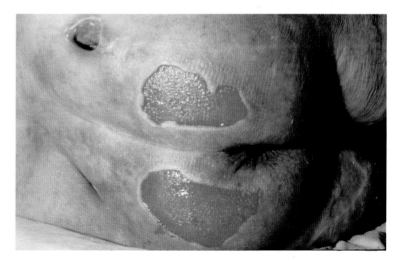

Fig. 12.31 Pressure sores on buttocks.

Lower legs
Chronic erythematous rash/lesions
Ulcerated surface
Unusual causes
Consider if there is no evidence of venous disease and the patient has normal foot pulses and sensation

In a Negro consider **Sickle cell disease**, p. 351.
If there has been recent foreign travel consider:–
Ecthyma *see* p. 164, **Tropical ulcers** p. 351,
Leishmaniasis *see* p. 122.

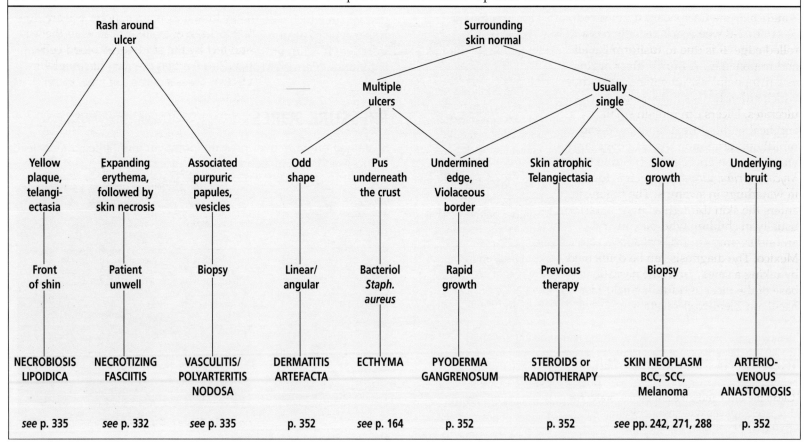

Rash around ulcer					**Surrounding skin normal**			
				Multiple ulcers		**Usually single**		
Yellow plaque, telangi-ectasia	Expanding erythema, followed by skin necrosis	Associated purpuric papules, vesicles	Odd shape	Pus underneath the crust	Undermined edge, Violaceous border	Skin atrophic Telangiectasia	Slow growth	Underlying bruit
Front of shin	Patient unwell	Biopsy	Linear/ angular	Bacteriol *Staph. aureus*	Rapid growth	Previous therapy	Biopsy	
NECROBIOSIS LIPOIDICA	NECROTIZING FASCIITIS	VASCULITIS/ POLYARTERITIS NODOSA	DERMATITIS ARTEFACTA	ECTHYMA	PYODERMA GANGRENOSUM	STEROIDS or RADIOTHERAPY	SKIN NEOPLASM BCC, SCC, Melanoma	ARTERIO-VENOUS ANASTOMOSIS
see p. 335	*see* p. 332	*see* p. 335	p. 352	*see* p. 164	p. 352	p. 352	*see* pp. 242, 271, 288	p. 352

TROPICAL & BURULI ULCERS

A **tropical phagadenic ulcer** is a fast growing painful ulcer on the lower legs and feet in malnourished children from Africa, India, SE Asia, Central & South America or the Caribbean. It can grow 5+ cm in 2–3 weeks and usually has a rolled edge. It is due to fusiform bacilli and treponemes. A **Buruli ulcer** begins as a firm, painless, subcutaneous nodule which either heals spontaneously or ulcerates. Ulcers can remain small and heal without treatment, or spread rapidly undermining the skin over large areas, even an entire limb. It is due to *Mycobacterium ulcerans*, which is found in waterbugs in swamps. The organism enters the skin through a cut or abrasion, usually in children who play in and around swamps in tropical Africa or Mexico. The diagnosis can be confirmed by taking a smear from the necrotic base of the ulcer and finding acid-fast bacilli on Ziehl-Neilson stain.

TREATMENT TROPICAL ULCER

Clean the ulcer and give antibiotics orally for 1–2 weeks (phenoxymethyl-penicillin, erythromycin or metronidazole).

TREATMENT BURULI ULCERS

Early (non-ulcerated) lesions can be healed with oral rifampicin. Ulcerated lesions need surgical excision.

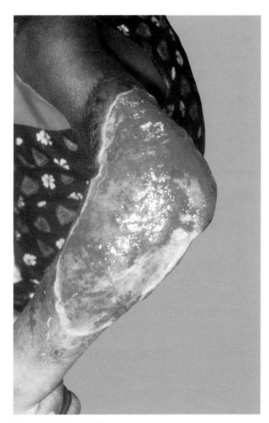

Fig. 12.32 Buruli ulcer.

SICKLE CELL ULCERS

Patients with sickle cell anaemia who are homozygous for the sickle cell gene develop ischaemic ulcers on the legs and feet in childhood and early adult life. They look like venous ulcers but are due to blockage of small arterioles in the legs and feet by the sickled red blood cells. Confirm the diagnosis by haemoglobin electrophoresis. Keep the ulcer clean until it heals.

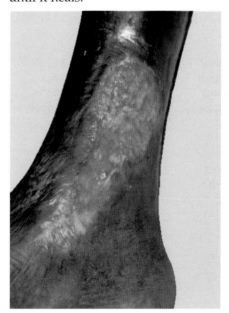

Fig. 12.33 Sickle cell ulcer over the lateral malleolus.

PYODERMA GANGRENOSUM

A rapidly growing ulcer with a violaceous overhanging edge and a yellow honey comb-like base should make you think of pyoderma gangrenosum. It is associated with ulcerative colitis, Crohn's disease, rheumatoid arthritis and multiple myeloma. In patients with ulcerative colitis, the activity of the pyoderma gangrenosum reflects the activity of the bowel problem, but with the other diseases the two conditions seem to behave independently of each other.

ARTERIO-VENOUS ANASTOMOSIS

This diagnosis is suggested in a large warm leg with an obvious bruit. It can be a congenital defect or follow a fracture. Treatment is difficult.

TREATMENT PYODERMA GANGRENOSUM

Patients with pyoderma gangrenosum should be referred urgently to a dermatologist or gastroenterologist for investigation of the underlying cause. The ulcer is treated with large doses of systemic steroids, beginning with 60mg prednisolone daily. Once the ulcer is healed the dose can gradually be reduced, and eventually the patient will be able to come off the steroids. Other immunosuppressive agents such as ciclosporin 3–5mg/kg/day or azathioprine 3mg/kg/day can also be tried in addition to or instead of oral steroids.

Other possible treatments are a very potent[UK]/group 1[USA] topical steroid such as 0.05% clobetasol propionate applied b.i.d. to the ulcer, oral clofazamine, dapsone or minocycline.

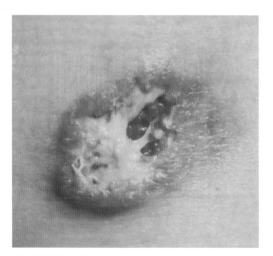

Fig. 12.34 Pyoderma gangrenosum: close up.

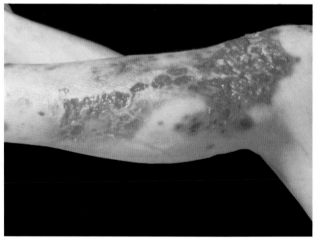

Fig. 12.35 Dermatitis artefacta.

STEROIDS or RADIOTHERAPY

Topical or systemic steroids used over a long period, or previous radiotherapy may result in thinning of dermal collagen and ulceration after minor trauma.

DERMATITIS ARTEFACTA

Any ulcer with straight edges (linear, square or triangular) is likely to be artefactual unless proven otherwise (*see* p. 227).

Lower legs (& trunk, arms)
Non-erythematous rash/lesions (including purpura)
Normal surface
Purple/orange/brown colour

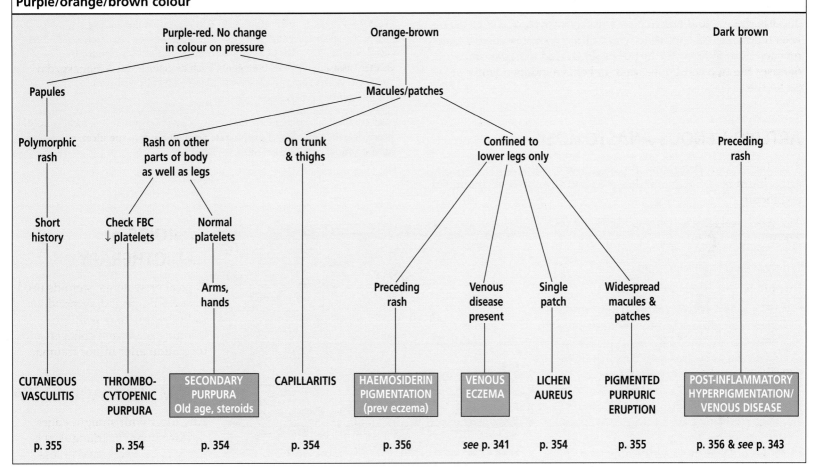

Purple-red. No change in colour on pressure

Orange-brown

Dark brown

Papules

Macules/patches

Polymorphic rash

Rash on other parts of body as well as legs

On trunk & thighs

Confined to lower legs only

Preceding rash

Short history

Check FBC ↓ platelets

Normal platelets

Arms, hands

Preceding rash

Venous disease present

Single patch

Widespread macules & patches

CUTANEOUS VASCULITIS

THROMBO-CYTOPENIC PURPURA

SECONDARY PURPURA Old age, steroids

CAPILLARITIS

HAEMOSIDERIN PIGMENTATION (prev eczema)

VENOUS ECZEMA

LICHEN AUREUS

PIGMENTED PURPURIC ERUPTION

POST-INFLAMMATORY HYPERPIGMENTATION/ VENOUS DISEASE

p. 355   p. 354   p. 354   p. 354   p. 356   *see* p. 341   p. 354   p. 355   p. 356 & *see* p. 343

PURPURA

Purpura is due to leakage of red blood cells from blood vessels into the skin. When compressed with the finger the red colour does not disappear as it would if the blood were still inside the blood vessels as in erythema (*see* p. 14). The extravasated blood is broken down to haemosiderin causing the colour to change from purple to orangy-brown. Purpura may be due to a platelet disorder (thrombocytopenic) or a vascular disorder (non-thrombocytopenic).

Thrombocytopenic purpura

If the platelet count falls below $50,000/mm^3$ bleeding may occur. In the skin this is seen as tiny purpuric macules and papules (petechiae) and larger patches (echymoses). There may be bleeding elsewhere too. Thrombocytopenia may be due to bone marrow disease (pancytopenia, leukaemia, drug induced marrow failure), systemic infections, splenomegaly or idiopathic thrombocytopenic purpura.

Non-thrombocytopenic purpura

This can be due to the following:–

- Leaky blood vessels (**capillaritis**). Uniformly small, orange-brown macules occur anywhere on the skin. The cause is unknown and no treatment is available. When this is localised to a single area it is known as **lichen aureus.**
- Lack of connective tissue support for blood vessels, occurring in old age (**senile purpura**) or after topical or systemic corticosteroid therapy. Bruising occurs after minor trauma. Large purpuric patches are seen especially on the forearms and dorsum of the hands.
- **Pigmented purpuric eruption** (*see* p. 355).
- **Cutaneous vasculitis** (*see* p. 355).

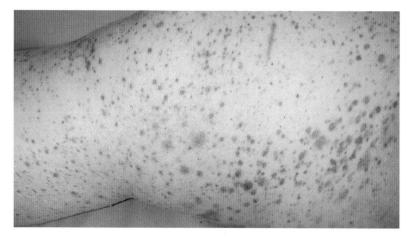

Fig. 12.36 Purpuric macules and papules on the leg.

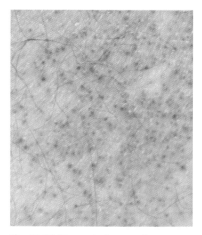

Fig. 12.37 Pigmented purpuric eruption.

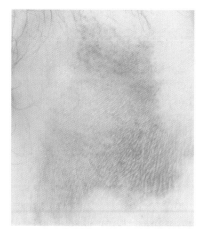

Fig. 12.38 Lichen aureus.

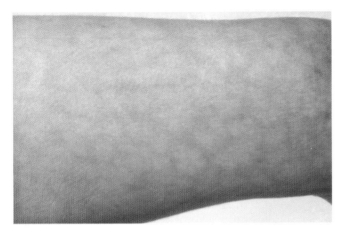

Fig. 12.39 Livedo reticularis. Annular mottling of skin. This can be a normal finding especially in the cold, or a sign of cutaneous polyarteritis nodosa.

PURPURIC DRUG RASH

Some drugs cause **thrombocytopenia** with purpura and larger echymoses. All such patients should be referred urgently to hospital for investigation. Drugs which can cause a fall in platelet count include:–

- all cytotoxic drugs
- co-trimoxazole
- gold
- rifampicin
- chlorpromazine
- frusemide
- indomethacin.

Other drugs cause a **non-thrombocytopenic** purpura, where there is an underlying vasculitis. This is is likely to be mainly on the lower legs. Drugs which do this include:–

- allopurinol
- carbimazole
- barbiturates
- thiazide diuretics.

PIGMENTED PURPURIC ERUPTION

This presents as rusty-brown pigmentation starting on the feet and gradually working its way up the lower leg over a period of months to years. If you look carefully you will see tiny purpuric macules within the pigmented areas which are the result of deposition of haemosiderin following the purpura. There is no obvious cause for the condition and no effective treatment.

VASCULITIS

Vasculitis is an inflammation of the blood vessels in the skin usually due to deposition of immune complexes in their walls. There are several different patterns dependent on the size and site of the vessels involved:–

- Capillaries in the superficial and mid dermis (**leucocytoclastic vasculitis; Henoch–Schönlein purpura**, *see* p. 356). There will be a polymorphic rash with palpable purpura as well as macules, papules, vesicles and pustules.
- Arteries at the junction of the dermis and subcutaneous fat (**cutaneous polyarteritis nodosa**). There will be livedo reticularis, nodules and/or ulceration on the lower legs.
- Arteries and veins in the subcutaneous fat (**nodular vasculitis; erythema nodosum**). There will be tender red nodules or plaques deep in the subcutaneous fat (*see* p. 335).

Causes of cutaneous vasculitis

- Distant focus of infection – e.g. streptococcal infection
- Collagen vascular disease (SLE, rheumatoid, systemic sclerosis)
- Plasma protein abnormality and cryoglobulinaemia
- Drugs – see left
- Idiopathic (no cause found).

TREATMENT CUTANEOUS VASCULITIS

Look for an underlying cause and treat this if possible. It is worth checking the urine for protein, blood and casts and the blood urea and creatinine to make sure that the kidneys are not involved. If there is renal damage specialist help should be sought because treatment with systemic steroids or cyclophosphamide may be needed. If no cause can be found the patient can be reassured that it is a self limiting condition which will get better after 3–6 weeks. Bed rest will stop new lesions from developing on the skin. Treatment is symptomatic, with analgesics for pain.

HENOCH–SCHÖNLEIN PURPURA

This form of leucocytoclastic vasculitis occurs mainly in young children and is associated with arthralgia and abdominal pain. Leucocytoclastic is a histological term describing dead white blood cells seen around blood vessels. The rash consists of erythematous and purpuric macules and papules together with vesicles and pustules. It should be thought of in any child with purpura and a normal platelet count. It may follow a streptococcal sore throat.

TREATMENT HENOCH–SCHÖNLEIN PURPURA

If it follows a streptococcal throat infection, treat with phenoxymethyl penicillin. Otherwise bed rest will stop new lesions from occurring, and most cases will get better spontaneously after 3–6 weeks. Use analgesics (paracetamol syrup) for the joint and abdominal pain. Renal involvement may be more serious. Proteinuria or microscopic haematuria without impairment of renal function will normally get better spontaneously in less than 4 weeks. If acute nephritis or progressive renal failure occurs the patient should be referred urgently to a renal physician.

POST-INFLAMMATORY HYPERPIGMENTATION

Post-inflammatory hyperpigmentation may follow any inflammatory condition of the epidermis. It commonly follows lichen planus or eczema. It is distinguished from haemosiderin pigmentation by being a darker brown colour. On the lower legs both may co-exist particularly in individuals with chronic venous disease (*see* p. 343).

HAEMOSIDERIN PIGMENTATION

Haemosiderin pigmentation is the orange-brown pigmentation in the dermis which follows purpura and is due to haemoglobin that has leaked into the skin being broken down. It is most commonly seen in chronic venous disease and pigmented purpuric eruption.

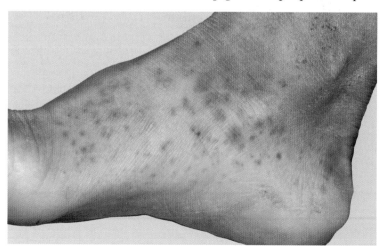

Fig. 12.40 Henoch–Schönlein purpura. Note polymorphic nature of lesions, macules, papules, vesicles and crusts.

Hands and feet

13

HANDS

Dorsum hand and wrist

Palm

Hand eczema/dermatitis

FEET

Dorsum foot

Soles

HANDS

Hands (dorsum & palms)
Acute erythematous rash/lesion(s)

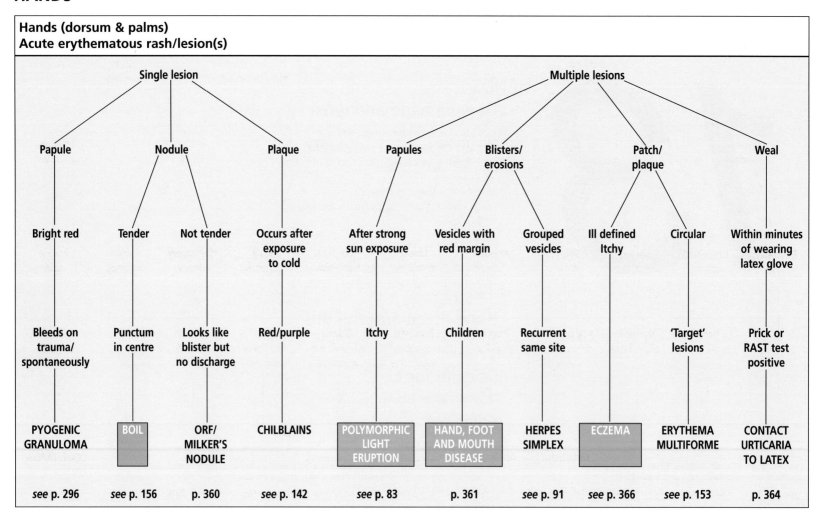

Single lesion				Multiple lesions			
Papule	Nodule		Plaque	Papules	Blisters/erosions		Patch/plaque	Weal

| Bright red | Tender | Not tender | Occurs after exposure to cold | After strong sun exposure | Vesicles with red margin | Grouped vesicles | Ill defined Itchy | Circular | Within minutes of wearing latex glove |

| Bleeds on trauma/spontaneously | Punctum in centre | Looks like blister but no discharge | Red/purple | Itchy | Children | Recurrent same site | | 'Target' lesions | Prick or RAST test positive |

| PYOGENIC GRANULOMA | BOIL | ORF/MILKER'S NODULE | CHILBLAINS | POLYMORPHIC LIGHT ERUPTION | HAND, FOOT AND MOUTH DISEASE | HERPES SIMPLEX | ECZEMA | ERYTHEMA MULTIFORME | CONTACT URTICARIA TO LATEX |

| *see* p. 296 | *see* p. 156 | p. 360 | *see* p. 142 | *see* p. 83 | p. 361 | *see* p. 91 | *see* p. 366 | *see* p. 153 | p. 364 |

Dorsum wrist/hand/fingers
Chronic erythematous rash/lesion(s)
Papules, plaques, erosions & blisters

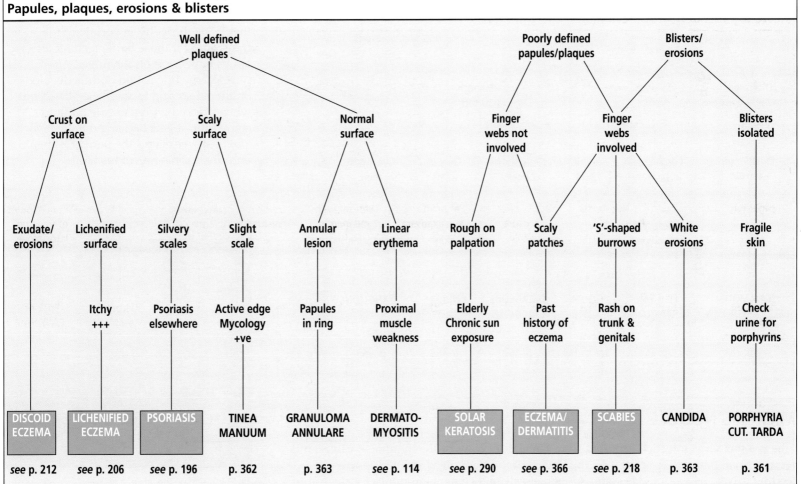

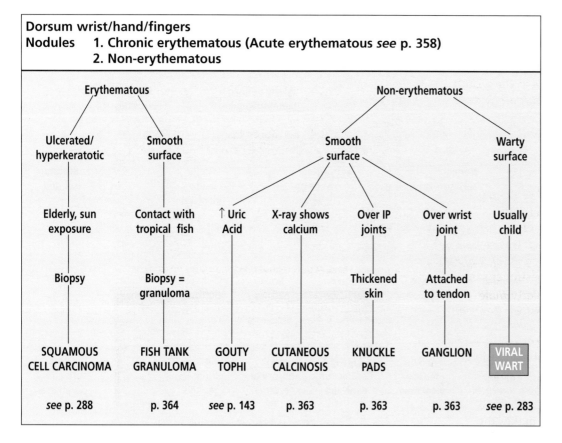

Dorsum wrist/hand/fingers
Nodules   1. **Chronic erythematous** (Acute erythematous *see* p. 358)
              2. **Non-erythematous**

Erythematous | Non-erythematous

Ulcerated/hyperkeratotic — Smooth surface | Smooth surface — Warty surface

Elderly, sun exposure | Contact with tropical fish | ↑ Uric Acid | X-ray shows calcium | Over IP joints | Over wrist joint | Usually child

Biopsy | Biopsy = granuloma | | | Thickened skin | Attached to tendon |

SQUAMOUS CELL CARCINOMA | FISH TANK GRANULOMA | GOUTY TOPHI | CUTANEOUS CALCINOSIS | KNUCKLE PADS | GANGLION | **VIRAL WART**

see p. 288 | p. 364 | *see* p. 143 | p. 363 | p. 363 | p. 363 | *see* p. 283

MILKER'S NODULE

This is a pox virus infection acquired from the teats of cows or the mouths of calves. It is seen as small papules or vesicles on the fingers of those involved in milking cows or feeding calves. Like orf it gets better spontaneously and confers immunity for the future.

ORF

Orf is a pox virus infection of lambs. It causes sores around the mouth so that they have difficulty in suckling. It is transmitted if those bottle feeding affected lambs have a cut on the finger. A red, purple, or white round nodule develops on the finger and looks like a blister, but when pricked with a needle no fluid comes out. It gets better spontaneously after 3–4 weeks and the patient is then immune for the rest of his life.

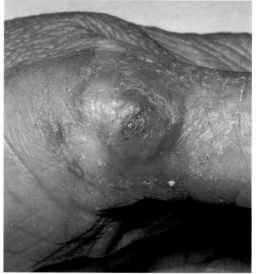

Fig. 13.01 Orf on the side of a finger.

HAND, FOOT AND MOUTH DISEASE

This is a mild infection due to Coxsackie A16 virus which occurs in children where small grey vesicles with a red halo occur on the fingers and toes together with small erosions in the mouth (Fig. 6.02, p. 125). It gets better spontaneously after a few days so no treatment is necessary.

PORPHYRIA CUTA TARDA (PCT)

This is an acquired porphyria and the one most likely to be seen in clinical practice. It is due to reduced levels of uroporphyrinogen decarboxylase in the liver resulting in increased levels of urophorphyrins in the urine and plasma. It is caused by excessive alcohol intake (2% of alcoholics develop PCT), hepatitis C, subclinical haemochromatosis or the use of oestrogens or HRT. The patient is usually a middle aged or elderly male (less common in females), who presents with blisters, scars and milia on sun exposed skin – dorsum hands and forearms, face and bald scalp. There may also be hypertrichosis on the face. The patient rarely associates the development of skin lesions with sunlight. The diagnosis is made by finding increased porphyrins in the urine. The urine can be screened using a Wood's (ultra-violet) lamp where a coral pink fluorescence is seen. Acidifying the urine or adding talc to it makes the fluorescence more obvious. Detailed analysis of the various porphyins by a specialist laboratory will confirm the type of porphyria. Check also the liver enzymes, hepatitis C antibodies, serum ferritin and look for the haemochromatosis gene mutation.

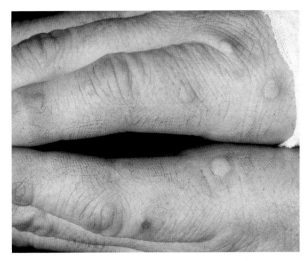

Fig. 13.02 Hand, foot & mouth disease: vesicles on fingers.

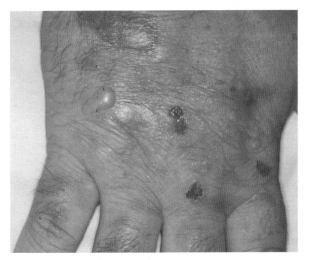

Fig. 13.03 Porphyria cuta tarda. Blisters and erosions on dorsum of hand.

TREATMENT PORPHYRIA CUTANEA TARDA

Stop alcohol or the contraceptive pill (the most likely causes). If symptoms do not improve remove 500ml blood fortnightly until the serum ferritin is back to normal or symptoms abate, usually after 2–3 months. The patient should avoid sun exposure (even through window glass – porphyrins absorb UVA radiation), wear a long sleeved shirt, hat and opaque sunscreen. Oral chloroquine 200mg twice a week improves the skin fragility within 6 months by complexing the porphyrins and promoting excretion.

TINEA MANUUM

Ringworm infection should be considered in any red scaly rash affecting only one hand. This can be confirmed or excluded by mycology (*see* p. 19). The source of the infection is often the patient's own toe webs or nails, so look at the feet as well. Three patterns of infection can occur. 1. An annular plaque on the dorsum of the hand (Fig. 13.04); 2. Fine scaling picking out the creases on one palm only (*see* Fig. 13.35, p. 379); 3. Scaling or vesicles on one hand only.

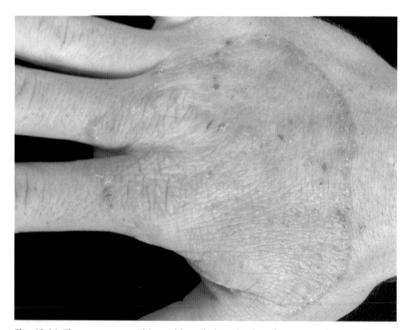

Fig. 13.04 Tinea manuum. This could easily be mistaken for eczema because it appears lichenified and has excoriations. The distinguishing feature is that it is unilateral and has a well defined edge.

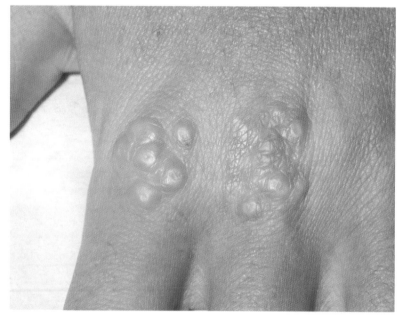

Fig. 13.05 Granuloma annulare.

NODULES ON DORSUM OF HAND

White hard papules or nodules containing calcium (**calcinosis cutis**) can occur on the fingers or dorsum of the hand in patients with scleroderma or dermatomyositis (*see also* p. 241). The diagnosis can be confirmed by X-ray. A **ganglion** is a synovial cyst associated with the wrist joint.

CANDIDA INFECTION OF FINGER WEBS

Infection with *Candida albicans* occurs in the finger webs as well as the toe webs especially if the hands are always in water. The finger webs become macerated and are usually white in colour.

GRANULOMA ANNULARE

Small skin coloured or mauvish-pink papules form rings on the dorsum of the fingers, hand or foot. It is usually asymptomatic although it can be tender if knocked. It is distinguished from ringworm by not being scaly (*see also* p. 177). **Knuckle pads** are thickened plaques that occur over the interphalangeal joints in young adults for no apparent reason.

TREATMENT CANDIDA

Dry the hands thoroughly after washing, especially in the finger webs. Apply a topical antifungal such as nystatin ointment, an imidazole cream or 0.5% Gentian violet paint b.i.d. until it is better.

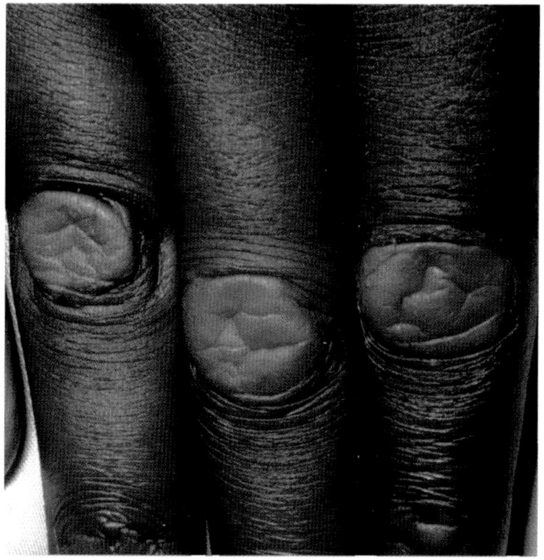

Fig. 13.06 Knuckle pads.

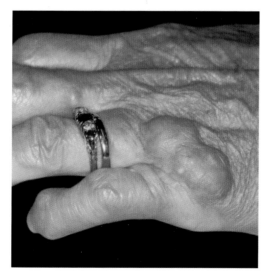

Fig. 13.07 Cutaneous calcinosis.

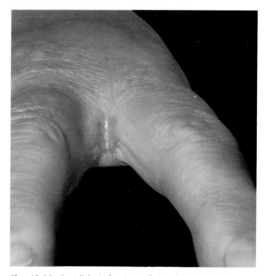

Fig. 13.08 Candida infection of the finger webs.

FISH TANK GRANULOMA

Tropical fish infected with *Mycobacterium marinum* die. In removing the dead fish the owner can scrape the back of his hand on the gravel at the bottom of the tank and so implant the atypical mycobacterium into the skin. Pink/purple nodules occur at the site of inplantation. Occasionally the lesions may be ulcerated. Similar lesions can occur proximally up the arm due to spread through the lymphatics.

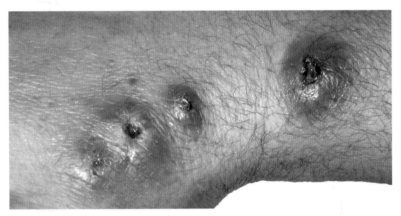

Fig. 13.09 Fish tank granuloma on dorsum of hand.

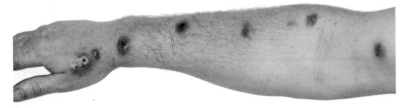

Fig. 13.10 Lesions spreading up the arm proximally (sporotrichoid spread).

TREATMENT FISH TANK GRANULOMA

Treatment is with co-trimoxazole 960mg twice a day, or minocycline 100mg twice a day until the skin heals (usually 6–12 weeks). Advise the patient to remove dead fish wearing rubber gloves in the future.

CONTACT URTICARIA TO LATEX

Natural latex is the sap from the rubber tree (*Hevea brasiliensis*). Latex gloves or condoms are made from water-based natural rubber latex (NRL) emulsions, and these can cause type I hypersensitivity (contact urticaria), angioedema, asthma or anaphylaxis. Powdered NRL gloves cause more problems than the non-powdered ones. Contact urticaria presents with itchy weals within a few minutes at the site of contact with the rubber. Patients who react in this way also get problems with bananas, avocado pears, Kiwi fruit and/or chestnuts. NRL is responsible for about 10% of all intra-operative anaphylactic reactions, and is due to the surgeon or nurse wearing NRL gloves. The diagnosis can be confirmed by a positive prick test, or if this is negative and the history is suggestive, by a 'use test' – wearing a finger from a NRL glove on wet skin for 15 minutes. Dry rubber latex (in household rubber gloves, elasticated bandages, balloons, shoes, car tyres etc.) cause a type IV hypersensitivity reaction, i.e. allergic contact dermatitis.

TREATMENT CONTACT URTICARIA TO LATEX

Avoid direct contact with NRL gloves and condoms. Use vinyl, neoprene, elastyren or nitrile gloves instead of latex gloves and use condoms made of polyurethane. It is essential to warn surgeons of the possibility of latex sensitivity before surgery is undertaken, and prick test such patients before surgery.

Palms
1. Chronic erythematous rash/multiple lesions (single/few lesions *see* Chapter 8, p. 169)
2. Non-erythematous rash with scaling, peeling or increased skin markings

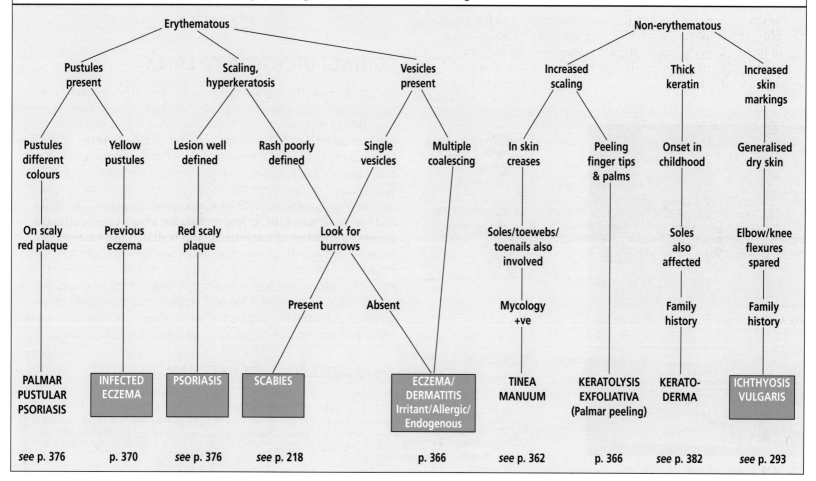

see p. 376   p. 370   *see* p. 376   *see* p. 218   p. 366   *see* p. 362   p. 366   *see* p. 382   *see* p. 293

KERATOLYSIS EXFOLIATIVA (Palmar peeling)

Peeling of the palms and fingers is common, often occurring about once a month. It is usually asymptomatic but there may be increased sensitivity to touch. The cause is not known and there is no specific treatment.

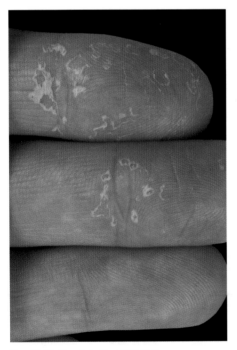

Fig. 13.11 Keratolysis exfoliativa.

HAND ECZEMA/DERMATITIS

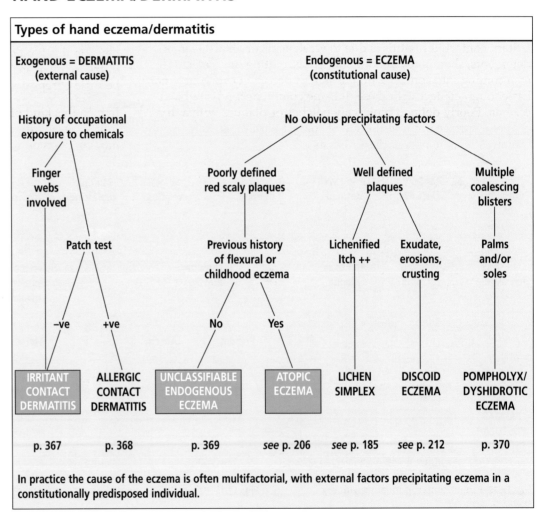

Types of hand eczema/dermatitis

Exogenous = DERMATITIS (external cause)

History of occupational exposure to chemicals

Finger webs involved

Patch test

−ve → IRRITANT CONTACT DERMATITIS (p. 367)

+ve → ALLERGIC CONTACT DERMATITIS (p. 368)

Endogenous = ECZEMA (constitutional cause)

No obvious precipitating factors

Poorly defined red scaly plaques

Previous history of flexural or childhood eczema

No → UNCLASSIFIABLE ENDOGENOUS ECZEMA (p. 369)

Yes → ATOPIC ECZEMA (see p. 206)

Well defined plaques

Lichenified Itch ++ → LICHEN SIMPLEX (see p. 185)

Exudate, erosions, crusting → DISCOID ECZEMA (see p. 212)

Multiple coalescing blisters

Palms and/or soles → POMPHOLYX/ DYSHIDROTIC ECZEMA (p. 370)

In practice the cause of the eczema is often multifactorial, with external factors precipitating eczema in a constitutionally predisposed individual.

DERMATITIS = EXOGENOUS ECZEMA

1. IRRITANT CONTACT DERMATITIS

Irritant contact dermatitis is due to weak acids or alkalis (e.g. in detergents, shampoos, cleaning materials, cutting oils, cement dust etc.) coming into contact with the skin. It occurs in everyone who has enough contact with these. It is the commonest type of hand eczema. Poorly defined pink scaly patches or plaques with a dry chapped surface occur at the site of contact with the irritant. Usually there are no vesicles or crusts.

In women detergents are the main culprit. The rash begins under a ring or in the finger webs where the alkaline detergent particles get trapped. A lot of young mothers will get dermatitis on their hands when their children are small. Hairdressers commonly develop this kind of eczema when they first begin work because of the frequent shampooing. Cooks and nurses are also at risk because of repeated hand washing.

In men this kind of eczema is mainly on the dorsum of the hands from contact with cement dust or soluble oils used for cooling the moving parts of machinery in the engineering industries.

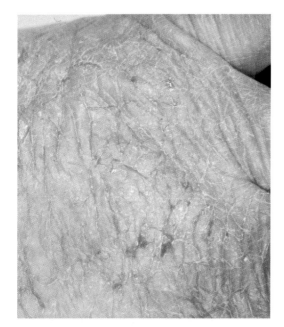

Fig. 13.12 Irritant contact dermatitis with dry chapped surface.

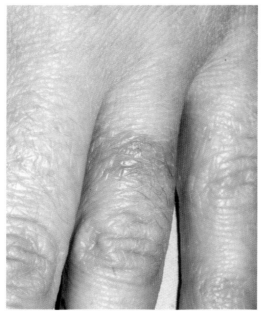

Fig. 13.13 Irritant contact dermatitis under a wedding ring.

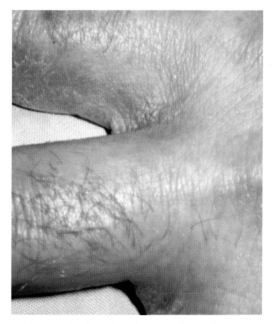

Fig. 13.14 Irritant contact dermatitis in the finger webs.

2. ALLERGIC CONTACT DERMATITIS

Allergic contact dermatitis is a type IV allergic reaction and affects only a very small proportion of the population. The rash occurs at the site of contact with the allergen, but on the hands it is difficult to predict the cause from the site involved because the hands come into contact with so many things during the day.

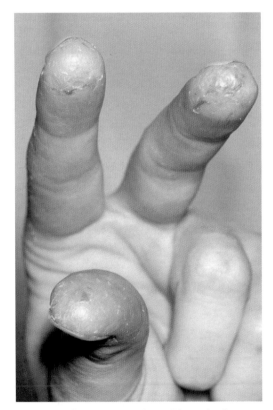

Fig. 13.15 Allergic contact dermatitis on the finger tips due to garlic (usually on the non-dominant hand).

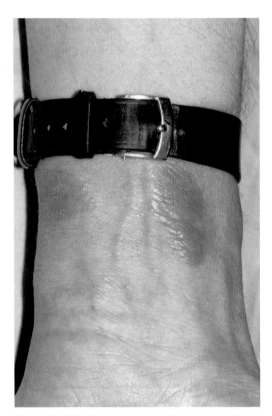

Fig. 13.16 Allergic contact dermatitis due to PTBP formaldehyde resin in a watch strap.

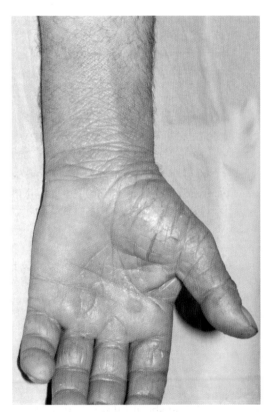

Fig. 13.17 Allergic contact dermatitis due to rubber gloves.

Nevertheless there are several well recognised patterns:–

- Finger tips – from formalin in laboratory workers and secretaries (from formaldehyde resins in cardboard folders), local anaesthetics in dentists, garlic & onion in cooks, Balsam of Peru in orange peel and tulip bulbs.
- Centre of palm and flexor aspects of fingers – from rubber, nickel or plastic handle grips.
- Whole hand (palm, dorsum and wrist) – from rubber gloves.
- Flexor aspect of wrist in lines – from the leaves of the indoor primula plant (*Primula obconica*), *see* p. 159.
- Flexor aspect of the wrist from nickel in watch buckle or PTBP formaldehyde resin in the watch strap.

It is probably wise to patch test (*see* p. 20) anyone with hand eczema who does not get better quickly with topical steroids.

Allergic contact dermatitis may develop explosively with vesicles, exudate and crusting. If it develops more slowly then the rash is a poorly defined red scaly rash just like eczema elsewhere.

Occupational dermatitis has medico-legal implications. The assessement of each patient depends on whether he/she could have reasonably expected to have developed eczema if they had not been engaged in that particular job or occupation.

ENDOGENOUS ECZEMA

Endogenous eczema can occur on both the palms and dorsum of the hand. You should think of this diagnosis if the patient has symmetrical eczema, particularly if there is a past history of atopic eczema in childhood. The eczema is itchy and continual

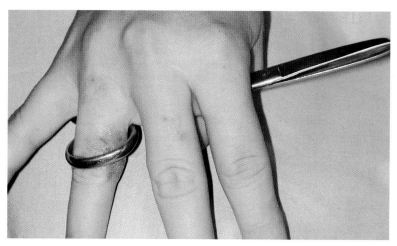

Fig. 13.18 Allergic contact dermatitis to nickel in scissors in a hairdresser.

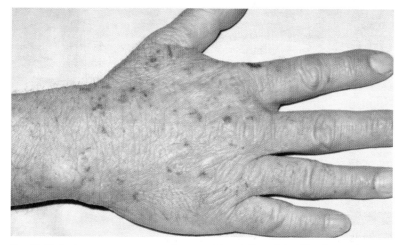

Fig. 13.19 Endogenous eczema on dorsum of hand. Note lichenification and excoriations.

scratching and rubbing will lead to lichenification. If it becomes secondarily infected with bacteria (*Staphylococcus aureus*), pustules may occur. On the palms this differs from pustular psoriasis because all the pustules are the same colour (yellow).

Acute eczema resulting in blistering on the palms and soles is termed **pompholyx** (or **dyshidrotic eczema**^{USA}). Because of the thickened stratum corneum, the epidermal blisters persist and appear as tiny grey-white 'grains' within the skin. Eventually they burst and erosions occur. Sometimes pompholyx can occur as an isolated episode which then resolves spontaneously.

Some hand eczema becomes hyperkeratotic resulting in fissures over the finger joints, along the skin creases and over finger tips. These are painful and can be very disabling.

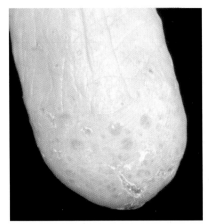

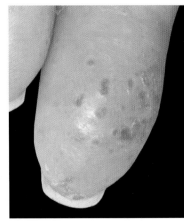

Fig. 13.21 Pompholyx on the finger tips.

Fig. 13.22 Pompholyx after blisters have burst.

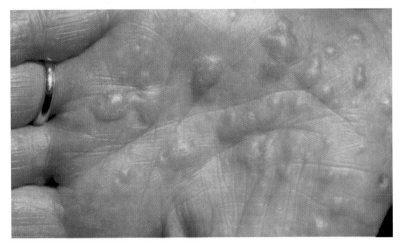

Fig. 13.20 Pompholyx. Intact vesicles under the thick stratum corneum of the palm.

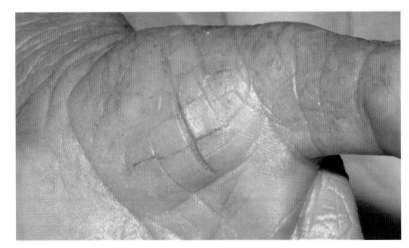

Fig. 13.23 Hyperkeratotic eczema on the palm with a fissure.

TREATMENT OF HAND AND FOOT ECZEMA

With eczema on the hands it is always worth doing patch tests, because the hands touch a lot of things during the course of a day. If the cause can be found and contact with it stopped, the eczema may be cured. Otherwise the patient will be condemned to using ointments or creams indefinitely.

1. **Acute weeping eczema.** Initially rest will be required to get the eczema better. For the hands stop washing up, cleaning, shampooing etc. Resting the feet in practice means bed rest. Dry up the exudate by soaking the hands/feet for 10 minutes twice a day in an astringent such as 1:10,000 potassium permanganate solution[UK] or aluminium acetate (Burow's solution[USA]), *see* p. 26. After drying the skin apply a moderate[UK]/group 4–5[USA] topical steroid ointment which does not contain lanolin. Always use an ointment rather than a cream until the cause of the eczema is sorted out. Once the eczema is better try to find the cause by patch testing (*see* p. 20).

2. **Chronic eczema.** The patient will require a moderate[UK]/group 4–5[USA] topical steroid ointment or cream applied once or twice a day. It will often be a question of trial and error to find the one which will suit this particular patient best. If the skin is very dry or there are a lot of fissures, start with an ointment. If it is not too scaly the patient may prefer to use a cream.

If the eczema is on the hands prevent further damage by wearing cotton gloves for doing housework, and rubber gloves or cotton-lined PVC gloves for all wet work. Manual labourers also will need to protect their hands from irritants as much as possible by wearing surgical latex gloves which should be provided at work. Often wearing gloves is not practicable, and it may be necessary to have time off work if the eczema will not settle down. In many cases once the dermatitis is established, it will not resolve without a change in occupation (e.g. trainee hairdressers, machine workers, chefs and nurses may have to change jobs). If the eczema is on the feet, white cotton socks and leather shoes are likely to be more comfortable than man-made fibres, unless of course the eczema is an allergic contact dermatitis due to chromate in leather.

3. **Hyperkeratotic eczema**. Both the eczema and the hyperkeratosis need treating. The thickened keratin will prevent applied topical steroids getting through the skin, and any fissures will be painful when the hyperkeratosis cracks.

For the hyperkeratosis the options include:–

i) 5% salicylic acid ointment, either applied alone or mixed with a topical steroid, e.g. *Diprosalic* ointment. If the salicylic acid is used alone, it can be applied either in the morning or at night, and a topical steroid ointment used alone the other time. One of the moderate[UK]/group 4–5[USA] steroid ointments will be required.

ii) 50% propylene glycol in water is applied under polythene occlusion at night (use plastic bags on the feet and either plastic bags or plastic gloves on the hands). In the morning a moderately potent[UK]/group 4–5[USA] topical steroid ointment can be applied.

Haelan tape (fludroxycortide 4µg/cm^2) may also be useful for hyperkeratotic or fissured eczema on the hands and feet. Patients like it because it is not messy. A strip of tape is applied to the area and left on for 12 hours at a time.

Failure of topical treatment

Severe disabling hand or foot eczema may require treatment with systemic immuno-suppresive agents such azathioprine or ciclosporin.

FEET

Dorsum of foot
Erythematous rash/lesions

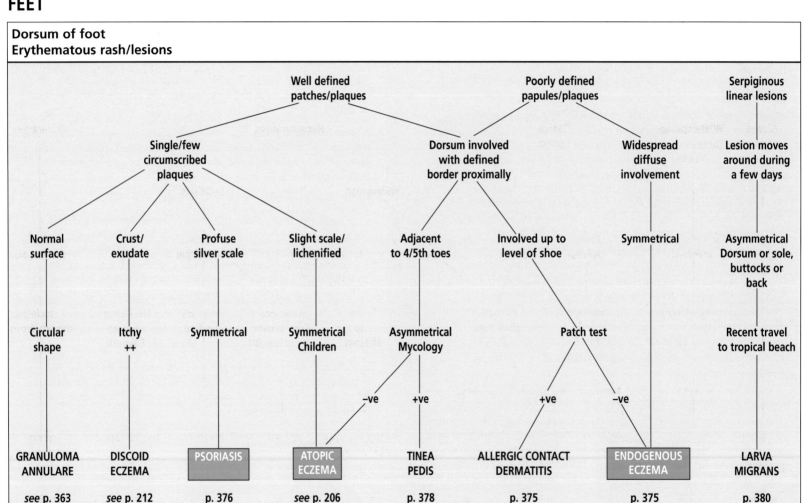

Soles – instep and weight bearing areas
Scaling/hyperkeratosis/maceration

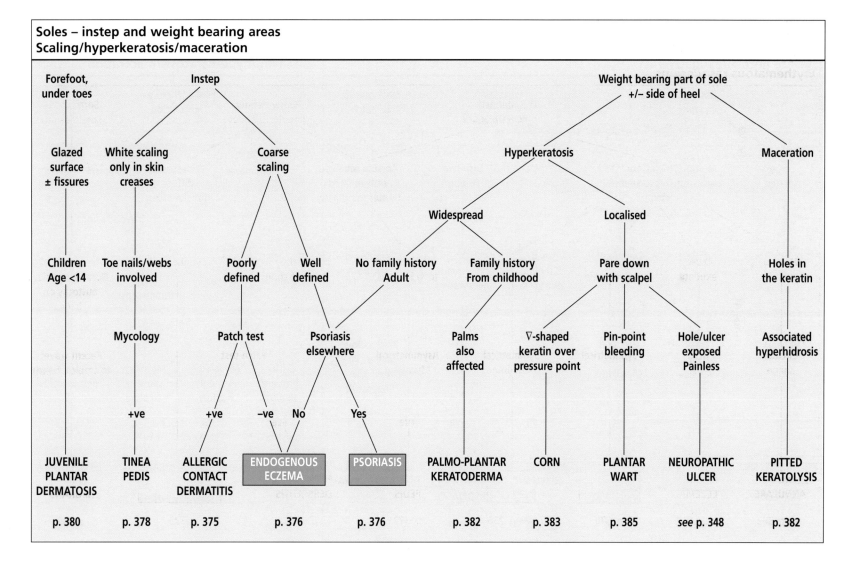

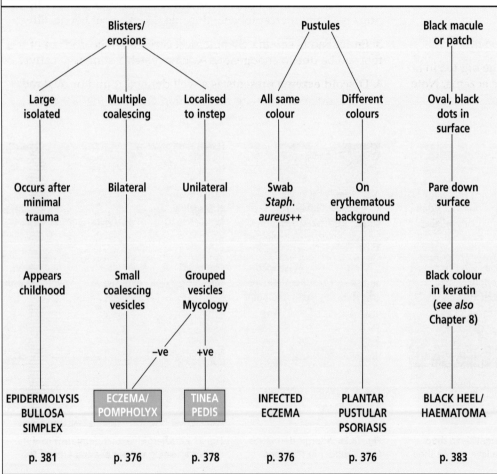

Soles
Vesicles/pustules/erosions (for ulcers *see* Chapter 12)
Surface normal/exudate/crust

Blisters/
erosions

- Large
  isolated
  - Occurs after
    minimal
    trauma
    - Appears
      childhood
      - **EPIDERMOLYSIS**
        BULLOSA
        SIMPLEX
        p. 381

- Multiple
  coalescing
  - Bilateral
    - Small
      coalescing
      vesicles
      - –ve → **ECZEMA/**
        POMPHOLYX
        p. 376

- Localised
  to instep
  - Unilateral
    - Grouped
      vesicles
      Mycology
      - +ve → **TINEA**
        PEDIS
        p. 378

Pustules

- All same
  colour
  - Swab
    Staph.
    aureus++
    - **INFECTED**
      ECZEMA
      p. 376

- Different
  colours
  - On
    erythematous
    background
    - **PLANTAR**
      PUSTULAR
      PSORIASIS
      p. 376

Black macule
or patch

- Oval, black
  dots in
  surface
  - Pare down
    surface
    - Black colour
      in keratin
      (*see also*
      Chapter 8)
      - **BLACK HEEL/**
        HAEMATOMA
        p. 383

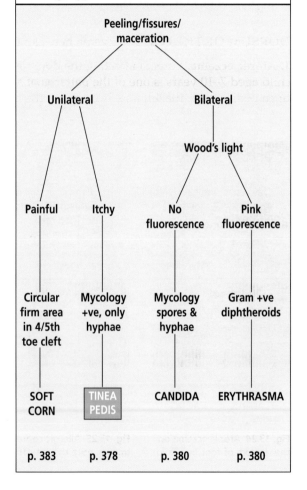

Soles – between 3rd/4th or 4th/5th toes
Plaques/nodules
Scaling/hyperkeratosis/maceration

Peeling/fissures/
maceration

- Unilateral
  - Painful
    - Circular
      firm area
      in 4/5th
      toe cleft
      - **SOFT**
        CORN
        p. 383
  - Itchy
    - Mycology
      +ve, only
      hyphae
      - **TINEA**
        PEDIS
        p. 378

- Bilateral
  - Wood's light
    - No
      fluorescence
      - Mycology
        spores &
        hyphae
        - **CANDIDA**
          p. 380
    - Pink
      fluorescence
      - Gram +ve
        diphtheroids
        - **ERYTHRASMA**
          p. 380

ECZEMA ON THE FOOT

A symmetrical red scaly rash on the foot in which vesicles have been present at some stage is likely to be eczema.

DORSUM OF THE FOOT – Eczema here can be due to:–

1. Atopic eczema. Eczema affecting the dorsum of the big toe in a child aged 7–10 years is one of the patterns of atopic eczema. Note tinea pedis affects the 4th and 5th toes not the big toe.

2. Allergic contact dermatitis. A rash up to the level of the shoe and sparing the toe webs is usually due to an allergic contact dermatitis to chrome in the leather of the shoe uppers, or azo dyes in nylon socks/stockings. A rash at the site of contact with flip flops is due to mercaptobenzothiazole (MTB), a rubber additive.

3. Endogenous eczema. Symmetrical eczema on the dorsum of the foot can be due to endogenous eczema. Patch testing is negative.

4. Discoid eczema presents as a well defined round or oval red scaly plaque with obvious vesiculation and crusting (*see* p. 212).

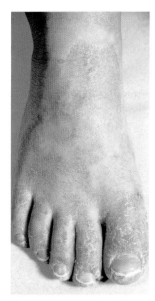

Fig. 13.24 Atopic eczema on the dorsum of foot in a child.

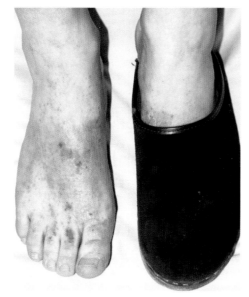

Fig. 13.25 Allergic contact dermatitis to shoe uppers, note the cut off at the level of the shoe.

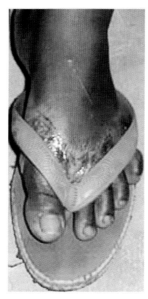

Fig. 13.26 Allergic dermatitis to the rubber in flip flops.

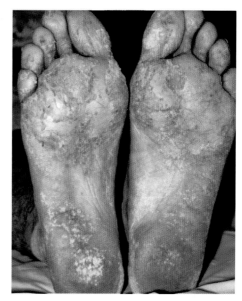

Fig. 13.27 Allergic contact dermatitis to shoe rubber affecting weight bearing area of the soles.

SOLE OF THE FOOT

Hyperkeratosis occurs when eczema affects the weight bearing areas of the soles. Painful fissures occur if the thickened keratin splits. The causes of eczema on the soles are:–

1. Allergic contact dermatitis. Symmetrical eczema on the weight bearing area of the soles (Fig. 13.27) is due to an allergic contact dermatitis until proven otherwise. It is usually due to rubber in the soles of shoes, PTBP formaldehyde resin (the glue used to stick layers of leather together) or the azo dyes in nylon socks/ stockings. The diagnosis can be confirmed by patch testing.

2. Endogenous eczema. An identical rash can occur in endogenous eczema or psoriasis. Because of the thick layer of keratin on the soles, rashes are much more difficult to distinguish from one another at this site. Eczema tends to have a less well defined border. There may be evidence of eczema or psoriasis elsewhere. Often both hands and feet are involved which suggests an endogenous cause.

3. Pompholyx (dyshidrotic eczema). Vesicles often remain intact for days or weeks on the soles and look like tapioca. When they are present alone with no redness or scaling it is called pompholyx (*see* hands, p. 370). This is usually due to endogenous or atopic eczema but can occur as a reaction to tinea between the toes ('id' reaction). Unilateral vesicles on one instep are usually due to tinea (*see* p. 379).

For treatment of foot eczema *see* p. 371.

PSORIASIS OF HANDS AND FEET

Psoriasis of the hands and feet can be of four different patterns:–

1. Plaque psoriasis. Just like psoriasis elsewhere – well defined, bright red scaly plaques with silver scaling (*see* p. 196).

2. Hyperkeratosis of the central palm or weight bearing area of the sole. There is no redness to give you a clue to the diagnosis, although the plaques are often well defined. Usually there is more typical psoriasis elsewhere.

3. Pustular psoriasis, where there are pustules of different colours. Individual pustules dry out as they pass through the keratin layer changing in colour from white to yellow to orangy-brown to dark brown before peeling off in the scale. There may or may not be a background erythema and scaling. It differs from eczema or tinea which has become secondarily infected because in these conditions the pustules will all be the same colour (yellow).

4. Rupioid psoriasis affects the ends of the fingers and toes. There are bright red thickened scaly plaques with involvement of the nails as well.

TREATMENT PSORIASIS OF HANDS AND FEET

1. **Ordinary plaque psoriasis** on the palms and soles. The treatment of this is the same as treatment of plaque psoriasis anywhere else (*see* p. 197).

2. **Thick hyperkeratotic psoriasis.** Treatment is the same as for hyperkeratotic eczema, *see* p. 371. Use the keratolytic agent at night, if necessary under occlusion and white soft paraffin/petrolatum in the daytime. Once the thick keratin has been removed, use a specific psoriatic agent during the day. You can try coal tar and salicylic acid ointment but the tar will make a mess so may not be tolerated. Alternatively try a vitamin D_3 analogue ointment (*see* p. 198), a potent[UK]/group 2–3[USA] topical steroid ointment or a combination of both (*Dovobet*).

3. **Pustular psoriasis** of the palms and soles. This is a very difficult condition to help. Start by trying any of the following:–

- Coal tar and salicylic acid ointment BP* applied at night with a pair of cotton gloves over it on the hands, or a pair of old socks over it on the feet, to keep the tar off the bedding. Most patients will find it helpful to apply white soft paraffin in the morning to keep the skin supple.
- 0.1% Dithrocream rubbed carefully into the psoriasis at night and covered with gloves and/or socks to keep it off the sheets. The strength can be gradually increased to 0.25% or 0.5% (provided the skin does not burn).

- A potent[UK]/group 2–3[USA] topical steroid ointment or cream applied twice a day. Alternatively use a topical steroid in the day with salicylic acid ointment at night, or they can be mixed together (*Diprosalic* ointment). A topical steroid and vitamin D_3 analogue (*Dovobet*) is a further alternative. When a topical steroid cream or ointment is applied to the palm or sole, some of it inevitably gets onto the thinner skin on the dorsum of the hand or foot where it can cause atrophy. It is important therefore not to go on using a potent topical steroid for too long.

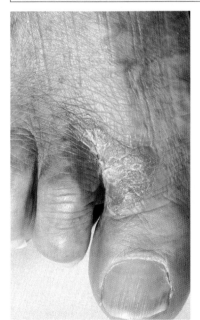

Fig. 13.28 Plaque psoriasis affecting the dorsum of the 1st toe and toe cleft. Tinea never occurs here.

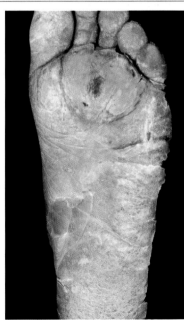

Fig. 13.29 Hyperkeratotic psoriasis.

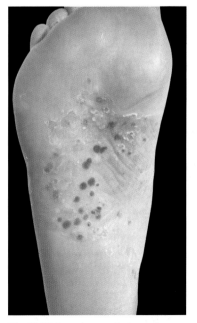

Fig. 13.30 Pustular psoriasis on the sole.

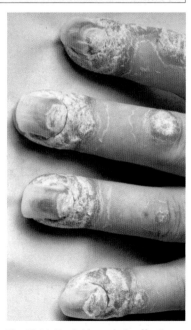

Fig. 13.31 Rupioid psoriasis affecting the ends of the fingers.

*Available from Martindale Pharmaceuticals in the UK. Tel: 0800 137627.

Failure of topical treatment for hand and foot psoriasis

Sometimes no topical agents will help patients with hand or foot psoriasis in which case either patients will learn to live with it or you will need to consider a systemic treatment:–

1. Acitretin – *see* p. 41.

2. PUVA. There are special hand and foot machines for PUVA with small banks of light tubes (emitting long-wave ultraviolet light) about the size of an X-ray viewing box. The patient takes the 8-methoxy psoralen as he would for ordinary PUVA treatment and 2 hours later puts the hands or feet on the box emitting the UVA. He will still need to protect both his eyes and his skin in the same way as if he had been irradiated all over, because of the circulating psoralens. For details about the precautions to be taken with PUVA and the side effects *see* p. 49.

3. Topical PUVA is an alternative. The hands and/or feet are soaked in a 1% solution of 5-methoxypsoralen for 15 minutes, patted dry and then irradiated with UVA using a hand and foot machine (*see* above).

4. One of the cytotoxic drugs – methotrexate, ciclosporin, azathioprine or hydroxycarbamide. Obviously the disease will need to be seriously interfering with the patient's life to consider using drugs like these. For how to use them *see* pp. 43–45.

TINEA PEDIS

There are five different patterns of tinea on the feet:–

1. Scaling or maceration between the toes, usually between the 4th and 5th toes. Here the web spaces are narrow and the humidity high. It begins on one foot only and results in itching. With time it may spread medially but never as far as the space between the 1st and 2nd toes. Later it may spread to the other foot and/or the toenails.

2. Typical plaques of tinea on the dorsum of one foot with a raised scaly edge (*see* Fig. 13.04). It usually starts laterally adjacent to the 4/5th toe cleft.

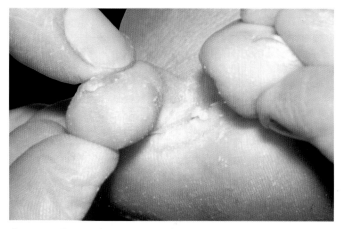

Fig. 13.32 Tinea pedis. Maceration between the 4/5th toe cleft. This pattern may also be due to candida or erythrasma.

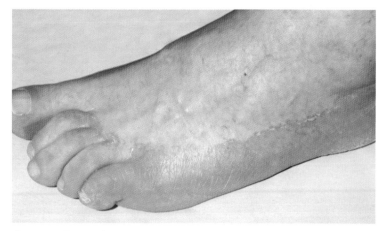

Fig. 13.33 Tinea pedis. 'Moccasin' pattern on the side of the foot.

3. White scaling on the soles. This may be unilateral or bilateral, and is often associated with discolouration and thickening of the toenails; it is due to one particular fungus, *Trichophyton rubrum*. It may be found by chance when examining a patient's feet, or the patient may complain of burning or itching of the soles. Rarely a similar pattern can be found on the palm, in which case it is usually on one side only.

4. Scaling on the sides of the foot in the shape of a 'moccasin' shoe.

5. Vesicles on the instep. Unilateral vesicles are due to tinea until proven otherwise. Sometimes they may be present on both feet, but usually there will be more on one foot than the other. The fungus is in the roof of the blisters. To confirm the diagnosis cut off the roof of the blister with a pair of fine scissors and examine under the microscope for fungal hyphae (*see* p. 299) or send the blister roof for mycology culture.

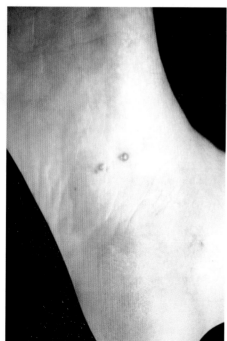

Fig. 13.34 Tinea pedis. Unilateral vesicles on instep.

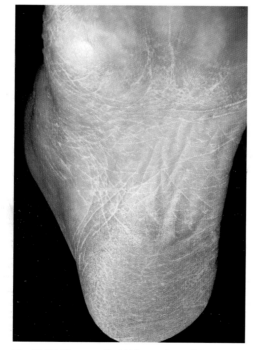

Fig. 13.35 Tinea pedis. White scaling of the skin creases due to *Trichophyton rubrum* infection.

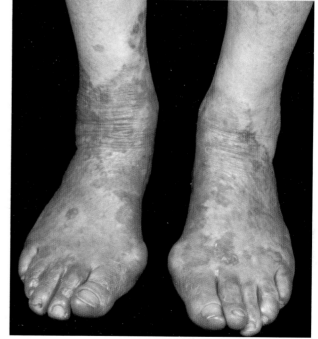

Fig. 13.36 Tinea incognito. Tinea treated with topical steroids giving a symmetrical red rash with a well-defined margin proximally.

TREATMENT TINEA PEDIS

For tinea **between the toes, plaques on the dorsum of the foot** or for **blisters on the instep,** use Whitfield's ointment twice a day for 3–4 weeks, an imidazole cream b.i.d. for 2 weeks, or 1% terbinafine cream daily for 7–10 days.

For the **white scaling** on the soles or the moccasin pattern due to *Trichophyton rubrum,* terbinafine 250mg orally once a day for 2 weeks should clear it up. Often the nails will be involved and these should be treated by continuing with terbinafine for a further 3 months.

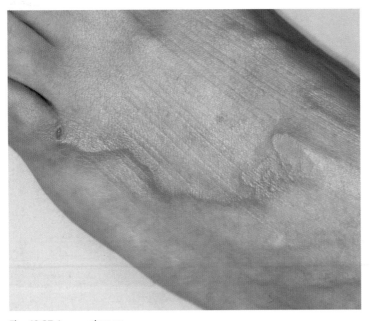

Fig. 13.37 Larva migrans.

CANDIDA & ERYTHRASMA

Symmetrical maceration or scaling between the lateral toe webs may be due to candida or erythrasma and not a dermatophyte fungus. Erythrasma will fluoresce bright pink under a Wood's (UV) light (*see* p. 18). If there is no fluorescence, then take scrapings to examine under the microscope (Fig. 10.12, p. 305) and for culture which will distinguish tinea from candida. (For treatment *see* pp. 304 & 308.)

LARVA MIGRANS

The larva of the dog hookworm (*Ankylostoma braziliense*) burrows into the skin and migrates under the skin producing a serpiginous track. Sometimes blistering can occur within the track. The patient notices itching and can see the track extend over a period of a few days. It is acquired by walking or sitting on a tropical beach where dogs have been defecating (Africa or West Indies usually). The tracks can be found on the feet, buttocks, back of legs or back.

TREATMENT LARVA MIGRANS

Oral albendazole 400mg daily for 4 days or a single dose of ivermectin (*Mectizan*) 200µg/kg body weight will cure it.

JUVENILE PLANTAR DERMATOSIS

This condition occurs only in children, usually between the ages of 7 and 14. The plantar surface of the forefoot is bright red and shiny, and children complain of itching or painful fissures. It is thought to be due to modern footwear, nylon socks and synthetic soles which do not allow sweat to escape through the shoe. It gets better spontaneously after puberty.

TREATMENT JUVENILE PLANTAR DERMATOSIS

Nylon socks and trainers should be discouraged, and cotton socks and leather shoes worn if possible. Charcoal or cork insoles inside the shoes will also help the sweat to evaporate. Medical treatment on the whole is unsatisfactory. Topical steroids are not usually of any help. We suggest trying one of the following:–

1. White soft paraffin applied two or three times a day. Alternatively use one of the less greasy moisturisers (*see* p. 24).
2. A mild keratolytic agent, e.g. 10% urea cream (*Calmurid*) or 2% salicylic acid ointment applied b.i.d.
3. 2% crude coal tar in *Unguentum M* or white soft paraffin (*Vaseline*) applied first just at night and later twice a day. This is very messy and may not be convenient for children to use.

EPIDERMOLYSIS BULLOSA SIMPLEX

Epidermolysis bullosa is a group of inherited conditions where blisters occur in response to trauma. There are three main types depending on where the site of the split is in the skin. EB simplex is the mildest form, and blisters appear on the feet spontaneously or after minimal trauma, e.g. a new pair of shoes or joining the Army and having to march. Junctional EB is usually lethal in the first two years of life. Dystrophic EB (*see* p. 227) results in recurrent blisters and erosions throughout life.

TREATMENT EPIDERMOLYSIS BULLOSA SIMPLEX

Apply a moisturiser such as aqueous cream to the feet b.i.d. to keep the skin soft. Gradually wear in new shoes and avoid excessive walking. Cotton socks are more comfortable than nylon ones. Patients usually can lead a normal life.

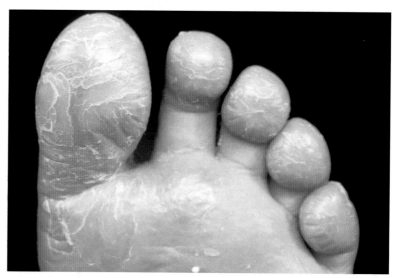

Fig. 13.38 Juvenile plantar dermatosis.

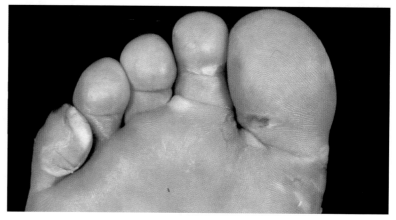

Fig. 13.39 Epidermolysis bullosa simplex showing blistering on toes.

PALMO-PLANTAR KERATODERMA

This is a genetically determined condition inherited as an autosomal dominant trait. Thickening of the keratin on the palms and soles is present from birth or early infancy. There are many variants of this condition, some with striate or punctate patterns.

TREATMENT PALMO-PLANTAR KERATODERMA

Salicylic acid ointment (5–20%) applied at night may keep the hyperkeratosis down. Regular chiropody will almost certainly be needed. If it is very severe it may be necessary to use acitretin by mouth. This is only available in hospitals. The dosage is the same as in psoriasis, *see* p. 41.

PITTED KERATOLYSIS

This a condition which only occurs in patients with sweaty feet. A corynebacterium eats into the keratin on the sole which becomes covered with shallow pits.

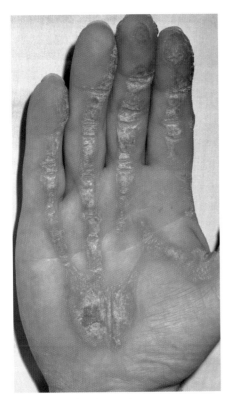

Fig. 13.40 Striate keratoderma.

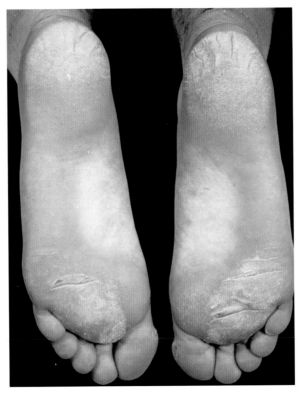

Fig. 13.41 Diffuse plantar keratoderma.

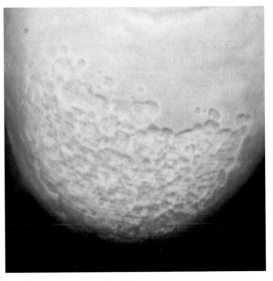

Fig. 13.42 Pitted keratolysis.

TREATMENT PITTED KERATOLYSIS

Treating the sweaty feet works better than specifically removing the causative organism. The feet should be soaked in a 5% solution of formaldehyde for 10–15 minutes once or twice a day. If this does not work apply 3% fusidic acid cream twice a day or clindamycin lotion (*Dalacin-T*).

CORN

A corn is a localised V-shaped area of hyperkeratosis over a pressure point on the foot. When pared down with a scalpel no bleeding points are seen (Fig. 13.45b).

SOFT CORN

Scaling between the 4th and 5th toes on one foot may be due to a soft corn (Fig. 13.47). If you remove the surface keratin with a scalpel you will quickly come to firmer keratin underneath just like a corn elsewhere. Soft corns are due to wearing shoes that are too tight around the toes. The problem can be explained very simply to the patient by making them stand on a piece of paper on the floor in their bare feet. Draw around the affected foot with a pencil and then put their shoe on the drawing. It will be immediately obvious that the shoe is too tight for the foot (*see* Fig. 13.46).

BLACK HEEL/HAEMATOMA

It is quite common for bleeding to occur into the skin on the back of the heel or the sole in teenagers and young adults engaged in sporting activities. It is due to rubbing from shoes or direct trauma. A painless dark red or black patch is seen over the heel. The sudden appearance may alarm the patient and make them think that they have a malignant melanoma. When pared down dried blood is seen within the keratin layer. Reassurance is all that is needed.

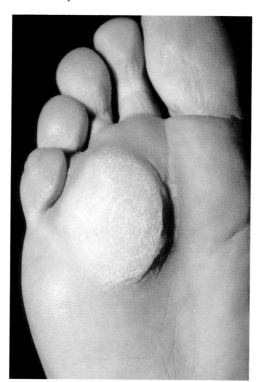

Fig. 13.43 Corn over metatarsal heads on sole of foot.

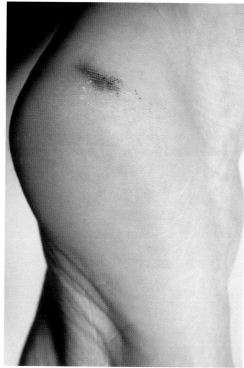

Fig. 13.44 Black heel due to bleeding into the keratin layer.

a) PLANTAR WART

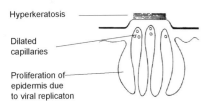

Hyperkeratosis

Dilated capillaries

Proliferation of epidermis due to viral replicaton

Paring down produces pin-point bleeding once the hyperkeratosis has been removed and the capillaries reached

b) CORN

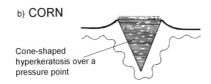

Cone-shaped hyperkeratosis over a pressure point

Paring down produces a decreasing cone of keratin with no capillary bleeding

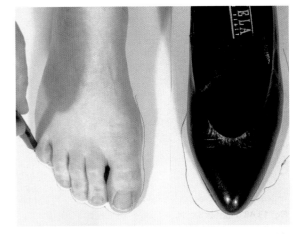

Fig. 13.46 Compare size of foot and shoe in a patient with a soft corn.

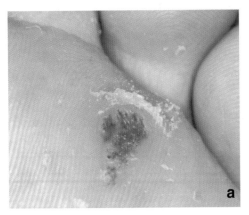

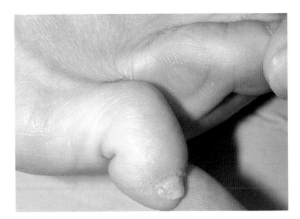

Fig. 13.45 Differentiation between plantar wart and corn by paring down the surface keratin.

a. Plantar wart showing bleeding points.

b. Corn showing cone of solid keratin in centre.

Fig. 13.47 Soft corn.

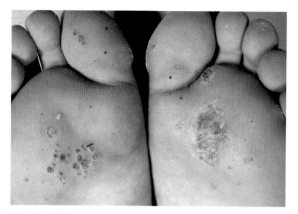

Fig. 13.48 Plantar warts.

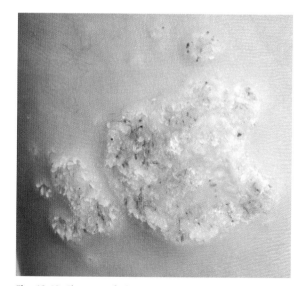

Fig. 13.49 Close up of plantar warts.

TREATMENT CORN

If a bony exostosis is present or there is an obvious anatomical abnormality of the foot, the help of an orthopaedic surgeon may be needed. The patient should wear shoes that fit properly.

The area of hyperkeratosis can be pared down regularly with a scalpel by the patient or a podiatrist and the central core of keratin removed. Alternatively 5–10% salicylic acid ointment can be applied every night to soften the keratin and make it easier to remove. Salicylic acid plasters left on for a week at a time will do the same thing. Wearing a corn pad or circle of orthopaedic felt around the corn will take the pressure off it and make walking more comfortable. Alternatively, a proper orthotic appliance can be made to fit into the shoe.

Soft corns. Keep the affected toes apart with a piece of foam or a silicone wedge to reduce the sideways pressure. Most importantly the patient must wear shoes that are not too small around the toes.

PLANTAR WART (VERRUCA)

Verruca is the proper name for a wart. In common usage, warts on the hands are called warts and those on the feet verrucae. On the feet individual lesions are discrete, round papules with a rough surface surrounded by a collar of hyperkeratosis. They may be very numerous and join together to form mosaic warts. If the diagnosis is in doubt, pare down the surface with a scalpel and very soon tiny bleeding points will be seen.

Two problems arise from warts on the feet:–

1. They hurt. This is not due to the wart growing into the foot when it is situated on weight bearing areas, but to the hyperkeratosis that occurs around the wart. This grows outward and causes pain just as a stone in the shoe does. Less commonly very severe pain occurs when the blood vessels in the wart thrombose – this causes the wart to go black and within a few days drop off.

2. Children with verrucae are not allowed to swim. This may be overcome by wearing a sock on the affected foot to prevent spread of virus from one person to another.

TREATMENT PLANTAR WARTS

SINGLE/FEW PLANTAR WARTS

Keratolytic agents

The most important thing is for the patient to pare down the hard skin every night with a scalpel or to rub it flat with a pumice stone so that it does not hurt. A wart paint or gel is then applied carefully just to the warts, left to dry and then covered with a plaster overnight. In the morning the plaster is removed to allow the wart to harden up again before the wart is pared down the next night.

Wart paints (suitable for use on the feet) are:–

- Salicylic acid/lactic acid mixtures in collodion (*Cuplex, Duofilm, Occlusal, Salactol, Salactac*).
- Podophyllotoxin preparations, e.g. podophyllin resin BP[UK] (15% in Tinc. Benz. Co), *Condyline*[UK] soln, *Condylox*[UK], *Podocon 25*[UK], *Warticon*[UK] cream.
- 10% glutaraldehyde solution (*Glutarol*).

Whichever paint (or gel) is chosen, it should be used each night before the patient goes to bed. A fair trial of a treatment is to use it for 12–16 weeks before giving up and changing to something else. If the plaster is left on for too long the wart becomes soggy and painful. If this occurs, treatment will have to be left off for a few days. One of the reasons why the treatment does not work is that the patient stops using it if the foot becomes sore.

Freezing with liquid nitrogen

This is not a good treatment for plantar warts, because you need to freeze for quite a long time to produce a blister (because of the thick layer of keratin on the sole of the foot) and this will be too painful for the patient.

Surgery

Any kind of surgery is contraindicated on the feet. The most likely outcome is recurrence of the wart, and there is always the risk that scarring will lead to the formation of permanent callosities, especially over pressure points.

MOSAIC WARTS

These do not respond as well to treatment as single warts. You can try:–

- One of the salicylic and lactic acid paints applied every night (*see left*).
- Formalin soaks. Get the patient to soak the affected part of the foot in a 5% solution of formaldehyde BP once a day. First apply a thickish layer of white soft paraffin (*Vaseline*) around the warts, so that the formalin does not make the normal skin sore. Then pour the formalin into a saucer or shallow bowl and soak the warts in it for 10 minutes each day. The next day rub down any hard skin on the surface with a pumice stone or foot scraper before repeating the treatment.
- Apply 40% salicylic acid plasters cut to the same size as the warts. These are stuck onto the warts shiny side down, taped securely in place with *Hypafix* (or something similar), and left for a week at a time. When they are removed the soggy keratin is removed with a sharp scalpel blade before putting on a new plaster. This can be done once a week by the nurse or podiatrist until no wart is left.

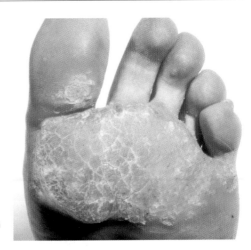

Fig. 13.50 Mosaic warts on forefoot.

Nails

14

ANATOMY OF THE NAIL

Nails are keratin produced by a modified epidermis called the nail matrix. From this grows the nail plate which lies on the nail bed. Nails protect the end of the digits and on the fingers are useful for picking up small objects and for scratching. Abnormalities can arise from any part of the nail apparatus.

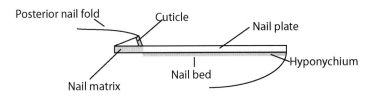

Fig. 14.01 Anatomy of the nail.

EXAMINATION OF THE NAIL

When looking at nails, examine the following in turn:–

1. The nail from above

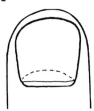

SURFACE OF NAIL
1. Pitting, p. 389
2. Transverse ridges, p. 389
3. Longitudinal ridges, p. 390
4. Shiny, *see* p. 206

COLOUR OF NAIL
1. Discolouration of nail bed, p. 391
2. Discolouration of nail plate, p. 392

NAIL FOLD & CUTICLE
1. Loss of cuticle – paronychia, p. 396
2. Nail fold telangiectasia, *see* p. 115

2. The nail from end on

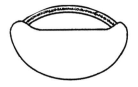

THICKNESS OF NAIL
1. Thickening of nail plate, p. 393
2. Splitting of nail plate, p. 395
3. Subungual hyperkeratosis, p. 395

DETACHMENT OF THE NAIL from nail bed
1. Onycholysis, p. 395

3. The nail from the side

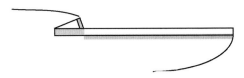

SHAPE OF NAILS
1. Over curvature, p. 397
2. Spoon shaped nails, p. 397
3. Wedge shaped nails, p. 397
4. Ingrowing toenails, p. 397

LOSS OF NAILS
1. Without scarring, p. 398
2. With scarring (permanent), p. 398

LUMPS AND BUMPS AROUND NAILS, p. 398

ABNORMALITIES OF NAIL MATRIX

PITTING

Inflammatory conditions affecting the matrix cause abnormal keratin to be formed, which becomes detached from the nail plate leaving pits or ridges. Pits are more easily seen in the finger nails than in toe nails.

Causes of pitting:–

1. **Psoriasis.** Small regular pits.
2. **Eczema.** Larger and more irregular pits; associated with eczema on the skin around the nail.
3. **Alopecia areata.** Small, regular pits may be a poor prognostic sign for regrowth of the hair.
4. **Normal finding.** Isolated pits may be found in normal nails.

TRANSVERSE RIDGING

Causes:–

1. **Eczema.** Some pits are so broad as to form transverse ridges.
2. **Chronic paronychia** due to pressure on the nail matrix (*see* p. 396).
3. **Beau's lines.** A single line at the same place in all the nails is due to cessation of growth of the nail matrix at the time of a severe illness. When this is over the matrix will begin to function normally again and the nail will grow out with a line in it. Finger nails grow at a rate of approximately 1mm/week (toenails at about a third of that speed) so you can tell how long ago the illness was (*see* Fig. 14.07).

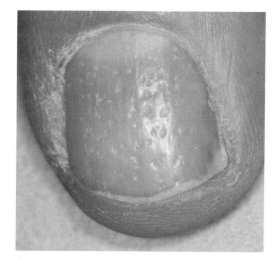

Fig. 14.02 Nail pitting in psoriasis.

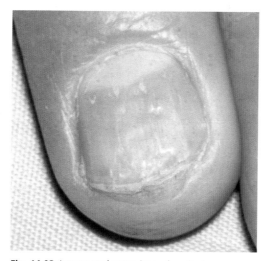

Fig. 14.03 Larger and more irregular pits in eczema.

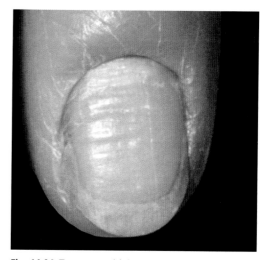

Fig. 14.04 Transverse ridging secondary to paronychia.

LONGITUDINAL RIDGING

Causes when all nails are affected:–

1. A few ridges are seen in normal nails.
2. **Lichen planus**. Fine regular lines (*see also* p. 398).
3. **Darier's disease**. Regular fine lines with 'V'-shaped notching at the end of the nails (*see also* p. 217).

Causes when a single nail is affected:–

1. **Median nail dystrophy** looks like an upside down Christmas tree. It is a temporary abnormality and gets better spontaneously after a few months. The cause is unknown.
2. **Habit tic deformity**. Here there is a broader groove made up of numerous concave transverse ridges. It is due to picking or biting the cuticle which damages the nail plate as it grows out.
3. A single wide groove may be due to **myxoid cyst** or **wart** over the posterior nail fold which presses on the underlying matrix (*see* p. 398).

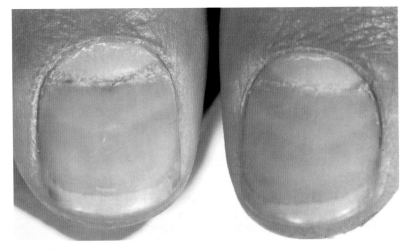

Fig. 14.07 Beau's lines.

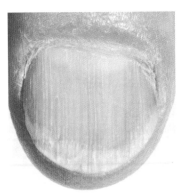

Fig. 14.05 Longitudinal ridging seen in lichen planus.

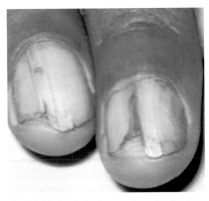

Fig. 14.06 Darier's disease. Longitudinal ridging with V-shaped notches.

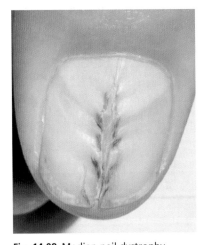

Fig. 14.08 Median nail dystrophy.

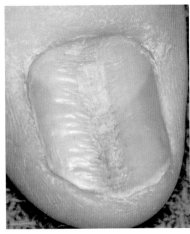

Fig. 14.09 Habit tic nail deformity on a thumb nail.

ABNORMALITIES OF NAIL BED

DISCOLOURATION UNDER THE NAIL

The nail bed is the epidermis underneath the nail. In normal circumstances it does not produce keratin. Problems in the nail bed cause areas of discolouration under the nail.

White Pallor of the nail bed occurs in hypoalbuminaemia or chronic renal failure.

Orangy-brown (called salmon patches) due to psoriasis.

Brown A round or oval area is a junctional naevus of the nail bed. If it is growing or made up of different colours consider a malignant melanoma (*see* p. 392).

Red/purple/black

1. **Splinter haemorrhages** are small red longitudinal streaks classically seen in subacute bacterial endocarditis. In fact they are very common so are an unreliable clinical sign.

2. **Subungual haematoma** results from bleeding under the nail following trauma. It can occur on finger or toe nails. Initially the area is exquisitely painful and dark red/purple in colour. With time, if the blood is not released immediately by puncturing the nail, the area is discoloured black or brown. It can be distinguished from a subungual malignant melanoma by making a small horizontal nick on the nail plate at the distal end of the discolouration and watching for a week. A subungual haematoma will grow out at the same rate as the nail so the nick will still be at the distal end of the discolouration; a melamona does not grow at such a regular rate.

Pink/mauve

A **glomus tumour** is a rare benign tumour that presents as a tender mauve area under the nail, particularly on pressure or in the cold.

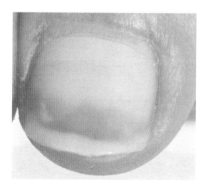

Fig. 14.10 White nail bed due to hypoalbuminaemia.

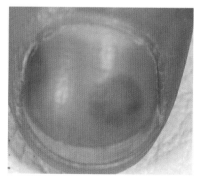

Fig. 14.11 Salmon patch due to psoriasis.

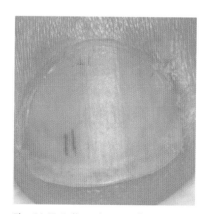

Fig. 14.12 Splinter haemorrhages.

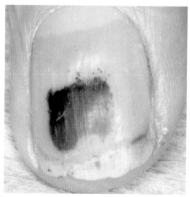

Fig. 14.13 Subungual haematoma.

ABNORMALITIES OF NAIL PLATE

DISCOLOURATION OF THE NAIL PLATE

Causes:–

1. **External staining**, especially from nicotine and medicaments (e.g. $KMnO_4$ [*see* p. 26] & dithranol). It can occur less commonly from hair dyes or tints in nail varnish.

2. **Drugs**. All the nails will be equally affected, e.g.:–
   - Chloroquine, AZT and gold stain nails blue-grey.
   - Penicillamine stains nails yellow.

3. **Brown lines** in a nail. A thin line down the entire length of the nail is due to a junctional naevus of the nail matrix. A broad line under the nail which is expanding in width or extending up through the nail should make you think of a malignant melanoma.

4. **White nails**
   i. Small white streaks due to minor trauma occur in most people at some time.
   ii. Familial leuconychia where the whole of the nail is white. This is inherited as an autosomal dominant trait.
   iii. White discolouration which affects nails irregularly is often due to tinea infection (*see* p. 393).

5. **Green** discolouration occurs with pseudomonas infection.

6. **Blue** discolouration occurs in patients with HIV/AIDS infection and this may be a useful indicator of the disease. Similar discolouration can be due to AZT.

7. **Yellow nails**
   i. **Yellow nail syndrome**. All the nails are yellow or green in colour and are excessively curved in both longitudinal and transverse directions. The rate of growth is slowed almost

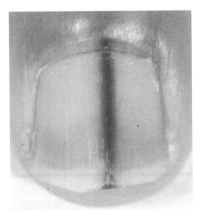

Fig. 14.14 Thin brown line due to a junctional naevus in the nail matrix.

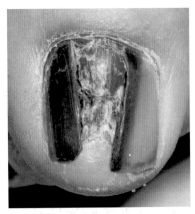

Fig. 14.15 Malignant melanoma arising in the nail matrix.

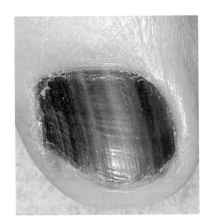

Fig. 14.16 Whole nail discoloured by a malignant melanoma in the matrix.

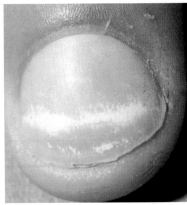

Fig. 14.17 White streaks probably related to trauma.

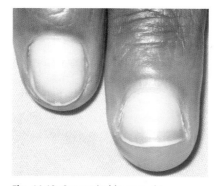

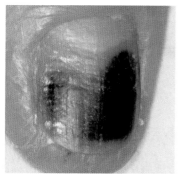

Fig. 14.18 Congenital leuconychia.

Fig. 14.19 Green staining due to infection with pseudomonas.

to a standstill and sometimes onycholysis can also occur. It is thought to be due to a congenital abnormality of the lymphatics although the nail changes do not occur until adult life and often not until middle or old age. There may be other abnormalities of the lymphatics such as lymphoedema of the legs or bilateral pleural effusions.

ii. Localised yellow/brown discolouration can be due to **tinea**.

THICKENING OF NAIL PLATE

1. **Tinea unguium**. Dermatophyte fungi live on keratin so multiply within the nail plate causing it to become thickened and discoloured white or yellow. They can only become established in nails that are growing slowly so affect toenails much more readily than finger nails. Once established the rate of growth slows down even more so that cutting the affected nails becomes an infrequent necessity.

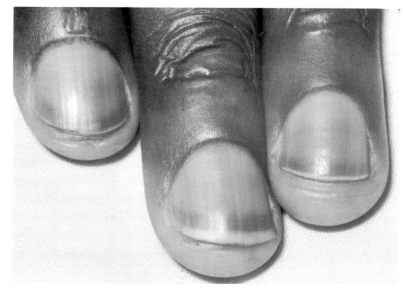

Fig. 14.20 Blue nails in a patient with HIV infection.

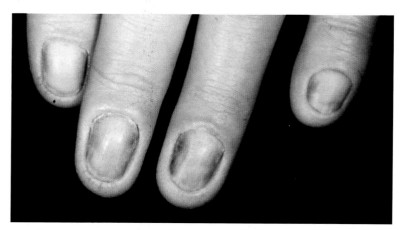

Fig. 14.21 Yellow nail syndrome.

It can be difficult on the feet to distinguish clinically between thickening of the nails due to tinea, and onycholysis and sub-ungual hyperkeratosis due to psoriasis. First look at the finger nails; the changes of psoriasis will be more obvious there with associated pits, salmon patches and onycholysis. If the finger nails are not involved tinea is more likely. On the toes tinea does not affect all the nails and usually affects one foot before the other. You can also look between the toes or on the instep for other evidence of tinea of the feet (*see* p. 378). Nail clippings for direct microscopy (*see* Fig. 10.03, p. 299) or fungal culture will confirm the diagnosis.

2. **Chronic trauma** to toe nails (in patients who play football, tennis etc.) can produce thickened nails.

3. In **old age** the nails become thickened, curved and difficult to cut.

4. Wedge shaped nails occur in **pachyonychia congenita** (*see* p. 397).

TREATMENT TINEA UNGUIUM

Many patients have tinea of their toe nails without being aware of it. Treatment is only needed if the patient is complaining of the problem or he is getting recurrent tinea infections elsewhere (feet, groin, body).

If there are only 1 or 2 nails involved, paint with 5% amorolfine (Loceryl) nail lacquer once or twice a week. Amorolfine also works for toenail infections with the saprophytic moulds *Hendersonula toruloidea* and *Scopulariopsis brevicalis*.

If there are more than 2 or 3 nails involved, it is better to use terbinafine 250mg once daily by mouth for 3 months. An alternative is itraconazole 100mg orally/day for 6 months. This can be given continuously or pulsed (1 week on and 3 weeks off). The efficacy of oral therapy can be improved by combination with amorolfine topically. Failure of oral treatment necessitates the removal of the affected toenail(s) plus oral terbinafine 250mg daily for 3–6 months.

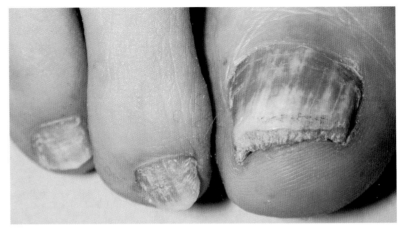

Fig. 14.22 Tinea unguium showing a thickened and discoloured nail plate.

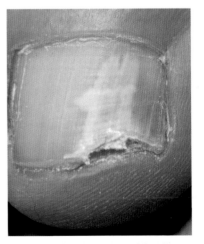

Fig. 14.23 Tinea unguium with yellow discolouration.

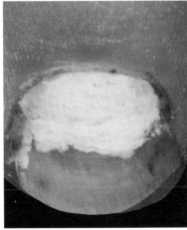

Fig. 14.24 Tinea unguium: white nails.

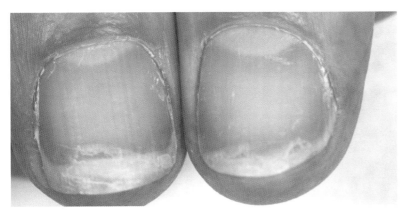

Fig. 14.25 Lamellar splitting at distal end of nail plate.

SPLITTING OF THE ENDS OF THE NAILS

1. **Lamellar splitting** occurs when the distal portion of the nail plate splits into horizontal layers. It is mainly seen in women who have their hands wet for long periods of time. The keratin is damaged by water and detergents. It is treated by keeping the hands out of water and wearing rubber gloves.

2. **Longitudinal splitting** may occur along a longitudinal ridge, especially in Darier's disease (*see* Fig. 14.06, p. 390).

ABNORMALITIES OF THE HYPONYCHIUM

ONYCHOLYSIS

Onycholysis is separation of the nail plate from the nail bed. It is due to an abnormality of the hyponychium where the nail plate is less firmly stuck down onto the nail bed. It can be due to:–

1. **Trauma**. On the hands the commonest cause is over manicuring. The hyponychium is damaged by cleaning underneath the nails with a nail file. On the feet it usually follows a subungual haematoma.

2. **Psoriasis**. Onycholysis is more obvious on finger nails (Fig. 14.26) than toe nails. Once the nail has lifted off subungual hyperkeratosis occurs and it may be difficult to distinguish from thickening of the nail plate due to tinea.

3. **Poor peripheral circulation**.

4. **Thyrotoxicosis**.

5. **Allergic contact dermatitis** to substances which penetrate through the nail plate, e.g. methacrylate used as a glue for sticking on artificial nails.

6. **Doxycycline** taken orally can cause a photo-onycholysis in the summer. The patient experiences severe pain in all finger nails, and then the nails lift off. This is becoming more common since doxycycline is being used for malaria prophylaxis.

SUBUNGUAL HYPERKERATOSIS

This is a build up of keratin under the end of the nail (Fig. 14.27). It needs to be distinguished from nail thickening. The cause is usually **psoriasis**.

TREATMENT PSORIASIS OF THE NAILS

There is no topical treatment which will help psoriatic nail changes (pitting, salmon patches, onycholysis or subungual hyperkeratosis). Coloured nail varnish will hide onycholysis in a woman, and keeping the nails cut short will stop onycholysis getting worse. Fortunately patients do not often ask for treatment for their nails. If the skin psoriasis is bad enough to be treated with a systemic agent (*see* p. 197), the nails will also improve.

ABNORMALITIES OF THE CUTICLE

The cuticle is an area of keratin joining the posterior nail fold to the nail plate preventing bacteria and yeasts from getting into the soft tissues around the nail. If the cuticle is lost (usually due to chronic trauma to hands that are continually wet, or to eczema), infection can occur under the posterior or lateral nail folds to cause paronychia. There are two types:–

Acute paronychia. This is due to infection with *Staphylococcus aureus* (less commonly *Streptococcus pyogenes*). There is exquisite pain, a bright red swelling and pus formation. Rarely herpes simplex may be the cause, but grouped vesicles over the distal phalanx will be seen.

Chronic paronychia. *Candida albicans* produces a more chronic infection with less swelling, a duller red colour and no pus. The nail plate may show transverse or longitudinal ridges from chronic pressure on the matrix (*see* Fig. 14.04, p. 389).

TREATMENT PARONYCHIA

Acute. Flucloxacillin or erythromycin, 250mg four times a day for 7 days. If there is obvious pus present, it should be lanced to let it out.

Chronic. The real cause is the loss of the cuticle. The paronychia will only get better permanently if a new cuticle can be induced to grow. The patient must keep the hands dry by wearing rubber or cotton-lined rubber or PVC gloves for all wet work until a new cuticle has grown (3–4 months). A protective film of Vaseline can be applied around the nail several times a day to keep water out.

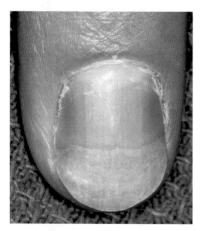

Fig. 14.26 Onycholysis.

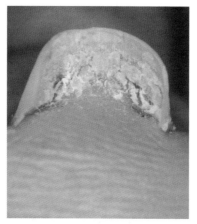

Fig. 14.27 Subungual hyperkeratosis.

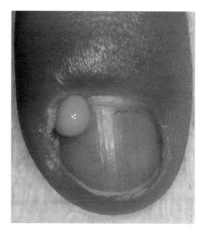

Fig. 14.28 Acute paronychia.

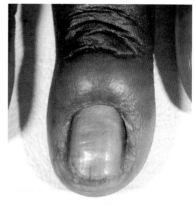

Fig. 14.29 Chronic paronychia.

ABNORMALLY SHAPED NAILS

1. OVER CURVATURE can be due to:–

i. **Clubbing.** This is an apparent over curvature of the nail due to loss of the angle between the posterior nail fold and the nail plate. If there is any doubt put the distal phalanges of the two thumbs together; there should be a diamond-shaped gap between them. This disappears if the nails are clubbed. Clubbing is due to chronic chest disease, carcinoma of the bronchus or congenital heart disease.

ii. Resorption of the distal phalanx in **hyperparathyroidism** – the nail curves over the end of the finger.

iii. **Yellow nail syndrome,** *see* p. 392.

2. SPOON SHAPED NAILS (Koilonychia)

Most often seen in association with iron deficiency anaemia (although most patients with iron deficiency do not have this change). It may be a normal finding in young children.

3. WEDGE SHAPED NAILS

Pachyonychia congenita is a rare genetic abnormality present from birth. The nail grows both vertically and horizontally causing a thick wedge shaped nail which is unsightly on the fingers and causes pain from pressure of shoes on the toes.

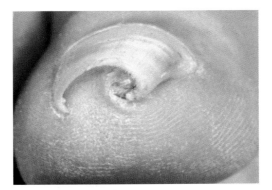

Fig. 14.30 Ingrowing toe nail.

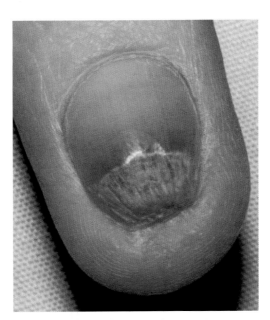

Fig. 14.31 Pachyonychia congenita.

4. INGROWING TOENAILS

Penetration of the lateral nail fold by the nail itself or a spicule of the nail causes redness, tenderness, pus formation and later granulation tissue. The great toe nail is most commonly involved. It is due to wearing shoes that are too tight and cutting the nails in a half-circle instead of straight across. Similar changes occur as a side effect of the retinoid drugs.

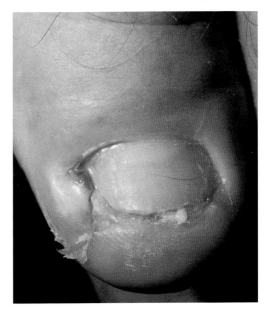

Fig. 14.32 Ingrowing toe nail.

LOSS OF NAILS

WITHOUT SCARRING (temporary)

i. **Trauma**, especially to the great toe nails. It can occur to finger nails too after a large subungual haematoma.

ii. **Beau's lines** after a severe illness. The nail may break off at the line (*see* p. 389).

WITH SCARRING (permanent)

i. In **Lichen planus** the cuticle grows down, over and through the nail plate resulting in permanent scarring. This is called pterygium.

ii. **Genetic** abnormalities: all rare.

TREATMENT NAIL LICHEN PLANUS

> Longitudinal ridging (p. 390) needs no treatment. If pterygium occurs, which will cause permanent scarring of the nails, prednisolone 30mg/day started as soon as possible will often switch it off. Give this dose for 2 weeks and then gradually tail it off over the next month.

LUMPS & BUMPS AROUND THE NAIL

1. **Viral warts**. Small skin coloured/grey/brown papules with a rough warty surface may occur on the skin around the nail.

2. **Mucous/myxoid cyst**. A round skin coloured papule on the dorsal surface of the distal phalanx. If pricked it discharges a sticky clear fluid.

If warts or cysts occur over the nail matrix the pressure on the matrix can cause a longitudinal groove in the nail plate.

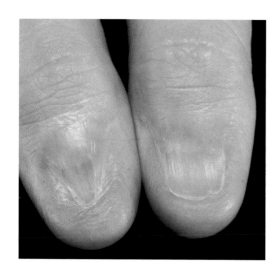

Fig. 14.33 Pterygium.

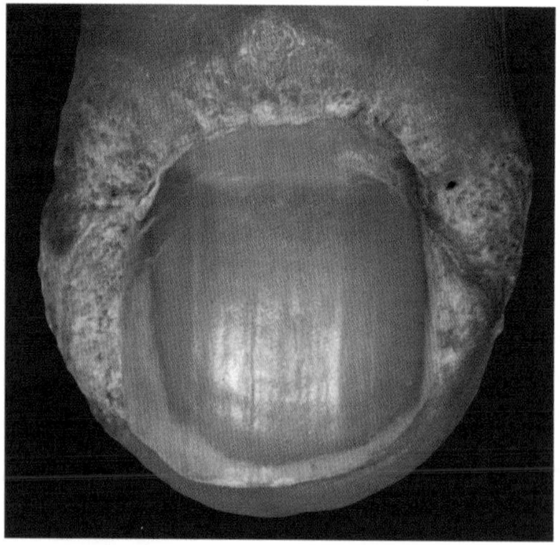

Fig. 14.34 Viral warts around nail fold.

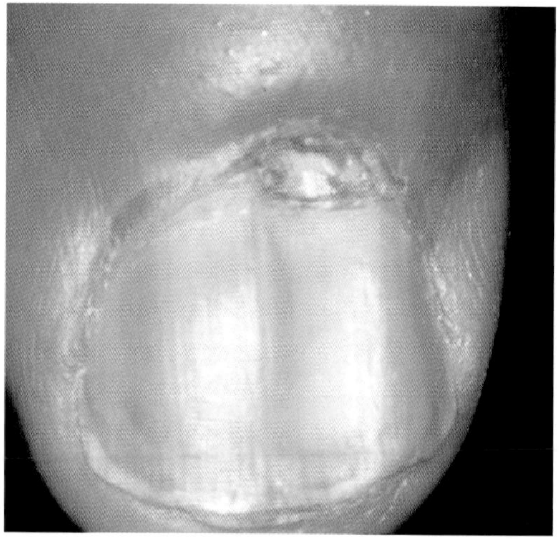

Fig. 14.35 Myxoid cyst causing a groove in the nail.

3. **Subungual and periungual fibroma**. Small firm pink/skin coloured papules protruding from the posterior nail fold or from under the nail occur in patients with tuberous sclerosis. They appear after puberty.

4. **Subungual exostosis**. This is a localised outgrowth of bone which presents as a subungual skin coloured papule. If in doubt X-ray the digit.

5. **Tumours**. Rarely squamous cell carcinoma and malignant melanoma can occur around the nail. Any inflammatory condition around a single nail which does not improve with treatment is an indication for biopsy.

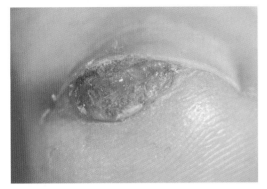

Fig. 14.36 Subungual fibroma.

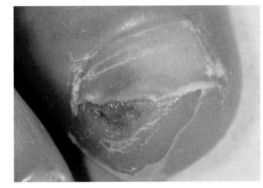

Fig. 14.38 Subungual exostosis.

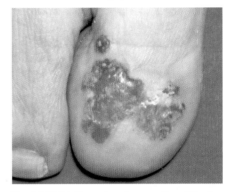

Fig. 14.40 Malignant melanoma in nail bed.

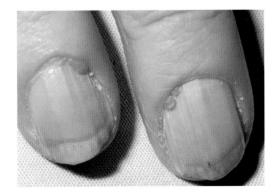

Fig. 14.37 Periungual fibromas in patient with tuberous sclerosis (*see also* p. 232).

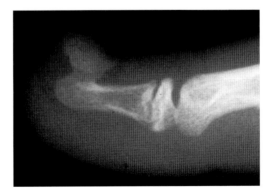

Fig. 14.39 X-ray of subungual exostosis.

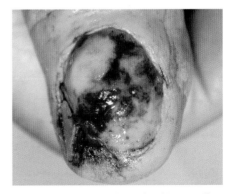

Fig. 14.41 Tumour under nail. A biopsy will be needed to make a diagnosis.

List of drugs and associated drug reactions

Acitretin	Dry lips, nose and eyes	**Carbamazepine**	Erythrodermic	**Frusemide**	Exanthematous
	Hair loss		Exanthematous		Phototoxic
ACTH	Acne	**Carbimazole**	Hair loss	**Gold**	Erythrodermic
Allopurinol	Erythrodermic		Purpura		Lichenoid
	Purpura		Toxic epidermal necrolysis		Pigmentation of face
	Toxic epidermal necrolysis	**Chloroquine**	Erythrodermic		(blue/grey)
	Vasculitis		Lichenoid		Purpura
Aminophylline	Eczematous		Hyperpigmentation of skin		(thrombocytopenia)
Ampicillin	Erythrodermic		Bleaching of hair		Vasculitis
	Exanthematous	**Chlorpromazine**	Erythrodermic	**Heparin**	Hair loss
	Vasculitis		Photoallergic		Vasculitis
Androgens	Acne		Purpura	**Hydralazine**	Lupus erythematosus
Amiodarone	Hyperpigmentation		(thrombocytopenia)		Vasculitis
	Phototoxic	**Chlorpropamide**	Eczematous	**Iodides**	Acne
Aspirin	Histamine release		Lichenoid	**Isoniazid**	Acne
	(urticaria)	**Ciclosporin**	Hypertrichosis		Erythrodermic
Barbiturates	Erythrodermic	**Cimetidine**	Erythrodermic		Pellagra
	Fixed drug reaction	**Clofazimine**	Pigmentation – red/pink	**Lithium**	Acne
	Purpura	**Codeine**	Histamine release		Psoriasis
	Toxic epidermal necrolysis		(urticaria)	**Nalidixic acid**	Erythrodermic
β-blockers	Lichenoid	**Contraceptives**	Erythema nodosum		Phototoxic reaction
	Psoriasis		Pigmentation of face	**Nitrofurantoin**	Serum sickness (urticaria)
β-carotene	Orange discolouration		(chloasma)	**NSAIDs**	Erythema multiforme
Benzodiazepines	Exanthematous	**Coumarins**	Skin necrosis		Exanthematous
	Fixed drug eruption	**Cytotoxics**	Hair loss		Fixed drug reaction
Bromides	Acne		Purpura		Toxic epidermal necrolysis
Busulphan	Hyperpigmentation		(thrombocytopenia)		Vasculitis
Captopril	Erythrodermic	**Dapsone**	Pigmentation – blue/grey	**Mepacrine**	Lichenoid
	Exanthematous	**Diazoxide**	Hypertrichosis		Yellow discolouration of
	Pemphigus	**Diclofenac**	Pemphigoid		skin

Methyl dopa	Lichenoid	**Phenytoin**	Acne	**Tetracyclines**	Phototoxic
Minocycline	Pigmentation of skin (blue/grey)		Erythrodermic		Photo-onycholysis
			Hyperpigmentation	**Thiazides**	Eczematous
	SLE		Toxic epidermal necrolysis		Exanthematous
Minoxidil	Hypertrichosis	**Procainamide**	Lupus erythematosus		Lichenoid
Opiates	Histamine release (urticaria)	**Promethazine**	Photoallergic		Purpura
		Psoralens	Hypertrichosis		Serum sickness (urticaria)
Penicillins	Exanthematous		Phototoxic		Vasculitis
	Anaphylaxis (urticaria)	**Rifampicin**	Pemphigus	**Thioureas**	Hair loss
	Serum sickness (urticaria)		Purpura (thrombocytopenia)		Vasculitis
Penicillamine	Hypertrichosis			**Warfarin**	Hair loss
	Lichenoid	**Sulphonamides**	Eczematous		Skin necrosis
	Pemphigus		Erythrodermic		
Phenolphthalein	Fixed drug eruption		Exanthematous		
Phenothiazines	Exanthematous		Fixed drug eruption		
	Phototoxic		Lichenoid		
	Serum sickness		Purpura		
			Serum sickness (urticaria)		
			Toxic epidermal necrolysis		
			Vasculitis		

General index

Classification of topical steroids by potency

	Weak[UK]/Group 6–7[USA] Potency = 1% hydrocortisone	Moderately potent[UK]/Group 4–5[USA] Potency = 2.5 × 1% hydrocortisone	Potent[UK]/Group 2–3[USA] Potency = 10 × 1% hydrocortisone	Very potent[UK]/Group 1[USA] Potency = 50 × 1% hydrocortisone
Available in UK	Fluocinolone acetonide 0.0025% (Synalar 1:10) Hydrocortisone 0.5–2.5% (Dermacort, Dioderm, Efcortelan, Hc 45, Mildison)	Betamethasone valerate 0.025% (Betnovate RD) Clobetasone butyrate 0.05% (Eumovate) Flurandrenolone 0.0125% (Haelan) Fluocinolone acetonide 0.00625% (Synalar 1:4)	Beclometasone dipropionate 0.025% (Propaderm) Betamethasone valerate 0.1% (Betnovate) Diflucortolone valerate 0.1% (Nerisone) Fluocinolone acetonide 0.025% (Synalar)	Diflucortolone valerate 0.3% (Nerisone forte) Halcinonide 0.1% (Halciderm)
Available in UK/USA	Aclometasone dipropionate 0.05% (Modrasone/Aclovate) Hydrocortisone 0.5–2.5%	Desoxymetasone 0.05% (Stiedex LP/Topicort-LP) Hydrocortisone 17-butyrate 0.1% (Locoid)	Betamethasone dipropionate cream 0.05% (Diprolene AF) Fluocinonide 0.05% (Metosyn/Lidex) Fluticasone propionate 0.005% (Cutivate) Halcinonide 0.1% (Halciderm/Halog) Mometasone furoate 0.1% (Elocon)	Clobetasol propionate 0.05% (Dermovate/Temovate)
Available in USA	Desonide 0.05% (Desowen/Tridesilon) Dexamethasone 0.1% (Decadron phosphate) Methylprednisolone 1% (Medrol)	Betamethasone benzoate 0.025% (Benisone, Uticort) Clocortalone 0.1% (Cloderm) Fluocinolone acetonide 0.025% (Synalar) Flurandrenolide 0.05% (Cordran) Halcinonide 0.025% (Halog) Hydrocortisone valerate 0.2% (Westcort) Predincarbate 0.1% (Dermatop) Triamcinolone acetonide 0.1% & 0.25% (Kenalog/Aristocort)	Amicinonide 0.1% (Cyclocort) Betamethasone valerate 0.1% (Valisone) Desoximetasone 0.25% (Topicort) Diflorasone diacetate 0.05% (Florone, Maxiflor) Triamcinolone acetonide 0.5% (Kenalog) Triamcinolone acetate 0.5% (Aristocort-HP)	Betamethasone diproprionate ointment 0.05% (Diprolene) Halbetosol propionate 0.05% (Ultravate)

Note: ointment or cream base may result in differing groups for same molecule

Index of algorithms

ERYTHEMATOUS LESIONS

Surface changes	Type of lesion	Number/size of lesions	Face/ bald scalp	Trunk/arms thighs	Axilla/ groin	Lower legs	Dorsum hand	Dorsum foot
Acute erythematous lesions/rash								
Normal/ smooth	Macules/patches/ papules/plaques	Progressive rash	146	146	146	146	146	146
		Multiple lesions/rash	82	149	149	330	358	330
		Transient lesions	82	150	150	150	150	150
	Papules/nodules	Single/few (2–5)	155	155	155	155	358	155
	Generalised rash		166	166	166	166	166	166
Crust/ exudate	Vesicles/bullae		87	157	157	157/330	358	157/330
	Pustules		161	161	161	161	161	161
	Erosions/ulcers		87	163	163	163	163	163
Chronic erythematous lesions/rash								
Normal/ smooth	Macules		94	188	188	188	188	188
	Papules	Single/few (2–5)	230	230	230	230	230	230
		Multiple lesions/rash	96	170	298	333	359	372
	Pustules		96	174	174	333	359	333
	Patches & plaques	Lesions <2cm	108/113	188	188	333	359	372
		Lesions >2cm	108/113	175	298	333	359	333
	Nodules		180	180	305	333	360	360
Scaly/ hyperkeratotic	Papules		116	188	188	188	359	372
	Patches & plaques	Single/few (2–5)	116	184	298	184	359	372
		Multiple lesions *all* <2cm size	116	188	298	188	359	372
		Multiple lesions *some* >2cm size	116	195	298	339	359	372
	Nodules		287	287	287	287	287	287
	Generalised rash		214	214	214	214	214	214
Crust/ exudate/ excoriated	Papules, plaques & small erosions (no blisters present)		120	215	298	339/215	359	372
	Vesicles/bullae/large erosions		223	223	298	223	223/359	223
	Nodules		120/295	295	295	295	295	295
	Ulcers		120	350	350	342/350	350	342/350